Nurse
Practitioner's
Clinical
Companion

Nurse Practitioner's
Clinical
Companion

Springhouse Corporation ■ Springhouse, Pennsylvania

STAFF

Vice President
Matthew Cahill

Publisher
Judith A. Schilling McCann, RN, MSN

Clinical Manager
Joan Robinson, RN, MSN, CCRN

Creative Director
Jake Smith

Design Director
John Hubbard

Executive Editor
H. Nancy Holmes

Clinical Editors
Gwynn Sinkinson, RN, MSN, CRNP (clinical project manager); Joanne Bartelmo, RN, MSN, CCRN; Collette Bishop Hendler, RN, CCRN

Editors
Rachel A. Bedard, Margaret Eckman, Peter H. Johnson, Vijay S. Kothare

Copy Editors
Brenna H. Mayer (manager), Mary T. Durkin, Jake Marcus-Cipolla, Jaime Stockslager, Pamela Wingrod

Designers
Arlene Putterman (associate design director), Kate Nichols (book designer), Linda Franklin (project manager), Joseph John Clark, Donna A. Morris, Jeff Sklarow

Desktop Services
Diane Paluba (manager), Joyce Rossi Biletz

Manufacturing
Deborah Meiris (director), Patricia K. Dorshaw (manager), Otto Mezei (book production manager)

Editorial and Design Assistants
Tom Hasenmayer, Beverly Lane, Liz Schaeffer

Indexer
Barbara E. Hodgson

Printed in the United States of America.

03 02 01 00   10 9 8 7 6 5 4 3 2 1

Library of Congress Cataloging-in-Publication Data

Nurse practitioner's clinical companion.
    p. ; cm.
    Includes bibliographical references and index.
    1. Nurse practitioners. 2. Clinical medicine.
    I. Springhouse Corporation.
    [DNLM: 1. Nurse Practitioners. 2. Clinical Medicine. 3. Nursing Care. WY 128 N97325 2000]
RT82.8 .N8635 2000
610.73'06'92—dc21   99-052581
ISBN 1-58255-006-9 (alk. paper)

Contents

Contributors and consultants

Debora Bukey, BSN, MSN, CRNP
Family Nurse Practitioner
Boyertown (Pa.) Medical Associates
Pottstown (Pa.) Medical Specialists Inc.

Janice T. Chussil, MSN, RN,C, ANP, DNC
Nurse Practitioner
Dermatology Associates
Portland, Ore.

Beverly Sigl Felten, MS, RN,CS, APNP
President, Gero-Psych Nursing, SC
Lannon, Wis.

Ellie Z. Franges, MSN, CNRN, CCRN
Director, Neuroscience Services
Sacred Heart Hospital
Allentown, Pa.

Susan F. Galiczynski, RN, MSN, CRNP
Nurse Practitioner
Temple University Hospital
Philadelphia

Susan J. Kimble, RN,CS, MSN, APN
Nurse Practitioner
Seaport Family Practice
Clinical Instructor
UMKC School of Nursing
Liberty, Mo.

Karen Landis, RN, MS, CRNP
Family Nurse Practitioner
Private Practice
Allentown, Pa.

David Pipher, RPh, PharmD
Pharmacy Director
Forbes Regional Hospital
Monroeville, Pa.

Cynthia Possanza, MSN, CRNP
Nurse Practitioner, Cardiology
Albert Einstein Medical Center
Philadelphia

Constance L. Seymour, RN, BSN, CIC
Nurse Epidemiologist-Consultant
Hatboro, Pa.

Gwynn Sinkinson, RNC, CRNP
Clinical Editor
Springhouse Corporation
Adult Nurse Practitioner
St. Vincent de Paul's Clinic
Philadelphia

Sylvia J. Smith, RN, CRNP
OB/GYN Nurse Practitioner
Rosedale Women's Care, P.C.
Pottstown, Pa.

Courtney Barilar Vose, MSN, RN, CRNP
Nurse Practitioner for Neuroscience Services
Sacred Heart Hospital
Allentown, Pa.

Foreword

Advanced practice nurses (APNs) play a crucial role in the provision of health services in the United States. Health-related issues, such as an aging society, excessive health care costs, increasing use of technology, and lack of preventive care, have mandated the need for change in our health care system. The traditional roles filled by physicians are now being supplemented by APNs. Studies show that patient satisfaction with the APNs' care is high. Other studies confirm that APN practice achieves a high level of safety, competence, cost-effectiveness, and improved health status for patients.

The role of the APN was developed to provide health service to individuals, families, and communities. The growing demand for viable alternatives to traditional health care options has opened many doors for APNs. Our communities are seeking competent providers who will focus on disease prevention and health education.

The focus of care by APNs — providing care on a continuum through sickness and health — has attracted the support of other health care providers, insurers, third party payors and, most importantly, the patients themselves.

Nurse Practitioner's Clinical Companion was developed to provide APNs with a comprehensive resource for essential facts and guidelines that will help them provide cost-effective, quality care. The book provides the latest information on medical disorders, associated diagnoses, and appropriate treatments. Information on common drug therapy is provided, including adverse drug reactions and drug overdoses, interactions, and hazards.

Nurse Practitioner's Clinical Companion also contains chapters developed to assist the APN with interpreting electrocardiograms (ECGs), including normal ECGs and arrhythmias; laboratory test values; dermatology evaluation and treatment; and common X-ray findings. Primary care procedures and management of trauma and emergencies are also included. Finally, the book includes chapters on clinical and legal issues and health promotion over the lifespan.

The book's accessible two-column format promotes quick retrieval of information that is useful for developing a plan of care. Graphic logos highlight clinical warnings, times when collaboration is needed, teaching tips, and pediatric, geriatric, and pregnancy-related pointers.

Appendices include normal and crisis laboratory values and a guide to simplified charting.

APN students will find *Nurse Practitioner's Clinical Companion* invaluable for use during clinical rotation and as they grow into practice. It will help them develop their diagnosis and treatment skills. Furthermore, practicing APNs will find *Nurse Practitioner's Clinical Companion* an essential addition to their daily practice. The vital information contained in this book will provide the APN with the details needed to deliver safe, competent, holistic care.

Geriann Bernadette Gallagher, ND, APRN
Gerontological Nurse Practitioner
St. Frances Care
Rehabilitation Hospital of Connecticut
Hartford
Guest Lecturer, Yale University School of Nursing
New Haven, Conn.

Assessment findings

Arriving at a differential diagnosis

Review of normal findings

To distinguish between health and disease, you must be able to recognize normal assessment findings in each part of the body. When you perform a physical examination, use this head-to-toe roster of normal findings as a reference. It's designed to help you quickly zero in on physical abnormalities and evaluate your patient's overall condition.

Head and neck

Inspection

• Symmetrical, lesion-free skull
• Symmetrical facial structures with no cyanosis or vascular lesions
• Unrestricted range of motion in the neck
• Ability to shrug the shoulders, a sign of an adequately functioning cranial nerve XI (accessory nerve)
• No bulging of the thyroid
• Symmetrical, unswollen lymph nodes

Palpation

• No lumps or tenderness on the head
• Symmetrical strength in the facial muscles, a sign of adequately functioning cranial nerves V and VII (trigeminal and facial nerves)
• Symmetrical sensation when stroked with a wisp of cotton on each cheek
• Mobile, soft lymph nodes less than ½″ (1 cm) with no tenderness
• Symmetrical pulses in the carotid arteries
• Palpable, symmetrical, lesion-free thyroid and absence of thyroid tenderness

• Midline location of the trachea and absence of tracheal tenderness
• No crepitus, tenderness, or lesions in the cervical spine
• Symmetrical muscle strength in the neck

Eyes

Inspection

• No edema, scaling, or lesions on the eyelids
• Eyelids completely covering the corneas when closed
• Eyelid color same as surrounding skin color
• Palpebral fissures of equal height
• Margin of upper lid falling between the superior pupil margin and the superior limbus
• Symmetrical, lesion-free upper eyelids that don't lag or droop when the patient opens his eyes
• Evenly distributed eyelashes that curve outward
• Globe of eye neither protruding from nor sunken into the orbit
• Eyebrows with equal size, color, and distribution
• Clear conjunctiva with visible small blood vessels and no signs of drainage
• White sclera visible through the conjunctiva
• Symmetrical irises of the same color
• Transparent anterior chamber that contains no visible material when a penlight is shone into the side of the eye
• Transparent, smooth, and bright cornea with no visible irregularities or lesions
• Closing of the lids of both eyes when each cornea is stroked with a wisp of cotton, a test of cranial nerve V (trigeminal nerve)
• Round, equal-sized pupils that react normally to light and accommodation

- Constriction of both pupils when a light is shone on one eye
- Lacrimal structures free of exudate, swelling, and excessive tearing
- Proper eye alignment
- Parallel eye movement in each of the six cardinal fields of gaze

Palpation

- Absence of eyelid swelling and tenderness
- Globes that are equally firm without feeling overly hard or spongy
- Lacrimal sacs that don't regurgitate fluid

Ears

Inspection

- Bilaterally symmetrical, proportionately sized auricles that have a vertical measurement between 1½" and 4" (4 and 10 cm)
- Lip of ear crossing eye-occiput line (an imaginary line extending from the lateral aspect of the eye to the occipital protuberance)
- Long axis of ear perpendicular to (or no more than 10 degrees from perpendicular to) the eye-occiput line
- Color match between the ears and facial skin
- No signs of inflammation, lesions, or nodules
- No cracking, thickening, scaling, or lesions behind the ear when the auricle is bent forward
- No visible discharge from auditory canal
- Patent external meatus
- Skin color on the mastoid process that matches the skin color of the surrounding areas
- No redness or swelling

Palpation

- No masses or tenderness on the auricle

- No tenderness on the auricle or tragus during manipulation
- Either small, nonpalpable lymph nodes on the auricle or discrete, mobile lymph nodes with no signs of tenderness
- Well-defined, bony edges on the mastoid process with no signs of tenderness

Nose and mouth

Inspection

- Symmetrical, lesion-free nose with little or no deviation of the septum or discharge
- Little or no nasal flaring
- Nonedematous frontal and maxillary sinuses
- Ability to identify familiar odors
- Pinkish red nasal mucosa with no visible lesions and no purulent drainage
- No evidence of foreign bodies or dried blood in the nose
- Pink lips with no dryness, cracking, lesions, or cyanosis
- Symmetrical facial structures
- Ability to purse the lips and puff out the cheeks, sign of an adequately functioning cranial nerve VII (facial nerve)
- Ability to easily open and close the mouth
- Light pink, moist oral mucosa with no ulcers or lesions
- Visible salivary ducts with no inflammation
- White hard palate
- Pink soft palate
- Pink gums with no tartar, inflammation, or hemorrhage
- All teeth intact with no signs of occlusion, caries, or breakage
- Pink tongue with no swelling, coating, ulcers, or lesions
- Tongue that moves easily and without tremor, sign of a properly functioning cranial nerve XII (hypoglossal nerve)

• No swelling or inflammation on anterior and posterior arches
• No lesions or inflammation on posterior pharynx
• Lesion-free tonsils that are the right size for the patient's age
• Uvula that moves when the patient says "ah" and a gag reflex when a tongue blade touches the posterior pharynx, signs of properly functioning cranial nerves IX (glossopharyngeal) and X (vagus)

Palpation

• No structural deviation, tenderness, or swelling in the external nose
• No tenderness or edema on the frontal and maxillary sinuses
• Lips free from pain and induration
• No lesions, unusual color, tenderness, or swelling on the posterior and lateral surfaces of the tongue
• No tenderness, nodules, or swelling on the floor of the mouth

Lungs

Inspection

• Side-to-side symmetrical chest configuration
• Anteroposterior diameter less than the transverse diameter, with a 1:2 to 5:7 ratio in an adult
• Normal chest shape with no deformities, such as a barrel chest, kyphosis, retraction, sternal protrusion, and depressed sternum
• Costal angle less than 90 degrees with the ribs joining the spine at a 45-degree angle
• Quiet, unlabored respirations with no use of accessory neck, shoulder, or abdominal muscles; no intercostal, substernal, or supraclavicular retractions
• Symmetrically expanding chest wall during respiration
• Normal adult respiratory rate of 16 to 20 breaths/minute; some variation

expected, depending on the patient's age
• Regular respiratory rhythm with expiration taking about twice as long as inspiration (Men and children breathe diaphragmatically, whereas women breathe thoracically.)
• Skin color that matches the rest of the body's complexion

Palpation

• Warm, dry skin
• No tender spots or bulges in the chest

Percussion

• Resonant percussion sounds over the lungs

Auscultation

• Loud, high-pitched breath sounds over the trachea
• Intense, medium-pitched bronchovesicular breath sounds over the mainstem bronchi, between the scapulae, and below the clavicles
• Soft, breezy, low-pitched vesicular breath sounds over most of the peripheral lung fields

Heart

Inspection

• No visible pulsations, except at the point of maximal impulse (PMI)
• No lifts (heaves) or retractions in the four valve areas of the chest wall

Palpation

• No detectable vibrations or thrills
• No lifts
• No pulsations, except at the PMI and epigastric area (At the PMI, a tapping pulse that is less than ½″ [1.25 cm] in diameter [localized] may be felt at the start of systole. In

the epigastric area, pulsation from the abdominal aorta may be palpable.)

Auscultation

• S_1 sound, which is the "lub" sound heard best with the diaphragm of the stethoscope over the mitral area when the patient is in a left lateral position (It sounds longer, lower, and louder there than S_2 sounds. S_1 splitting may be audible in the tricuspid area.)
• S_2 sound, which is the "dub" sound heard best with the diaphragm of the stethoscope in the aortic area while the patient sits and leans over (It sounds shorter, sharper, higher, and louder there than S_1 sounds. Normal S_2 splitting may be audible in the pulmonic area on inspiration.)
• S_3 sound, which is normal in children and slender, young adults with no cardiovascular disease (It usually disappears when adults reach ages 25 to 35. In an older adult, it may signify heart failure. S_3 may be heard best over the mitral area with the patient supine and exhaling. It sounds short, dull, soft, and low.)
• Murmurs, which may be functional in children and young adults but are abnormal in older adults (Innocent murmurs are soft and short and vary with respirations and patient position. They occur in early systole and are best heard in pulmonic or mitral positions with the patient supine.)

Abdomen

Inspection

• Skin free from vascular lesions, jaundice, surgical scars, and rashes
• Faint venous patterns (except in thin patients)
• Flat, round, or scaphoid abdominal contour
• Symmetrical abdomen
• Umbilicus positioned midway between the xiphoid process and the symphysis pubis with a flat or concave hemisphere
• No variations in the color of the patient's skin
• No apparent bulges
• Abdominal movement apparent with respiration
• Pink or silver-white striae from pregnancy or weight loss

Auscultation

• High-pitched, gurgling bowel sounds heard every 5 to 15 seconds through the diaphragm of the stethoscope
• Vascular sounds heard through the bell of the stethoscope
• Venous hum over the inferior vena cava
• No bruits, murmurs, friction rubs, or other venous hums

Percussion

• Tympany predominantly over hollow organs, including the stomach, intestines, bladder, abdominal aorta, and gallbladder
• dullness over solid masses, including the liver, spleen, pancreas, kidneys, uterus, and full bladder

Palpation

• No tenderness or masses
• Abdominal musculature free from tenderness and rigidity
• No guarding, rebound tenderness, distention, or ascites
• Unpalpable liver except in children (If palpable, liver edge is regular, sharp, and nontender and is felt no more than ¾" [2 cm] below the right costal margin.)
• Unpalpable spleen
• Unpalpable kidneys except in thin patients or those with a flaccid abdominal wall (Right kidney is felt more commonly than left.)

Arms and legs

Inspection

• No gross deformities
• Symmetrical body parts
• Good body alignment
• No involuntary movements
• Smooth gait
• Active range of motion (ROM) in all muscles and joints
• No pain with active ROM
• No visible swelling or inflammation of joints or muscles
• Equal bilateral limb length and symmetrical muscle mass

Palpation

• Normal shape with no swelling or tenderness
• Equal bilateral muscle tone, texture, and strength
• No involuntary contractions or twitching
• Equally strong bilateral pulses

Exploring the most common chief complaints

A patient's chief complaint is the starting point for almost every initial assessment. To evaluate the complaint thoroughly, you'll need to ask the right health history questions, conduct a physical examination based on the history data you collect, and analyze possible causes of the problem.

This alphabetized list examines the 22 complaints most frequently encountered in nursing practice. For each one, you'll find a concise description, detailed questions to ask during the history, areas on which to focus during the physical examination, and common causes to consider.

Abdominal pain

Usually, abdominal pain results from GI disorders, but it can also stem from reproductive, genitourinary, musculoskeletal, or vascular disorders; from drug use; or from the effects of toxins. Abdominal pain may originate in the abdominopelvic viscera, the parietal peritoneum, or the capsules of the liver, kidneys, and spleen. The pain may be acute or chronic, diffuse or localized.

Health history

• When did the pain begin? What does it feel like? How long does it last? Where exactly is it? Does it radiate to other areas, such as the chest or back? Does it get better or worse when you change position, move, exert yourself, cough, eat, or have a bowel movement?
• Does fever occur during episodes of pain? Do you have appetite changes, constipation, diarrhea, nausea, pain with urination, pink or cloudy urine, vomiting, or urinary frequency or urgency?
• Do you have a history of adrenal disease, heart disease, recent infection, or recent blunt trauma to the abdomen, flank, or chest? Have you had any condition that could predispose you to emboli or that could narrow an arterial lumen? Have you recently undergone a urinary tract procedure or surgery? Have you traveled to a foreign country recently?
• For women of childbearing age: what was the date of your last menses? Has your menstrual pattern changed? Could you be pregnant?
• Have you ever used I.V. drugs? Do you drink alcohol? If so, how much and how often? What prescription drugs do you take?

Physical examination

After assessing the patient's level of consciousness, observe his skin for diaphoresis, jaundice, and turgor. Then check for coolness, discoloration, and edema of the arms and legs. Inspect the abdomen and chest for signs of trauma; a bluish discoloration around the umbilicus (Cullen's sign) or around the flank area (Turner's sign) can indicate blunt trauma. Obtain and record a baseline measurement of abdominal girth at the umbilicus.

After inspecting for neck vein distention, observe the rate and depth of respirations, noting any abnormal patterns. Observe the color and odor of the patient's urine.

Because palpation and percussion can affect the frequency and intensity of bowel sounds, auscultate the abdomen first. Listen for bowel sounds in each quadrant, noting whether the sounds are high-pitched and tinkling, hyperactive, or absent.

Then, listen to the patient's heart and breath sounds for abnormalities. Be sure to monitor his blood pressure and pulse pressure.

As you systematically palpate the abdominal, pelvic, flank, and epigastric areas, note any enlarged organs, masses, rigidity, tenderness, rebound tenderness, and tenderness with guarding. Check the patient's peripheral pulses for rate, rhythm, and intensity.

Percuss each abdominal quadrant, noting tenderness, increased pain, and percussion sounds. Dull percussion sounds indicate free fluid; hollow sounds indicate air.

Causes

Abdominal aortic aneurysm (dissecting)
Constant, dull upper abdominal pain radiating to the lower back typically accompanies rapid aneurysm enlargement and may herald a rupture. Palpation may reveal an epigastric mass that pulsates before rupture. On auscultation, you may detect a systolic bruit over the aneurysm. You may also note abdominal rigidity, increasing abdominal girth, and signs of hypovolemic shock.

Abdominal trauma
The patient may have generalized or localized abdominal pain along with abdominal ecchymosis, abdominal tenderness, or vomiting. If he's hemorrhaging into the peritoneal cavity, you may note abdominal rigidity, dullness on percussion, and increasing abdominal girth. You may hear hollow bowel sounds if an abdominal organ has been perforated, or bowel sounds may be absent. Bowel sounds heard in the chest cavity usually signal a diaphragmatic tear.

Appendicitis
The patient with appendicitis may have sudden pain in the epigastric or umbilical region that increases over a few hours or days, along with flulike symptoms. Anorexia, constipation or diarrhea, nausea, and vomiting precede the pain, which may be dull or severe. Pain localizes at McBurney's point in the right lower quadrant. Abdominal rigidity and rebound tenderness may also occur.

Ectopic pregnancy
Lower abdominal pain may be sharp, dull, or cramping and either constant or intermittent. The pain may be accompanied by breast tenderness, nausea, vaginal bleeding, vomiting, and urinary frequency. The patient typically has a 1- to 2-month history of amenorrhea. Rupture of the fallopian tube produces lower abdominal pain, which may radiate to the shoulders and neck and become extreme on cervical or adnexal palpation.

ABDOMINAL PAIN: SPELL OUT THE CAUSES

Use the following mnemonic device to help you remember the possible causes of abdominal pain.

Altered bowel motility
Bloodless (vascular insufficiency)
Distant (referred pain)
Obstruction (bowel, gallbladder, liver, pancreas)
Metabolic (diabetic gastroparesis)
Irritation in the perineum
Nerve injury
Abdominal wall insufficiency (hernia)
Linings of organs (capsular distention)

Hepatitis
Liver enlargement from any type of hepatitis causes discomfort or dull pain and tenderness in the right upper quadrant.

Intestinal obstruction
With an intestinal obstruction, short episodes of intense, colicky, cramping pain alternate with pain-free periods.

Pancreatitis
The characteristic symptom of pancreatitis is fulminating, continuous upper abdominal pain that may radiate to both flanks and to the back.

Renal calculi
Depending on the location of the calculi, the patient may experience severe abdominal or back pain. However, the classic symptom of renal calculi is colicky pain that travels from the costovertebral angle to the flank, the suprapubic region, and the external genitalia.

Other causes
Abdominal pain may result from adrenal crisis, cholecystitis, heart failure, diabetic ketoacidosis, diverticulitis, hepatic abscess, mesenteric artery ischemia, myocardial infarction, ovarian cyst, perforated ulcer, peritonitis, pneumonia, pneumothorax, pyelonephritis, renal infarction, and splenic infarction. Also, salicy-

lates and nonsteroidal anti-inflammatory drugs can produce abdominal pain. (See *Abdominal pain: Spell out the causes.*)

 SPECIAL POPULATIONS Because a child often has difficulty describing abdominal pain, pay close attention to nonverbal cues — wincing, lethargy, or unusual positioning (such as a side-lying position with knees flexed to the abdomen).

In children, abdominal pain can signal a disorder with greater severity or different associated signs than in adults. Remember, too, that a child's complaint of abdominal pain may reflect an emotional need, such as the wish to avoid school or to gain adult attention.

Back pain

Back pain may be acute, chronic, constant, or intermittent. It also may remain localized in the back or radiate along the spine or down one or both legs. A patient's pain may be exacerbated by activity (most commonly, stooping and lifting) and alleviated by rest. Or it may be unaffected by either.

Intrinsic back pain results from muscle spasm, nerve root irritation, fracture, or a combination of these causes. It usually occurs in the lower back or lumbosacral area. Back pain may also be referred from the abdomen, possibly signaling a life-threatening disorder.

Health history

• When did the pain first occur? What does it feel like? Is it mild, moderate, or severe? Is it constant or intermittent? Where exactly is it? Is it associated with activity? What relieves or exacerbates it? For women of childbearing age: Does the pain occur before or during your menses?
• Have you had recent episodes of abdominal tenderness or rigidity, fever, nausea, or vomiting? Do you feel any unusual sensations in your legs? Have you had urinary frequency or urgency or painful urination?
• Do you have a history of trauma, back surgery, or urinary tract surgery, procedures, obstructions, or infections?
• What medications are you taking?

Physical examination

Observe the rate and depth of respirations, noting any breathing difficulty or abnormal breathing patterns. Check the skin for diaphoresis, discoloration, edema, mottling, and pallor. Then inspect the back, legs, and abdomen for signs of trauma. After checking for abdominal distention, take a baseline abdominal girth measurement.

Because palpation and percussion can affect the frequency and intensity of bowel sounds, auscultate the abdomen first. Listen for bowel sounds in each quadrant. Then listen over the abdominal aorta for bruits and over the lungs for crackles. Be sure to monitor the patient's blood pressure and pulse pressure.

Palpate the abdominal, epigastric, and pelvic areas for abdominal rigidity, enlarged organs, masses, and tenderness. If you feel any pulsations, don't palpate deeply. Check the peripheral pulses for rate, rhythm, and intensity. Then gently palpate the painful area, noting contractions, excessive muscle tone, and spasm.

Finally, percuss each abdominal quadrant, noting any abnormal sounds, increased pain, and tenderness.

Causes

Abdominal aortic aneurysm (dissecting)

Low back pain and dull upper abdominal pain often accompany a rapidly enlarging aneurysm and may indicate the early stages of rupture. On palpation, you may detect tenderness over the aneurysm area and a pulsating epigastric mass. Other signs include absent femoral and pedal pulses, mottling of the skin below the waist, and signs of hypovolemic shock.

Pancreatitis

Fulminating, continuous abdominal pain that may radiate to the back and both flanks characterizes pancreatitis. You may also note abdominal tenderness, rigidity, and distention; fever; hypoactive bowel sounds; pallor; tachycardia; and vomiting. The history may include alcohol abuse, use of thiazide diuretics, gallbladder disease, trauma.

Pyelonephritis (acute)

The patient with acute pyelonephritis has progressive back pain or tenderness in the flank area, accompanied by costovertebral angle pain and abdominal pain in one or two quadrants. Associated signs and symptoms include dysuria, high fever, hematuria, nocturia, shaking chills, vomiting, and urinary frequency and urgency. The history may reveal a recent urinary tract procedure, urinary tract infection or obstruction, compromised renal function, or neurogenic bladder.

Other causes
Back pain may also result from appendicitis, cholecystitis, a lumbosacral sprain, osteoporosis, a perforated ulcer, renal calculi, tumors, and vertebral osteomyelitis.

Chest pain

Patients describe chest pain in many ways. They may report a dull ache, a sensation of heaviness or fullness, a feeling of indigestion, or a sharp, shooting pain. The pain may be constant or intermittent, may radiate to other body parts, and may arise suddenly or gradually. Patients may say that stress, anxiety, exertion, deep breathing, or certain foods seem to trigger the pain.

Chest pain may indicate several acute and life-threatening cardiopulmonary and GI conditions. But it can also result from musculoskeletal and hematologic disorders, anxiety, and certain drugs.

Health history

• When did the chest pain begin? Did it develop suddenly or gradually? Is the pain localized or diffuse? Does it radiate to the neck, jaw, arms, or back? Is the pain sharp and stabbing or dull and aching? Is it constant or intermittent? Does breathing, changing positions, or eating certain foods exacerbate or relieve the pain?
• Do you have any other symptoms, such as coughing, shortness of breath, headache, nausea, palpitations, vomiting, or weakness?
• Have you ever had cardiac or respiratory disease, cardiac surgery,

chest trauma, or intestinal disease? Do you have a family history of cardiac disease?
• Do you drink alcohol or use any illicit drugs? What medications are you taking?

Physical examination

Assess the patient's skin temperature, color, and general appearance, noting coolness, cyanosis, diaphoresis, mottling below the waist, pallor, peripheral edema, and prolonged capillary refill time. Also look for facial edema, jugular vein distention, and tracheal deviation. Note any signs of altered level of consciousness, anxiety, dizziness, or restlessness.

Then observe the rate and depth of the patient's respirations, noting abnormal patterns or breathing difficulty. If the patient has a productive cough, examine the sputum.

Palpate the patient's neck, chest, and abdomen. Note asymmetrical chest expansion, masses, subcutaneous crepitation, tender areas, tracheal deviation, and tactile fremitus. Also, palpate his peripheral pulses, and record their rate, rhythm, and intensity.

As you percuss over an affected lung, note any dullness. Then auscultate the lungs to identify crackles, diminished or absent breath sounds, pleural friction rubs, rhonchi, and wheezes. Auscultate the heart for clicks, gallops, murmurs, and pericardial friction rub. To check for abdominal bruits, apply the bell of the stethoscope over the abdominal aorta. Be sure to monitor the patient's blood pressure closely.

Causes

Angina
Anginal pain usually begins gradually, builds to a peak, and then slowly subsides. The pain can last from 2 to

10 minutes. It occurs in the retrosternal region and radiates to the neck, jaw, and arms. Associated signs and symptoms include diaphoresis, dyspnea, nausea, vomiting, palpitations, and tachycardia. On auscultation, you may detect an atrial gallop (S_4 heart sound) or a murmur. Attacks may occur at rest or be provoked by exertion, emotional stress, or a heavy meal.

Aortic aneurysm (dissecting)

A patient with a dissecting aortic aneurysm complains of sudden, excruciating, tearing pain in the chest and neck, radiating to the upper back, lower back, and abdomen. Other signs and symptoms include abdominal tenderness; heart murmurs; jugular vein distention; systolic bruits; tachycardia; weak or absent femoral or pedal pulses; and pale, cool, diaphoretic, mottled skin below the waist.

Cholecystitis

With this disorder, the patient has sudden epigastric or right upper quadrant pain, which may be steady or intermittent, radiate to the back, and be sharp or intense. Other signs and symptoms include chills, diaphoresis, nausea, and vomiting. Palpation of the right upper quadrant may reveal distention, rigidity, tenderness, and a mass.

Myocardial infarction

Usually the patient has severe, crushing substernal pain that radiates to the left arm, jaw, or neck. The pain may be accompanied by anxiety, clammy skin, diaphoresis, dyspnea, a feeling of impending doom, nausea, vomiting, pallor, and restlessness. The patient may have an atrial gallop (or S_4 heart sound), crackles, hypotension or hypertension, murmurs, and a pericardial friction rub. A history of heart disease, hypertension,

hypercholesterolemia, or cocaine abuse is common.

Peptic ulcer

A sharp, burning pain arising in the epigastric region, usually hours after eating, characterizes peptic ulcer. Other signs and symptoms include epigastric tenderness, nausea, and vomiting. Food or antacids usually relieve the pain.

Pneumothorax

A collapsed lung produces a sudden, sharp, severe chest pain that's often unilateral and increases with chest movement. You may detect decreased breath sounds, hyperresonant or tympanic percussion sounds, and subcutaneous crepitation. Other signs and symptoms include accessory muscle use, anxiety, asymmetrical chest expansion, nonproductive cough, tachycardia, and tachypnea. The history may include chronic obstructive pulmonary disease, lung cancer, diagnostic or therapeutic procedures involving the thorax, or thoracic trauma.

Pulmonary embolism

Typically, the patient experiences sudden dyspnea with an intense anginalike or pleuritic ischemic pain aggravated by deep breathing and thoracic movement. Other findings include anxiety, cough with blood-tinged sputum, crackles, dull percussion sounds, restlessness, and tachycardia. If the embolism is large, the cardiovascular, pulmonary, and neurologic systems may be compromised. The patient's history may reveal thrombophlebitis, a hip or leg fracture, acute myocardial infarction, heart failure, pregnancy, or the use of oral contraceptives.

Other causes

Chest pain may also result from abrupt withdrawal of beta-adrenergic blockers, acute bronchitis, anxiety, esophageal spasm, lung abscess, muscle strain, pancreatitis, pneumonia, a rib fracture, or tuberculosis.

Cough, nonproductive

A nonproductive cough is a noisy, forceful expulsion of air from the lungs that doesn't yield sputum or blood. One of the most common symptoms of a respiratory disorder, a nonproductive cough can be ineffective and cause damage, such as airway collapse, rupture of the alveoli, and blebs.

A nonproductive cough that later becomes productive is a classic sign of a progressive respiratory disease. An acute nonproductive cough has a sudden onset and may be self-limiting. A nonproductive cough that persists beyond 1 month is considered chronic; often, such a cough results from cigarette smoking.

Health history

• When did the cough begin? Does any body position or specific activity relieve or exacerbate it? Does it get better or worse at certain times of the day? How does the cough sound? Does it occur often? Is it paroxysmal?
• Is the cough accompanied by pain?
• Have you noticed any recent changes in your appetite, energy level, exercise tolerance, or weight? Have you had surgery recently? Do you have any allergies? Do you smoke? Have you been exposed recently to fumes or chemicals?
• What medications are you taking?

Physical examination

Note whether the patient appears agitated, anxious, confused, diaphoretic, flushed, lethargic, nervous, pale, or restless. Is his skin cold or warm, clammy or dry?

Observe the rate and depth of his respirations, noting abnormal patterns. Then examine his chest configuration and chest wall motion.

Check the patient's nose and mouth for congestion, drainage, inflammation, and signs of infection. Then inspect his neck for vein distention and tracheal deviation.

As you palpate the patient's neck, note any enlarged lymph nodes or masses. Next, percuss his chest while listening for dullness, flatness, and tympany. Finally, auscultate his lungs for crackles, decreased or absent breath sounds, pleural friction rubs, rhonchi, and wheezes.

Causes

Asthma

Typically, an asthma attack occurs at night, starting with a nonproductive cough and mild wheezing. Then, it progresses to audible wheezing, chest tightness, a cough that produces thick mucus, and severe dyspnea. Other signs include accessory muscle use, cyanosis, diaphoresis, flaring nostrils, flushing, intercostal and supraclavicular retractions on inspiration, prolonged expirations, tachycardia, and tachypnea.

Interstitial lung disease

With this disorder, the patient has a nonproductive cough and progressive dyspnea. He may also be cyanotic and fatigued and have fine crackles, finger clubbing, chest pain, and recent weight loss.

Other causes

A nonproductive cough may stem from airway occlusion, atelectasis, common cold, hypersensitivity pneumonitis, pericardial effusion, pleural effusion, pulmonary embolism, *Hantavirus* infection, or sinusitis. Also, incentive spirometry, intermittent positive-pressure breathing, and suctioning can bring on a nonproductive cough.

 SPECIAL POPULATIONS A nonproductive cough can be difficult to evaluate in infants and young children because it can't be voluntarily induced and must be observed. Remember that psychogenic coughing may occur when the child is under stress, emotionally stimulated, or seeking attention.

Cough, productive

With productive coughing, the airway passages are cleared of accumulated secretions that normal mucociliary action doesn't remove. The sudden, forceful, noisy expulsion contains sputum, blood, or both.

Usually caused by a pulmonary disorder, productive coughing typically stems from an acute or a chronic infection that causes inflammation, edema, and increased mucus production in the airways. Such coughing can also result from inhaling antigenic or irritating substances; in fact, its most common cause is cigarette smoking.

Health history

• When did the cough begin? How much sputum do you cough up daily? Is sputum production associated with time of day, meals, activities, or environment? Has it increased since coughing began? What are the color, odor, and consistency of the sputum? How does the cough sound and feel? Have you ever had a productive cough before?
• Have you noticed recent changes in your appetite or weight?
• Do you have a history of recent surgery or allergies? Do you smoke or drink alcohol? If so, how much? Do you work around chemicals or respiratory irritants?
• What medications are you taking?

Physical examination

As you examine the patient's mouth and nose for congestion, drainage, and inflammation, note his breath odor. Then inspect his neck for vein distention. As he breathes, observe the chest for accessory muscle use, intercostal and supraclavicular retractions, and uneven expansion.

Palpate his neck for enlarged lymph nodes, masses, and tenderness. Next, percuss his chest, listening for dullness, flatness, and tympany. Finally, auscultate for abnormal breath sounds, crackles, pleural friction rubs, rhonchi, and wheezes.

Causes

Bacterial pneumonia
With this disorder, an initially dry cough becomes productive. Rust-colored sputum appears in pneumococcal pneumonia; brick red or currant-jelly sputum, in *Klebsiella* pneumonia; salmon-colored sputum, in staphylococcal pneumonia; and mucopurulent sputum, in streptococcal pneumonia.

Lung abscess
The cardinal sign of a ruptured lung abscess is coughing that produces copious amounts of purulent, foul-smelling and, possibly, blood-tinged sputum. A ruptured abscess can also cause anorexia, diaphoresis, dyspnea, fatigue, fever with chills, halitosis, headache, inspiratory crackles, pleuritic chest pain, tubular or amphoric breath sounds, and weight loss.

Other causes
A productive cough can result from acute bronchiolitis, aspiration and chemical pneumonitis, bronchiecta-

sis, common cold, cystic fibrosis, lung cancer, pertussis, pulmonary embolism, pulmonary edema, and tracheobronchitis. Also, expectorants, incentive spirometry, and intermittent positive-pressure breathing can cause a productive cough.

 SPECIAL POPULATIONS Because his airway is narrow, a child with a productive cough can quickly develop airway obstruction and respiratory distress from thick or excessive secretions.

Diplopia

Also called double vision, diplopia occurs when the extraocular muscles fail to work together, causing images to fall on noncorresponding parts of the retina. Diplopia can result from orbital lesions, eye surgery, or impaired function of the cranial nerves that supply the extraocular muscles.

Classified as binocular or monocular, diplopia is usually intermittent at first and affects near or far vision exclusively. Binocular diplopia usually results from ocular deviation or displacement or from retinal surgery. Monocular diplopia may result from an early cataract, retinal edema or scarring, or poorly fitting contact lenses. Diplopia may also occur with hysteria or malingering.

Health history

• When did you first notice your double vision? Are the images side by side (horizontal), one above the other (vertical), or both? Is the diplopia intermittent, or constant? Are both eyes affected or just one? Is near or far vision affected? Does the diplopia occur only when you gaze in certain directions? Has the problem worsened, remained the same, or subsided? Does it worsen as the day progresses? Can you correct the problem by tilting your head? If so, ask the patient to show you, and note the direction of the tilt.
• Do you have eye pain?
• Have you had recent eye surgery? Do you wear contact lenses?
• Have you had previous vision problems? Has anyone in your family had vision problems?
• What medications are you taking?

Physical examination

Observe the patient for conjunctival infection, exophthalmos, lid edema, ocular deviation, and ptosis. Have him occlude one eye at a time; if he sees double with only one eye, he has monocular diplopia. Test his visual acuity and extraocular muscle function. (See *Testing extraocular muscles.*)

Causes

Botulism

Hallmark signs and symptoms of botulism are diplopia, dysarthria, dysphagia, and ptosis. Early findings include diarrhea, dry mouth, sore throat, and vomiting. Later, descending weakness or paralysis of extremity and trunk muscles causes dyspnea and hyporeflexia.

Intracranial aneurysm

A life-threatening disorder, intracranial aneurysm initially produces diplopia and eye deviation, perhaps accompanied by a dilated pupil on the affected side and ptosis. Other findings include a decreased level of consciousness; dizziness; neck and spinal pain and rigidity; a severe, unilateral, frontal headache, which becomes violent after rupture of the aneurysm; tinnitus; unilateral muscle weakness or paralysis; and vomiting.

Other causes

Alcohol intoxication, brain tumors, diabetes mellitus, encephalitis, eye

TESTING EXTRAOCULAR MUSCLES

The coordinated action of six muscles controls eyeball movements. To test the function of each muscle and the cranial nerve (CN) that innervates it, ask the patient to look in the direction controlled by that muscle. The six directions you can test make up the *cardinal fields of gaze*. The patient's inability to turn the eye in the designated direction indicates muscle weakness or paralysis.

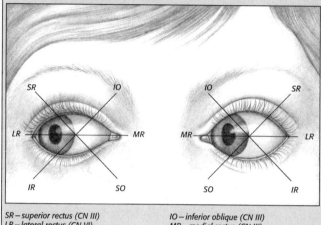

SR – superior rectus (CN III)
LR – lateral rectus (CN VI)
IR – inferior rectus (CN III)

IO – inferior oblique (CN III)
MR – medial rectus (CN III)
SO – superior oblique (CN IV)

surgery, head injury, migraine, multiple sclerosis, and orbital tumors may also cause diplopia.

SPECIAL POPULATIONS
Strabismus, a congenital disorder or one acquired at an early age, produces diplopia; however, in young children, the brain rapidly compensates for double vision by suppressing one image, so diplopia is a rare complaint. School-age children who complain of double vision require a careful examination to rule out serious disorders, such as a brain tumor.

Dizziness

A common symptom, dizziness is a sensation of imbalance or faintness sometimes associated with blurred or double vision, confusion, and weakness. Dizziness may be mild or severe, have an abrupt or a gradual onset, and be aggravated by standing up quickly and alleviated by lying down. Episodes are usually brief.

Dizziness typically results from inadequate blood flow and oxygen supply to the cerebrum and spinal cord. It may occur with anxiety, respiratory and cardiovascular disorders, and postconcussion syndrome. Dizziness is also a key symptom of certain serious disorders, such as hypertension and vertebrobasilar artery insufficiency.

Health history

• When did the dizziness start? How severe is it? How often does it occur, and how long does each episode last? Does the dizziness abate spontaneously? Is it triggered by standing up suddenly or bending over?

• Do you have blurred vision, chest pain, a chronic cough, diaphoresis, a headache, or shortness of breath?
• Have you ever had hypertension or another cardiovascular disorder? What about diabetes mellitus, anemia, respiratory or anxiety disorders, or a head injury?
• What medications are you taking?

Physical examination

Assess the patient's level of consciousness, respirations, and body temperature. As you observe his breathing, look for accessory muscle use and barrel chest. Look also for finger clubbing, cyanosis, dry mucous membranes, and poor skin turgor. Then, evaluate the patient's motor and sensory functions and reflexes.

Palpate the extremities for peripheral edema and capillary refill. Then, auscultate the patient's heart rate and rhythm and his breath sounds. Take his blood pressure while he's lying down, sitting, and standing. If the diastolic pressure exceeds 100 mm Hg, notify the doctor immediately and have the patient lie down.

Causes

Cardiac arrhythmias

Dizziness lasts for several minutes or longer and may precede fainting. Other signs and symptoms include blurred vision; confusion; hypotension; palpitations; paresthesia; weakness; and an irregular, rapid, or thready pulse.

Hypertension

Dizziness may precede fainting but may be relieved by rest. Other findings include blurred vision; elevated blood pressure; headache; and retinal changes, such as hemorrhage, exudate discharge, and papilledema.

Transient ischemic attack

Dizziness of varying severity occurs during a transient ischemic attack. Lasting from a few seconds to 24 hours, an attack may be triggered by turning the head to the side and typically signals an impending cerebrovascular accident. During an attack, blindness or visual field deficits, diplopia, hearing loss, numbness, paresis, ptosis, and tinnitus may also occur.

Other causes

Dizziness may result from anemia, generalized anxiety disorder, orthostatic hypotension, panic disorder, and postconcussion syndrome. Also, dizziness may be an adverse reaction to certain drugs, including antianxiety agents, central nervous system depressants, narcotic analgesics, decongestants, antihistamines, antihypertensives, and vasodilators.

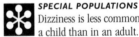 **SPECIAL POPULATIONS**
Dizziness is less common in a child than in an adult. Often the child has difficulty describing this symptom and instead complains of tiredness, stomachache, or feeling sick. If you suspect dizziness, assess for vertigo as well. A more common symptom, vertigo may result from vision disorders, ear infections, and the effects of antibiotics.

Dysphagia

Difficulty swallowing, or dysphagia, is the most common — and sometimes the only — symptom of esophageal disorders. This symptom may also result from oropharyngeal, respiratory, and neurologic disorders and from exposure to toxins. Patients with dysphagia have an increased risk of aspiration and choking and of malnutrition and dehydration.

Health history

• When did you start having trouble swallowing? Is swallowing painful? If so, is the pain constant, or intermittent? Can you point to the spot where you have the most trouble swallowing? Does eating alleviate or aggravate the problem? Do you have more trouble swallowing solids or liquids? Does the problem disappear after you try to swallow a few times? Is swallowing easier if you change position?

• Have you or has anyone in your family ever had an esophageal, oropharyngeal, respiratory, or neurologic disorder? Have you recently had a tracheotomy or been exposed to a toxin?

Physical examination

Evaluate the patient's swallowing and his cough and gag reflexes. As you listen to his speech, note signs of muscle, tongue, or facial weakness; aphasia; or dysarthria. Is his voice nasal or hoarse? Check his mouth for dry mucous membranes and thick secretions.

Causes

Airway obstruction

A life-threatening condition, upper airway obstruction is marked by respiratory distress. Dysphagia occurs along with gagging and dysphonia.

Esophageal carcinoma

Typically, painless dysphagia accompanies rapid weight loss. As the carcinoma advances, dysphagia becomes painful and constant. The patient complains of a cough with hemoptysis, hoarseness, sore throat, and steady chest pain.

Esophagitis

A patient with corrosive esophagitis has dysphagia accompanied by excessive salivation, fever, hematemesis, intense pain in the mouth and anterior chest, and tachypnea. Monilial esophagitis produces dysphagia and sore throat. In reflux esophagitis, dysphagia is a late symptom that usually accompanies stricture.

Hiatal hernia

The patient with a hiatal hernia may complain of belching, dysphagia, dyspepsia, flatulence, heartburn, regurgitation, and retrosternal or substernal chest pain aggravated by lying down or bending over.

Other causes

Dysphagia results from botulism, esophageal diverticula, external esophageal compression, hypocalcemia, laryngeal nerve damage, and Parkinson's disease. Radiation therapy and tracheotomy may also cause dysphagia.

 SPECIAL POPULATIONS In looking for dysphagia in an infant or a young child, be sure to pay close attention to his sucking and swallowing ability. Coughing, choking, or regurgitation during feeding suggest dysphagia.

Dyspnea

Patients typically describe dyspnea as shortness of breath, but this symptom also refers to difficult or uncomfortable breathing. Its severity varies greatly and is often unrelated to the seriousness of the underlying cause. Dyspnea may arise suddenly or slowly and may subside rapidly or persist for years.

Health history

• When did the dyspnea first occur? Did it begin suddenly or gradually? Is it constant or intermittent? Does it occur during activity or while you're

resting? Does anything seem to trigger, exacerbate, or relieve it? Have you ever had dyspnea before?
• Do you have a productive or nonproductive cough or chest pain?
• Have you recently had an upper respiratory tract infection or experienced trauma? Do you smoke? If so, how much and for how long? Have you been exposed to any allergens? Do you have any known allergies?
• What medications are you taking?

Physical examination

Observe the patient's respirations, noting their rate and depth, and breathing difficulties or abnormal respiratory patterns. Check, too, for flaring nostrils, grunting respirations, inspiratory stridor, intercostal retractions during inspiration, and pursed-lip expirations.

Also examine the patient for barrel chest, diaphoresis, neck vein distention, finger clubbing, and peripheral edema. Note the color, consistency, and odor of any sputum.

Palpate his chest for asymmetrical expansion, decreased diaphragmatic excursion, tactile fremitus, and subcutaneous crepitation. Also check the rate, rhythm, and intensity of his peripheral pulses.

As you percuss the lung fields, note dull, hyperresonant, or tympanic percussion sounds. Auscultate the lungs for bronchophony, crackles, decreased or absent unilateral breath sounds, egophony, pleural breath sounds, pleural friction rubs, rhonchi, whispered pectoriloquy, and wheezing. Then auscultate the heart for abnormal sounds or rhythms, such as ventricular or atrial gallop, and for pericardial friction rubs and tachycardia. Be sure to monitor the patient's blood pressure and pulse pressure.

Causes

Adult respiratory distress syndrome

In adult respiratory distress syndrome (ARDS), acute dyspnea is followed by accessory muscle use, crackles, grunting respirations, progressive respiratory distress, rhonchi, and wheezes. In the late stages, anxiety, cyanosis, decreased mental acuity, and tachycardia occur. Severe ARDS can produce signs of shock, such as cool, clammy skin and hypotension. The typical patient has no history of underlying cardiac or pulmonary disease but has sustained a recent pulmonary or systemic insult.

Airway obstruction (partial)

Inspiratory stridor and acute dyspnea occur as the patient tries to overcome the obstruction. Related findings include accessory muscle use, anxiety, asymmetrical chest expansion, cyanosis, decreased or absent breath sounds, diaphoresis, hypotension, and tachypnea. The patient may have aspirated vomitus or a foreign body or been exposed to an allergen.

Asthma

Acute dyspneic attacks occur along with accessory muscle use, apprehension, dry cough, flushing or cyanosis, intercostal retractions, tachypnea, and tachycardia. On palpation, you'll detect decreased tactile fremitus. Hyperresonance occurs on chest percussion. On auscultation, you'll note wheezing and rhonchi or, during a severe episode, decreased breath sounds.

Heart failure

Dyspnea usually develops gradually or occurs as chronic paroxysmal nocturnal dyspnea. In ventricular failure, dyspnea occurs with basilar crackles, dependent peripheral edema, distended neck veins, fatigue, orthopnea, tachycardia, ventricular or atrial gallop, and weight gain. The patient may have a history of cardiovascular disease or may be taking drugs that can precipitate heart failure, such as amiodarone (Cordarone), certain beta-adrenergic blockers, and corticosteroids.

Myocardial infarction
Sudden dyspnea occurs with crushing substernal chest pain that may radiate to the back, neck, jaw, and arms. The patient's history may include heart disease, hypertension, hypercholesterolemia, or use of drugs that can precipitate a myocardial infarction, such as cocaine, dextrothyroxine sodium (Choloxin), estramustine phosphate sodium (Emcyt), and aldesleukin (Proleukin).

Pneumonia
Dyspnea occurs suddenly, usually accompanied by fever, pleuritic chest pain that worsens with deep inspiration, and shaking chills. The patient also has a dry or productive cough, depending on the stage and type of pneumonia. Sputum may be discolored and foul-smelling. Crackles, decreased breath sounds, dullness on percussion, and rhonchi may also be present. The history may include exposure to a contagious organism, hazardous fumes, or air pollution.

Pulmonary edema
In this disorder, severe dyspnea is often preceded by signs of heart failure, such as crackles in both lung fields, cyanosis, tachycardia, tachypnea, and marked anxiety. The patient may have a dry cough or one that produces copious amounts of pink, frothy sputum. The history may reveal cardiovascular disease, cyanosis, fatigue, and pallor.

Pulmonary embolism
Severe dyspnea occurs with intense angina-like or pleuritic pain aggravated by deep breathing and thoracic movement. Other findings include crackles, cyanosis, diffuse wheezing, dull percussion sounds, low-grade fever, nonproductive cough, pleural friction rubs, restlessness, tachypnea, and tachycardia. The patient's history may include acute myocardial infarction, heart failure, hip or leg fracture, oral contraceptive use, pregnancy, thrombophlebitis, or varicose veins.

Other causes
Dyspnea may also result from anemia, anxiety, cardiac arrhythmias, cor pulmonale, inhalation injury, lung cancer, pleural effusion, and sepsis.

 SPECIAL POPULATIONS
Normally, an infant's respirations are abdominal, gradually changing to costal by age 7. Suspect dyspnea in an infant who breathes costally, in an older child who breathes abdominally, or in any child who uses his neck or shoulder muscles to help him breathe.

Earache

Usually, earache results from disorders of the external and middle ear associated with infection, obstruction, or trauma. Its severity ranges from a feeling of fullness or blockage to deep, boring pain; at times, it may be difficult to locate precisely. This common symptom may be intermittent or continuous and may develop suddenly or gradually.

Health history
• How long have you had the earache? Is it intermittent or continuous?
• Is the earache painful or slightly annoying?
• Can you localize the exact site of the ear pain?

- Do you have pain in other areas such as the jaw?
- Does swimming or showering trigger the ear pain?
- Have you had any recent ear injury or other trauma?
- Is the earache associated with itching? If so, when is the itching most intense and when did it begin?
- Have you noticed any ear drainage, and if so, what does it look like?
- Do you have ringing or noise in the ears?
- Have you been dizzy or had vertigo? If so, does it worsen when you change position?
- Do you have difficulty swallowing, hoarseness, neck pain or pain from opening your mouth?
- Did you recently have a head cold or problems with your eyes, mouth, teeth, jaws, sinuses, or throat?

Physical examination

Begin your physical examination by inspecting the external ear for redness, drainage, swelling, and deformity. Then apply pressure to the mastoid process and the tragus to elicit tenderness. Using an otoscope, examine the external auditory canal for lesions, bleeding or discharge, impacted cerumen (earwax), foreign bodies, tenderness, and swelling. Examine the tympanic membrane. Is it intact? Is it pearly gray (normal)? Look for tympanic membrane landmarks: the cone of light, umbo, pars tensa, and the handle and short process of the malleus. Perform the watch tick, whispered voice, Rinne, and Weber's tests to assess for hearing loss. (See *Using an otoscope correctly*.)

Causes

Barotrauma (acute)

Earache associated with barotrauma ranges from mild pressure to severe pain. Tympanic membrane ecchymosis or bleeding into the tympanic cavity may occur, producing a blue drumhead; usually, the eardrum isn't perforated.

Cerumen impaction

Impacted cerumen may cause a plugged, blocked, or full sensation in the ear. Additional features include partial hearing loss, itching and, possibly, dizziness.

Otitis externa

Earache characterizes both types of otitis externa. Acute otitis externa begins with mild to moderate ear pain that occurs with tragus manipulation. The pain may be accompanied by low-grade fever, sticky yellow or purulent ear discharge, partial hearing loss, and a feeling of blockage. Later, ear pain intensifies, causing the entire side of the head to ache and throb. The temperature may reach 104° F (40° C). Examination reveals swelling of the tragus, external meatus, and external canal; tympanic membrane erythema; and lymphadenopathy. The patient also complains of dizziness and malaise.

Malignant otitis externa abruptly causes ear pain that's aggravated by moving the auricle or tragus. The pain is accompanied by intense itching, parotid gland swelling, and trismus. Examination reveals a swollen external canal with exposed cartilage and temporal bone. Cranial nerve palsy may occur.

Otitis media (acute)

This middle ear inflammation may be serous or suppurative. Acute serous otitis media may cause a feeling of fullness in the ear, hearing loss, and

USING AN OTOSCOPE CORRECTLY

When the patient reports an earache, use an otoscope to inspect the ear structure closely. Follow these techniques to obtain the best view and ensure patient safety.

Young children
To inspect an infant's or a young child's ear, grasp the lower part of the auricle and pull it down and back to straighten the upward S-curve of the external canal. Then gently insert the otoscope into the canal no more than ½" (1.3 cm).

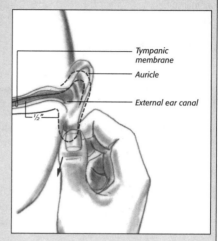

Adults and older children
To inspect an adult's ear, grasp the upper part of the auricle and pull it up and back to straighten the external canal. Then insert the otoscope about 1" (2.5 cm). Use this technique for children over age 3.

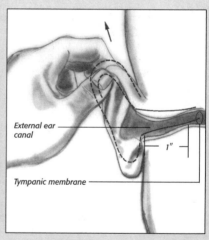

a vague sensation of top-heaviness. The tympanic membrane may be slightly retracted, amber-colored, and marked by air bubbles and a meniscus, or it may be blue-black from hemorrhage.

Severe, deep, throbbing ear pain; hearing loss; and a temperature that may reach 102° F (38.9° C) characterize acute suppurative otitis media. The pain increases steadily over several hours or days and may be aggravated by pressure on the mastoid antrum.

Perforation of the tympanic membrane is possible. Before rupture, the tympanic membrane appears bulging and fiery red. Rupture causes purulent drainage and relieves the pain.

Temporomandibular joint infection

Typically unilateral, this infection produces ear pain that's referred from the jaw joint. The pain is aggravated by pressure on the jaw with jaw movement; commonly, it radiates to the temporal area or the entire side of the head.

Fatigue

A common symptom, fatigue is a feeling of excessive tiredness, lack of energy, or exhaustion accompanied by a strong desire to rest or sleep. Fatigue differs from weakness, which involves the muscles, but may accompany it.

A normal response to physical overexertion, emotional stress, and sleep deprivation, fatigue can also result from psychological and physiologic disorders, especially viral infections and endocrine, cardiovascular, or neurologic disorders.

Health history

• When did the fatigue begin? Is it constant or intermittent? If it's intermittent, when does it occur? Does the fatigue worsen with activity and improve with rest or vice versa? (The former usually signals physiologic disorder; the latter, a psychological disorder.)
• Have you experienced any recent stressful changes at home or work?
• Have you changed your eating habits? Have you recently lost or gained weight?

• Have you or has anyone in your family been diagnosed with cardiovascular, endocrine, or neurologic disorder? What about viral infections or psychological disorders?
• What medications are you taking?

Physical examination

Observe the patient's general appearance for signs of depression and organic illness. Is he unkempt? Expressionless? Tired or unhealthy looking? Is he slumped over? Assess his mental status, noting especially any agitation, attention deficits, mental clouding, or psychomotor impairment.

Causes

Anemia

Fatigue after mild activity is often anemia's first symptom. Other signs and symptoms typically include dyspnea, pallor, and tachycardia.

Cancer

Unexplained fatigue is often the earliest indication of cancer. Related signs and symptoms reflect the type, location, and stage of the tumor and usually include abnormal bleeding, anorexia, nausea, pain, a palpable mass, vomiting, and weight loss.

Chronic infection

In a patient with a chronic infections, fatigue is usually the most prominent symptom — and sometimes the only one.

Depression

Chronic depression is almost always accompanied by persistent fatigue that's unrelated to exertion. The patient may also complain of anorexia, constipation, headache, and sexual dysfunction.

Diabetes mellitus

The most common symptom in this disorder, fatigue may begin insidiously or abruptly. Related findings include polydipsia, polyphagia, polyuria, and weight loss.

Heart failure

Persistent fatigue and lethargy are characteristic symptoms of heart failure. Left-sided heart failure produces exertional and paroxysmal nocturnal dyspnea, orthopnea, and tachycardia. Right-sided heart failure causes neck vein distention and, sometimes, a slight but persistent nonproductive cough.

Myasthenia gravis

The cardinal symptoms of this disorder are easy fatigability and muscle weakness that worsen with exercise and abate with rest. These symptoms are related to the specific muscle groups affected.

Other causes

Fatigue can be caused by anxiety, myocardial infarction, rheumatoid arthritis, systemic lupus erythematosus, pregnancy, and malnutrition. Certain drugs — notably antihypertensives and sedatives — and most types of surgery also cause fatigue.

Fever

An abnormal elevation of body temperature above 98.6° F (37° C), fever (or pyrexia) is a common sign arising from disorders that affect virtually every body system. As a result, fever alone has little diagnostic value. However, persistently high fever is a medical emergency.

Fever can be classified as low (oral reading of 99° to 100.4° F [37.2° to 38° C]), moderate (100.5° to 104° F [38.1° to 40.1° C]), or high (above 104° F [40° C]). A temperature above 108° F (42.2° C) causes unconsciousness and, if prolonged, brain damage.

Health history

- When did the fever begin? How high did it reach? Is the fever constant, or does it disappear and then reappear later?
- Do you also have chills, fatigue, or pain?
- Have you had any immunodeficiency disorders, infections, recent trauma or surgery, or diagnostic tests? Have you traveled recently?
- What medications are you taking? Have you recently received an anesthetic?

Causes

Infectious and inflammatory disorders

Fever may be low, as in Crohn's disease and ulcerative colitis, or extremely high, as in bacterial pneumonia. It may be remittent, as in infectious mononucleosis; sustained, as in meningitis; or relapsing, as in malaria. The temperature may rise abruptly, as in Rocky Mountain spotted fever, or gradually, as in mycoplasmal pneumonia. Typically, it accompanies a self-limiting disorder such as the common cold.

Medications

Fever and rash commonly result from hypersensitivity to quinidine, methyldopa (Aldomet), procainamide hydrochloride (Pronestyl), phenytoin (Dilantin), anti-infectives, barbiturates, iodides, and some antitoxins. Fever can also result from the use of chemotherapeutic agents and medications that decrease sweating, such as anticholinergics. Plus, toxic doses of salicylates, amphetamines, and tricyclic antidepressants can cause fever.

Other causes

Fever may also result from an injection of contrast media used in diagnostic tests, from surgery, and from blood transfusion reactions.

 SPECIAL POPULATIONS Infants and young children experience higher and more prolonged fevers, more rapid temperature increases, and greater temperature fluctuations than do older children and adults.

Hematuria

A cardinal sign of renal and urinary tract disorders, hematuria is the presence of blood in the urine. Hematuria may be evident or confirmed by a urine test for occult blood.

The bleeding may be continuous or intermittent, is often accompanied by pain, and may be aggravated by prolonged standing or walking. Dark or brownish blood indicates renal or upper urinary tract bleeding; bright red blood, lower urinary tract bleeding.

Health history

• When did you first notice blood in your urine? Does it occur every time you urinate? Are you passing any clots? Have you ever had this problem before?
• Do you have any pain? If so, does the pain occur only when you urinate, or is it continuous?
• Do you have bleeding hemorrhoids? Have you had any recent trauma or performed any strenuous exercise? Do you have a history of renal, urinary, prostatic, or coagulation disorders? For women patients: Are you menstruating?
• What medications are you taking?

Physical examination

Check the urinary meatus for bleeding and abnormalities. Then palpate the abdomen and flanks, noting pain and tenderness. Finally, percuss the abdomen and flanks, especially the costovertebral angle, to elicit tenderness.

Causes

Bladder cancer

A primary cause of gross hematuria in men, bladder cancer may produce pain in the bladder, rectum, pelvis, flank, back, or legs. You may also note signs of urinary tract infection.

Calculi

Both bladder and renal calculi produce hematuria, which may be accompanied by signs and symptoms of urinary tract infection. Bladder calculi usually produce gross hematuria, pain referred to the penile or vulvar area and, in some patients, bladder distention. Renal calculi may produce either microscopic or gross hematuria.

Glomerulonephritis

Usually, acute glomerulonephritis begins with gross hematuria. It may also produce anuria or oliguria, flank and abdominal pain, and increased blood pressure. Chronic glomerulonephritis typically causes microscopic hematuria accompanied by generalized edema, increased blood pressure, and proteinuria.

Nephritis

Acute nephritis causes fever, a maculopapular rash, and microscopic hematuria. In chronic interstitial nephritis, the patient may have dilute, almost colorless urine along with polyuria.

Pyelonephritis (acute)

A typical sign of pyelonephritis is microscopic or macroscopic hematuria that progresses to grossly bloody hematuria. After the infection resolves, microscopic hematuria may persist for a few months. Other findings include flank pain, high fever, and signs and symptoms of a urinary tract infection.

Renal infarction

Patients with renal infarction usually have gross hematuria. Other signs and symptoms include anorexia; costovertebral angle tenderness; and constant, severe flank and upper abdominal pain.

Other causes

Hematuria may result from benign prostatic hyperplasia, bladder trauma, obstructive nephropathy, polycystic kidney disease, renal trauma, and urethral trauma. Also, diagnostic tests, such as cystoscopy and renal biopsy; drugs such as anticoagulants; and some chemotherapeutic agents, such as aldesleukin(interleukin 2), BCG intravesical (TheraCys), ifosfamide (IFEX), and leuprolide (Lupron).

Hemoptysis

The expectoration of blood or bloody sputum from the lungs or tracheobronchial tree is known as hemoptysis. Usually resulting from a tracheobronchial tree abnormality, hemoptysis is associated with inflammatory conditions or lesions that cause erosion and necrosis of bronchial tissues and blood vessels.

Sometimes, hemoptysis is confused with bleeding from the mouth, throat, nasopharynx, or GI tract. Severe hemoptysis requires emergency endotracheal intubation and suctioning.

Health history

• When did you begin expectorating blood? How much blood or sputum are you expectorating? How often?
• Did you recently have a flulike syndrome? Have you had any recent invasive pulmonary procedures or chest trauma?
• Do you smoke? Did you ever smoke? If so, how much? Have you ever been diagnosed with a cardiac, respiratory, or bleeding disorder?
• What medications are you taking? Are you taking anticoagulants?

Physical examination

After assessing the patient's level of consciousness, examine his nose, mouth, and pharynx for sources of bleeding. Observe the rate and depth of his respirations, noting any breathing difficulty or abnormal breathing patterns. Also, as he breathes, look for abnormal chest movement, accessory muscle use, and retractions. Inspect the skin for central and peripheral cyanosis, diaphoresis, lesions, and pallor.

Palpate the rate, rhythm, and intensity of the peripheral pulses. Then feel the chest, noting abnormal pulsations, diaphragmatic tenderness, and fremitus. Check for respiratory excursion. If the patient has a history of trauma, carefully check the position of the trachea and note edema.

As you percuss over the lung fields, note any dullness, flatness, hyperresonance, or tympany. Then auscultate the lungs for crackles, rhonchi, and wheezes and the heart for bruits, gallops, murmurs, and pleural friction rubs. Be sure to monitor the patient's blood pressure and pulse pressure. (See *Identifying hemoptysis,* page 26.)

IDENTIFYING HEMOPTYSIS

These guidelines will help you distinguish hemoptysis, hematemesis, and brown, red, or pink sputum.

Hemoptysis

Often frothy because it's mixed with air, hemoptysis is typically bright red with an alkaline pH (tested with nitrazine paper). It's strongly suggested by the presence of respiratory signs and symptoms, including a cough, a tickling sensation in the throat, and blood produced from repeated coughing episodes. (You can rule out epistaxis because the patient's nasal passages and posterior pharynx are usually clear.)

Hematemesis

The usual site of hematemesis is the GI tract. The patient vomits or regurgitates coffee-ground material that contains food particles, tests positive for occult blood, and has an acid pH. However, he may vomit bright red blood or swallow blood from the oral cavity and nasopharynx. After an episode of hematemesis, the patient may have stools with traces of blood. Many patients with hematemesis also complain of dyspepsia.

Brown, red, or pink sputum

Brown, red, or pink sputum can result from oxidation of inhaled bronchodilators. Sputum that looks like old blood may result from rupture of an amebic abscess into the bronchus. Red or brown sputum may occur in a patient with pneumonia caused by the enterobacterium *Serratia marcescens*. "Currant jelly" sputum occurs with *Klebsiella* infections.

Causes

Bronchitis (chronic)

With this disorder, the patient usually has a productive cough that lasts at least 3 months and leads to expectoration of blood-streaked sputum. Other respiratory signs include dyspnea, prolonged expiration, scattered rhonchi, and wheezing.

Lung abscess

A patient with a lung abscess expectorates copious amounts of bloody, purulent, foul-smelling sputum. He also has anorexia, chills, diaphoresis, fever, headache, and pleuritic or dull chest pain. Lung auscultation may reveal tubular breath sounds or crackles. Percussion reveals dullness on the affected side. The patient may have a history of a recent pulmonary infection or evidence of poor oral hygiene with dental or gingival disease.

Lung cancer

Ulceration of the bronchus commonly causes recurring hemoptysis, which can vary from blood-streaked sputum to frank blood. Related findings include anorexia, chest pain, dyspnea, fever, a productive cough, weight loss, and wheezing.

Pulmonary edema

A patient with pulmonary edema may expectorate copious amounts of frothy, blood-tinged, pink sputum. He may also complain of dyspnea and orthopnea. On examination, you may detect diffuse crackles in both lung fields and a ventricular gallop.

Tracheal trauma

With tracheal trauma, the bleeding appears to come from the back of the throat. Accompanying signs and symptoms include airway occlusion, dysphagia, hoarseness, neck pain, and respiratory distress.

Other causes

Hemoptysis may also result from bronchiectasis, coagulation disorders, cystic fibrosis, lung or airway injuries from diagnostic procedures, and primary pulmonary hypertension.

Hoarseness

A rough or harsh-sounding voice, hoarseness can be acute or chronic. It may result from infections or inflammatory lesions or exudates in the larynx, from laryngeal edema, from compression or disruption of the vocal cords or recurrent laryngeal nerve damage, or from irritating polyps on the vocal cords. Hoarseness can also occur with aging because the laryngeal muscles and mucosa atrophy, leading to diminished control of the vocal cords. Hoarseness may be exacerbated by excessive alcohol intake, smoking, inhalation of noxious fumes, excessive talking, and shouting.

Health history

• When did the hoarseness start? Is it constant or intermittent? Does anything relieve or exacerbate it? Have you been overusing your voice?
• Have you also had a cough, a dry mouth, difficulty swallowing dry food, shortness of breath, or a sore throat?
• Have you ever had cancer or other disorders? Do you regularly drink alcohol or smoke? If so, how much?

Physical examination

Inspect the patient's mouth and throat for redness or exudate, possibly indicating an upper respiratory tract infection. Ask him to stick out his tongue; if he can't, the hypoglossal nerve (cranial nerve XII) may be impaired.

As the patient breathes, observe for asymmetrical chest expansion, intercostal retractions, nasal flaring, stridor, and other signs of respiratory distress.

Palpate the patient's neck for masses and the cervical lymph nodes and thyroid gland for enlargement. Then palpate the trachea to assess for deviation.

As you percuss the chest wall, note any dullness. Then auscultate the lungs for crackles, rhonchi, tubular sounds, and wheezes. To detect bradycardia, auscultate the heart.

Causes

Inhalation injury

Exposure to a fire or an explosion can cause an inhalation injury, which produces coughing, hoarseness, orofacial burns, singed nasal hair, and soot-stained sputum. Subsequent signs and symptoms include crackles, rhonchi, wheezes, and respiratory distress.

Laryngitis

Persistent hoarseness may be the only sign of chronic laryngitis. In acute laryngitis, hoarseness or a complete loss of voice develops suddenly. Related findings include cough, fever, pain (especially during swallowing or speaking), profuse diaphoresis, rhinorrhea, and sore throat.

Vocal cord injuries

With vocal cord injuries, a raspy hoarseness is the chief complaint. The patient may also have a chronic cough and a crackling voice.

Other causes

Hoarseness may result from hypothyroidism, pulmonary tuberculosis, rheumatoid arthritis, and laryngeal cancer (most common in men ages 50 to 70). Prolonged intubation, surgical severing of the recurrent laryngeal nerve, and tracheostomy may also produce hoarseness.

Nausea

A profound feeling of revulsion to food or a signal of impending vomiting, nausea is usually accompanied by anorexia, diaphoresis, hypersalivation, pallor, tachycardia, tachypnea, and vomiting. A common symptom of GI disorders, nausea may also result from electrolyte imbalances; infections; metabolic, endocrine, and cardiac disorders; early months of pregnancy; drug therapy; surgery; and radiation therapy. Also, severe pain, anxiety, alcohol intoxication, overeating, and ingestion of something distasteful can trigger nausea.

Health history

• When did the nausea begin? Is it intermittent or constant? How severe is it?
• Do you have other symptoms, such as abdominal pain, loss of appetite, changes in bowel habits, excessive belching or gas, weight loss, and vomiting?
• For female patients: Are you pregnant or could you be?
• Have you ever had any GI, endocrine, or metabolic disorders? Have you had any recent infections? Have you ever had cancer, radiation therapy, or chemotherapy?
• What medications are you taking?
• Do you drink alcohol and, if so, how much?

Physical examination

Examine the patient's skin for bruises, jaundice, poor turgor, and spider angiomas. Then inspect his abdomen for distention.

Auscultate the abdomen first, listening for bowel sounds in each quadrant. Then, using the bell of the stethoscope, listen for abdominal bruits. Next, palpate the abdomen for rigidity, tenderness, and rebound tenderness and palpate the liver for enlargement. Finally, percuss the abdomen and liver for abnormalities.

Causes

Appendicitis

The patient with appendicitis feels nauseated and may vomit. He'll also have vague epigastric or periumbilical discomfort that localizes in the right lower quadrant.

Cholecystitis (acute)

In this disorder, nausea commonly follows severe right upper quadrant pain that may radiate to the back or shoulders. Associated findings include abdominal tenderness, vomiting, abdominal rigidity and distention, diaphoresis, fever, and chills.

Gastritis

Patients with gastritis often have nausea, especially after ingestion of alcohol, aspirin, spicy foods, or caffeine. Belching, epigastric pain, fever, malaise, and vomiting of mucus or blood may also occur.

Other causes

Nausea may result from cirrhosis, electrolyte imbalances, labyrinthitis, metabolic acidosis, myocardial infarction, renal and urologic disorders, and ulcerative colitis. Use of anesthetics, antibiotics, antineoplastics, ferrous sulfate, oral potassium, and quinidine as well as overdoses of digitalis glycosides and theophylline, radiation therapy, and surgery—especially abdominal surgery—may also trigger nausea.

Palpitations

Defined as a person's conscious awareness of his own heartbeat, palpitations are usually felt over the precordium or in the throat or neck. The patient may describe his heart as pounding, jumping, turning, fluttering, flopping, or missing or skipping beats. Palpitations may be regular or irregular, fast or slow, and paroxysmal or sustained. Besides cardiac causes, palpitations may stem from anxiety, drug reactions, hypertension, thyroid hormone deficiency, and several other problems.

Health history

• When did the palpitations start? Where do you feel them? How would you describe them? What were you doing when they started? How long did they last? Have you ever had palpitations before?
• Do you have chest pain, dizziness, or weakness along with the palpitations?
• Are you under unusual stress at home or work? Have you recently undergone multiple blood transfusions or an infusion of phosphate?
• Have you ever had thyroid disease, calcium or vitamin D deficiency, malabsorption syndrome, bone cancer, renal disease, hypoglycemia, or cardiovascular or pulmonary disorders that may produce arrhythmias or hypertension?
• What medications are you taking? Are you taking an over-the-counter drug that contains caffeine or a sympathomimetic, such as a cough, cold, or allergy preparation? Do you smoke or drink alcohol? If so, how much?

Physical examination

Assess the patient's level of consciousness, noting anxiety, confusion, or irrational behavior. Check his skin for pallor and diaphoresis. Then observe the eyes for exophthalmos.

Note the rate and depth of his respirations, checking for abnormal patterns and breathing difficulty. Also, inspect the fingertips for capillary nail bed pulsations.

To check for thyroid gland enlargement, gently palpate the patient's neck. Then palpate his muscles for weakness and twitching. Evaluate his peripheral pulses, noting the rate, rhythm, and intensity. Assess his reflexes for hyperreflexia.

Auscultate the heart for gallops and murmurs and the lungs for abnormal breath sounds. Be sure to monitor blood pressure and pulse pressure.

Causes

Acute anxiety attack
Palpitations may be accompanied by diaphoresis, facial flushing, and trembling. The patient usually hyperventilates, which may lead to dizziness, syncope, and weakness.

Cardiac arrhythmias
Paroxysmal or sustained palpitations may occur with dizziness, fatigue, and weakness. Other signs and symptoms include chest pain; confusion; decreased blood pressure; diaphoresis; pallor; and an irregular, rapid, or slow pulse rate. The patient may be using drugs that can cause cardiac arrhythmias — for instance, antihypertensives, sympathomimetics, ganglionic blockers, anticholinergics, or methylxanthines.

Thyrotoxicosis
In this disorder, sustained palpitations may accompany diaphoresis, diarrhea, dyspnea, heat intolerance, nervousness, tachycardia, tremors, and weight loss despite increased appetite. Exophthalmos and an enlarged thyroid gland may also develop.

Other causes
Palpitations may also arise from anemia, aortic insufficiency, hypocalcemia, hypertension, hypoglycemia, mitral valve stenosis or prolapse, and pheochromocytoma.

Paresthesia

Paresthesia is an abnormal sensation that is commonly described as a numbness, prickling, or tingling felt along peripheral nerve pathways. It may develop suddenly or gradually and be transient or permanent. A common symptom of many neurologic disorders, paresthesia may also occur in certain systemic disorders and with the use of certain drugs.

Health history

• When did the paresthesia begin? What does it feel like? Where does it occur? Is it transient or constant?
• Have you had recent trauma, surgery, or an invasive procedure that may have injured peripheral nerves? Have you been exposed to industrial solvents or heavy metals? Have you had long-term radiation therapy? Do you have any neurologic, cardiovascular, metabolic, renal, or chronic inflammatory disorders, such as arthritis and lupus erythematosus?
• What medications are you taking?

Physical examination

Focus on the patient's neurologic status, assessing his level of consciousness and cranial nerve function. Also note his skin color and temperature. Test muscle strength and deep tendon reflexes in the extremities affected by paresthesia. Systematically evaluate light touch, pain, temperature, vibration, and position sensation. Then palpate his pulses.

Causes

Arterial occlusion (acute)

A patient with arterial occlusion may complain of sudden paresthesia and coldness in one or both legs. Aching pain at rest, intermittent claudication, and paresis are also characteristic. The leg becomes mottled, and a line of temperature and color demarcation develops at the level of the occlusion. Pulses are absent below the occlusion and capillary refill time is diminished.

Brain tumor

Tumors that affect the parietal lobe may cause progressive contralateral paresthesia accompanied by agnosia, agraphia, apraxia, homonymous hemianopia, and loss of proprioception.

Herniated disk

Herniation of a lumbar or cervical disk may cause acute or gradual paresthesia along the distribution pathways of the affected spinal nerves. Other neuromuscular effects include muscle spasms, severe pain, and weakness.

Herpes zoster

Herniation, an early symptom of herpes zoster, occurs in the dermatome supplied by the affected spinal nerve. Within several days, this dermatome is marked by a pruritic, erythematous, vesicular rash accompanied by sharp, shooting pain.

Spinal cord injury

Paresthesia may occur in a partial spinal cord transection after spinal shock resolves. The paresthesia may be unilateral or bilateral and occur at or below the level of the lesion.

Other disorders

Paresthesia may result from arthritis, cerebrovascular accident, migraine headache, multiple sclerosis, peripheral neuropathies, vitamin B_{12} deficiency, hypocalcemia, and heavy metal or solvent poisoning. Also, long-term radiation therapy, parenteral gold therapy, and certain drugs, such as chemotherapeutic agents, guanadrel (Hylorel), interferons, and isoniazid (Laniazid), may cause paresthesia.

Pyrosis

A substernal burning sensation that rises in the chest and may radiate to the neck or throat, pyrosis results from the reflux of gastric contents into the esophagus. Usually, it's accompanied by regurgitation. Because increased intra-abdominal pressure contributes to reflux, pyrosis commonly occurs with pregnancy, ascites, or obesity, but it may also be caused by GI disorders, connective tissue disease, and certain drugs.

In most cases, pyrosis develops after meals or when a person lies down, bends over, lifts heavy objects, or exercises vigorously. It usually worsens with swallowing and improves when the person sits upright or takes antacids. Some patients confuse pyrosis with a myocardial infarction (MI), but a patient who is having an MI typically has other symptoms besides a burning sensation.

When a patient complains of pyrosis, you'll obtain a health history, but you won't perform a physical examination.

Health history

• When did the pyrosis start? Do certain foods or beverages trigger it? Does stress or fatigue seem to aggravate it? Do movement, certain body positions, or very hot or cold liquids worsen or relieve it? Where exactly is the burning sensation? Does it radiate to other areas? Does it cause you to regurgitate sour- or bitter-tasting fluids? Have you ever had pyrosis before?
• Do you have a history of GI problems or connective tissue disease? For women of child-bearing age: are you pregnant?
• What medications are you taking?

Causes

Esophageal cancer
Pyrosis may be a sign of esophageal cancer. The first symptom is usually painless dysphagia that progressively worsens. Eventually, partial obstruction and rapid weight loss occur. The patient may complain of a feeling of substernal fullness, hoarseness, nausea, sore throat, steady pain in the posterior and anterior chest, and vomiting.

Gastroesophageal reflux
Severe, chronic pyrosis is the most common symptom of this disorder. The pyrosis usually occurs within 1 hour after eating and may be triggered by certain foods or beverages. It worsens when the person lies down or bends over and abates when he sits, stands, or ingests antacids. Other findings include a dull retrosternal pain that may radiate, dysphagia, flatulent dyspepsia, and postural regurgitation.

Peptic ulcer
Pyrosis and indigestion usually signal the onset of a peptic ulcer attack. Most patients experience a gnawing, burning pain in the left epigastrium, although some report sharp pain. The pain typically occurs when the stomach is empty and is often relieved by taking antacids. The pain may also occur after the patient ingests coffee, aspirin, or alcohol.

Scleroderma

A connective tissue disease, scleroderma may cause esophageal dysfunction, resulting in pyrosis, bloating after meals, odynophagia, the sensation of food sticking behind the sternum, and weight loss. Other GI effects include abdominal distention, constipation or diarrhea, and malodorous, floating stools.

Other causes

Pyrosis may be caused by esophageal diverticula, obesity, and several drugs, including aspirin, nonsteroidal anti-inflammatory drugs, anticholinergic agents, inhaled corticosteroids or inhaled beta-adrenergic agents, and drugs having anticholinergic effects.

Vision loss

Vision loss can occur suddenly or gradually, can be temporary or permanent, and may range from a slight impairment to total blindness. It may result from eye, neurologic, and systemic disorders as well as from trauma and reactions to certain drugs.

Health history

• When did the loss first occur? Did it occur suddenly or gradually? Does it affect one or both eyes? Does it affect all or part of the visual field?
• Are you experiencing blurred vision, halo vision, nausea, pain, photosensitivity, or vomiting with the vision loss?
• Have you had a recent facial or eye injury?
• Have you ever had cardiovascular or endocrine disorders, infections, or allergies? Does anyone in your family have a history of vision loss or other eye problems?
• What medications are you taking?

Physical examination

Observe the patient's eyes for conjunctival or scleral redness, drainage, edema, foreign bodies, and signs of trauma. With a flashlight, examine the cornea and iris. Observe the size, shape, and color of the pupils. Then test direct and consensual light reflexes and visual accommodation, extraocular muscle function, and visual acuity. Gently palpate each eye, noting any hardness. Then auscultate over the temple for carotid bruits.

Causes

Eye trauma

Sudden unilateral or bilateral vision loss may occur after an eye injury. The loss may be total or partial, permanent or temporary. The eyelids may be reddened, edematous, and lacerated.

Glaucoma

Acute angle-closure glaucoma may cause sudden blindness. Findings include halo vision, nonreactive pupillary response, photophobia, rapid onset of unilateral inflammation and pain, and reduced visual acuity. By contrast, chronic open-angle glaucoma progresses slowly. Usually bilateral, it causes aching eyes, halo vision, peripheral vision loss, and reduced visual acuity.

Other causes

Vision loss may also be caused by congenital rubella or syphilis, herpes zoster, Marfan's syndrome, a pituitary tumor, retrolental fibroplasia, and drugs such as digitalis glycosides, indomethacin (Indocin), ethambutol hydrochloride (Myambutol), quinine sulfate, and methanol.

Visual floaters

Particles of blood or cellular debris that move about in the vitreous humor appear as spots or dots when they enter the visual field. Chronic floaters commonly appear in elderly or myopic patients. But the sudden onset of visual floaters often signals retinal detachment, an ocular emergency.

Health history

• When did the floaters first appear? What do they look like? Did they appear suddenly or gradually? If they appeared suddenly, did you also see flashing lights and have a curtainlike loss of vision?
• Are you nearsighted, and do you wear corrective lenses?
• Do you have a history of eye trauma or other eye disorders, allergies, granulomatous disease, diabetes mellitus, or hypertension?
• What medications are you taking?

Physical examination

Inspect the eyes for signs of injury, such as bruising and edema. Then assess the patient's visual acuity, using the Snellen alphabet or "E" chart.

Causes

Retinal detachment

Floaters and light flashes appear suddenly in the portion of the visual field where the retina has detached. As retinal detachment progresses (a painless process), gradual vision loss occurs, with the patient seeing a "curtain" falling in front of his eyes. Ophthalmoscopic examination reveals a gray, opaque, detached retina with an indefinite margin. Retinal vessels appear almost black.

Vitreous hemorrhage

Rupture of retinal vessels produces a shower of red or black dots or a red haze across the visual field. Vision blurs suddenly in the affected eye, and visual acuity may be greatly reduced.

Other causes

Visual floaters may also result from posterior uveitis.

Weight loss

Weight loss can reflect decreased food intake, increased metabolic requirements, or a combination of the two. Its causes include endocrine, neoplastic, GI, and psychological disorders; nutritional deficiencies; infections; and neurologic lesions that cause paralysis and dysphagia. Weight loss may also accompany conditions that prevent sufficient food intake, such as painful oral lesions, ill-fitting dentures, and the loss of teeth. Weight loss may stem from poverty, adherence to fad diets, excessive exercise, and drug use.

Health history

• When did you first notice you were losing weight? How much weight have you lost? Was the weight loss intentional? If not, can you think of any reason for it?
• What do you usually eat in a day? Have your eating habits changed recently? Why?
• Have your stools changed recently? For instance, have you noticed bulky, floating stools or have you had diarrhea? What about abdominal pain, excessive thirst, excessive urination, heat intolerance, nausea, or vomiting?
• Have you felt anxious or depressed? If so, why?

• What medications are you taking? Do you take diet pills or laxatives to lose weight?

Physical examination

Record the patient's height and weight. As you take his vital signs, note his general appearance. Does he appear well-nourished? Do his clothes fit? Is muscle wasting evident?

Next, examine his skin for turgor and abnormal pigmentation, especially around the joints. Does he have jaundice or pallor? Examine his mouth, including the condition of his teeth or dentures. Also check his eyes for exophthalmos and his neck for swelling.

Finally, palpate the patient's abdomen for liver enlargement, masses, and tenderness.

Causes

Anorexia nervosa

A psychogenic disorder, anorexia nervosa is most common in young women and is characterized by a severe, self-imposed weight loss. This may be accompanied by amenorrhea, blotchy or sallow skin, cold intolerance, constipation, frequent infections, loss of fatty tissue, loss of scalp hair, and skeletal muscle atrophy.

Cancer

Weight loss is a common sign of cancer. Associated signs and symptoms reflect the type, location, and stage of the tumor and typically include abnormal bleeding, anorexia, fatigue, nausea, pain, a palpable mass, and vomiting.

Crohn's disease

Weight loss occurs with abdominal pain, anorexia, and chronic cramping. Other findings include abdominal distention, tenderness, and guarding; diarrhea; hyperactive bowel sounds; pain; and tachycardia.

Depression

In severe depression, weight loss may occur along with anorexia, apathy, fatigue, feelings of worthlessness, and insomnia or hypersomnia. Other signs and symptoms include incoherence, indecisiveness, and suicidal thoughts or behavior.

Leukemia

Acute leukemia causes a progressive weight loss accompanied by bleeding tendencies, high fever, and severe prostration. Chronic leukemia causes a progressive weight loss with anemia, anorexia, bleeding tendencies, an enlarged spleen, fatigue, fever, pallor, and skin eruptions.

Other causes

Weight loss may result from adrenal insufficiency, diabetes mellitus, gastroenteritis, cryptosporidiosis, lymphoma, ulcerative colitis, and thyrotoxicosis. Drugs such as amphetamines, chemotherapeutic agents, laxatives, and thyroid preparations can also cause weight loss.

ECGs

Interpreting them with ease and accuracy

Normal ECG

How to read any ECG: An 8-step guide

An electrocardiogram (ECG) waveform has three basic elements: a P wave, a QRS complex, and a T wave. They're joined by five other useful diagnostic elements: the PR interval, the U wave, the ST segment, the J point, and the QT interval. The diagram below shows how these elements are related.

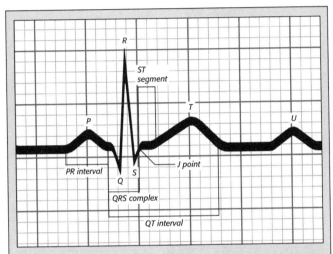

The following 8-step guide will enable you to read any ECG.

Step 1: Evaluate the P wave

Observe the P wave's size, shape, and location in the waveform. If the P wave consistently precedes the QRS complex, the electrical impulse is being initiated by the sinoatrial (SA) node, as it should be.

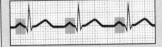

Step 2: Evaluate the atrial rhythm

The P wave should occur at regular intervals, with only small variations associated with respiration. Using a pair of calipers, you can easily measure the interval between P waves — the P-P interval. Compare the P-P intervals in several ECG cycles. Make sure the calipers are set at the same point — at the beginning of the wave or on its peak. Instead of lifting the calipers, rotate one of its legs to the next P wave, to ensure accurate measurements.

Step 3: Determine the atrial rate

To determine the atrial rate quickly, count the number of P waves in two 3-second segments. Multiply this number by 10. For a more accurate determination, count the number of small squares between two P waves, using either the apex of the wave or the initial upstroke of the wave. Each small square equals 0.04 second; 1,500 squares equal 1 minute (0.04 ×1,500 = 60 seconds). So, divide 1,500 by the number of squares you counted between the P waves. This gives you the atrial rate — the number of contractions per minute.

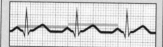

Step 4: Calculate duration of the PR interval

Count the number of small squares between the beginning of the P wave and the beginning of the QRS complex. Multiply the number of squares by 0.04 second. The normal interval is between 0.12 and 0.20 second, or between three and five small squares wide. A wider interval indicates delayed conduction of the impulse through the atrioventricular (AV) node to the ventricles. A short PR interval indicates the impulse originated in an area other than the SA node.

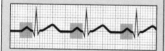

Step 5: Evaluate the ventricular rhythm

Use the calipers to measure the R-R intervals. Remember to place the calipers on the same point of the QRS complex. If the R-R intervals remain consistent, the ventricular rhythm is regular.

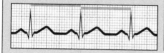

Step 6: Determine the ventricular rate

To determine the ventricular rate, use the same formula as in Step 3. In this case, however, count the number of small squares between two R waves to do the calculation. Also check that the QRS complex is shaped appropriately for the lead you're monitoring.

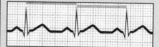

Step 7: Calculate the duration of the QRS complex

Count the number of squares between the beginning and the end of the QRS complex and multiply by 0.04 second. A normal QRS complex is less than 0.12 second, or less than three small squares wide. Some references specify 0.06 to 0.10 second as the normal duration for the QRS complex.

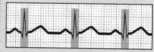

Step 8: Calculate the duration of the QT interval

Count the number of squares from the beginning of the QRS complex to the end of the T wave. Multiply this number by 0.04 second. The normal range is 0.36 to 0.44 second, or 9 to 11 small squares wide.

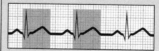

Normal sinus rhythm

When the heart functions normally, the sinoatrial (SA) node acts as the primary pacemaker, initiating the electrical impulses that set the rhythm for cardiac contractions. The SA node assumes this role because its automatic firing rate exceeds that of the heart's other pacemakers, allowing cells to depolarize spontaneously. Two factors account for increased automaticity. First, during the resting phase of the depolarization-repolarization cycle, SA node cells have the least negative charge. Second, depolarization actually begins during the resting phase.

Based on an electrical disturbance's location, arrhythmias can be classified as sinus, atrial, junctional, or ventricular arrhythmias or atrioventricular (AV) blocks. Functional disturbances in the SA node produce sinus arrhythmias. Enhanced automaticity of atrial tissue or reentry may produce atrial arrhythmias, the most common arrhythmias.

Junctional arrhythmias originate in the area around the AV node and His' bundle. These arrhythmias usually result from a suppressed higher pacemaker or blocked impulses at the AV node.

Ventricular arrhythmias originate in ventricular tissue below the bifurcation of the bundle of His. These rhythms may result from reentry or enhanced automaticity or after depolarization.

An AV block results from an abnormal interruption or delay of atrial impulse conduction to the ventricles. It may be partial or total and may occur in the AV node, bundle of His, or Purkinje system.

Characteristics and interpretation

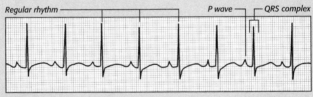

LEAD II

Atrial rhythm: regular
Ventricular rhythm: regular
Atrial rate: 60 to 100 beats/minute (80 beats/minute shown)
Ventricular rate: 60 to 100 beats/minute (80 beats/minute shown)
P wave: normally shaped (All P waves have similar size and shape; a P wave precedes each QRS complex.)
PR interval: within normal limits (0.12 to 0.20 second) and constant (0.20-second duration shown)

QRS complex: within normal limits (0.06 to 0.10 second) (All QRS complexes have the same configuration. The duration shown here is 0.12 second.)
T wave: normally shaped; upright and rounded (Each QRS complex is followed by a T wave.)
QT interval: within normal limits (0.36 to 0.44 second) and constant (0.44-second duration shown)

Arrhythmias
Sinus arrhythmia

In sinus arrhythmia, the heart rate stays within normal limits but the rhythm is irregular and corresponds to the respiratory cycle and variations in vagal tone. During inspiration, an increased volume of blood returns to the heart, reducing vagal tone and increasing sinus rate. During expiration, venous return decreases, vagal tone increases, and sinus rate slows.

Conditions unrelated to respiration may also produce sinus arrhythmia. These conditions include an inferior wall myocardial infarction, digitalis toxicity, and increased intracranial pressure.

Sinus arrhythmia is easily recognized in elderly, pediatric, and sedated patients. The patient's pulse rate increases with inspiration and decreases with expiration. Usually, the patient is asymptomatic.

Intervention

Treatment usually isn't necessary, unless the patient is symptomatic or the sinus arrhythmia stems from an underlying cause. When the patient is symptomatic, atropine may be administered if the heart rate falls below 40 beats/minute.

Characteristics and interpretation

Cyclic, irregular rhythm

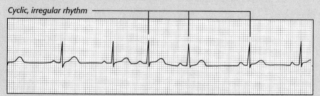

LEAD II

Atrial rhythm: irregular, corresponding to the respiratory cycle
Ventricular rhythm: irregular, corresponding to the respiratory cycle
Atrial rate: within normal limits; varies with respiration (60 beats/minute shown)
Ventricular rate: within normal limits; varies with respiration (60 beats/minute shown)
P wave: normal size and configuration (One P wave precedes each QRS complex.)

PR interval: within normal limits (0.16-second, constant interval shown)
QRS complex: normal duration and configuration (0.06-second duration shown)
T wave: normal size and configuration
QT interval: within normal limits (0.36- second interval shown)
Other: phasic slowing and quickening of the rhythm

Sinus bradycardia

Characterized by a sinus rate of less than 60 beats/minute, sinus bradycardia usually occurs as the normal response to a reduced demand for blood flow. It's common among athletes, whose well-conditioned hearts can maintain stroke volume with reduced effort. It may also be caused by drugs, such as digitalis glycosides, calcium channel blockers, and beta-adrenergic blockers. Sinus bradycardia may occur after an inferior wall myocardial infarction involving the right coronary artery, which provides the blood supply to the sinoatrial node. The rhythm may develop during sleep and in patients with increased intracranial pressure. It may also result from vagal stimulation caused by vomiting or defecating.

Pathological sinus bradycardia may occur with sick sinus syndrome.

The patient with sinus bradycardia is asymptomatic if he's able to compensate for the drop in heart rate by increasing stroke volume. If not, he may have signs and symptoms of decreased cardiac output, such as hypotension, syncope, confusion, and blurred vision.

Intervention

If the patient is asymptomatic, treatment isn't necessary. If he has signs and symptoms, treatment aims to identify and correct the underlying cause. The heart rate may be increased with such drugs as atropine and isoproterenol (Isuprel). A temporary or permanent pacemaker may be inserted if the bradycardia persists.

Characteristics and interpretation

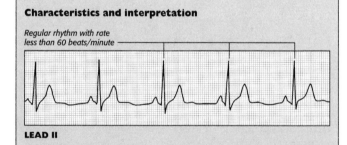

Regular rhythm with rate less than 60 beats/minute

LEAD II

Atrial rhythm: regular
Ventricular rhythm: regular
Atrial rate: less than 60 beats/minute (50 beats/minute shown)
Ventricular rate: less than 60 beats/minute (50 beats/minute shown)
P wave: normal size and configuration (One P wave precedes each QRS complex.)

PR interval: within normal limits and constant (0.14-second duration shown)
QRS complex: normal duration and configuration (0.08-second duration shown)
T wave: normal size and configuration
QT interval: within normal limits (0.40-second interval shown)

Sinus tachycardia

A normal response to cellular demands for increased oxygen delivery and blood flow commonly produces sinus tachycardia. Conditions that cause such a demand include heart failure, shock, anemia, exercise, fever, hypoxia, pain, and stress. Drugs that stimulate the beta receptors in the heart also cause sinus tachycardia. They include isoproterenol (Isuprel), aminophylline (Aminophyllin), and inotropic agents such as dobutamine. Alcohol, caffeine, and nicotine may also produce sinus tachycardia.

An elevated heart rate increases myocardial oxygen demands. If the patient can't meet these demands (for example, because of coronary artery disease), ischemia and further myocardial damage may occur. If tachycardia exceeds 140 beats/minute for longer than 30 minutes, the ECG may show ST-segment and T-wave changes, indicating ischemia.

Intervention

Treatment focuses on finding the primary cause. If it's high catecholamine levels, a beta-adrenergic blocker may slow the heart rate. After myocardial infarction, persistent sinus tachycardia may precede heart failure or cardiogenic shock.

Characteristics and interpretation

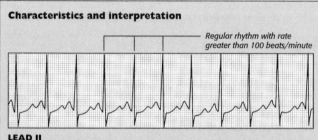

Regular rhythm with rate greater than 100 beats/minute

LEAD II

Atrial rhythm: regular
Ventricular rhythm: regular
Atrial rate: 100 to 160 beats/minute (110 beats/minute shown)
Ventricular rate: 100 to 160 beats/minute (110 beats/minute shown)
P wave: normal size and configuration (One P wave precedes each QRS complex. As the sinus rate reaches about 150 beats/minute, the P wave merges with the preceding T wave and may be difficult to identify. Examine the descending slope of the preceding T wave closely for notches, indicating the presence of the P wave. The P wave shown is normal.)
PR interval: within normal limits and constant (0.16-second duration shown)
QRS complex: normal duration and configuration (0.10-second shown)
T wave: normal size and configuration
QT interval: within normal limits and constant (0.36-second duration shown)
Other: gradual onset and cessation

Sinus arrest

Failure of the sinoatrial node to generate an impulse interrupts the sinus rhythm, producing "sinus pause" when one or two beats are dropped or "sinus arrest" when three or more beats are dropped. Such failure may result from an acute inferior wall myocardial infarction, increased vagal tone, or use of certain drugs (digitalis glycosides, calcium channel blockers, and beta-adrenergic blockers). The arrhythmia may also be linked to sick sinus syndrome. The patient has an irregular pulse rate associated with the sinus rhythm pauses. If the pauses are infrequent, the patient is asymptomatic. If they occur frequently and last for several seconds, the patient may have signs of decreased cardiac output.

Intervention

For a symptomatic patient, treatment focuses on maintaining cardiac output and discovering the cause of the sinus arrest. If indicated, atropine may be given or a temporary or permanent pacemaker may be inserted.

Characteristics and interpretation

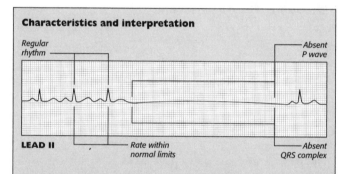

Regular rhythm — Absent P wave

LEAD II — Rate within normal limits — Absent QRS complex

Atrial rhythm: regular, except for the missing complex
Ventricular rhythm: regular, except for the missing complex
Atrial rate: within normal limits but varies because of the pauses (94 beats/minute shown)
Ventricular rate: within normal limits but varies because of pauses (94 beats/minute shown)
P wave: normal size and configuration (One P wave precedes each QRS complex but is absent during a pause.)

PR interval: within normal limits and constant when the P wave is present; not measurable when the P wave is absent (0.20-second duration shown on all complexes surrounding the arrest)
QRS complex: normal duration and configuration; absent during a pause (0.08-second duration shown)
T wave: normal size and configuration; absent during a pause
QT interval: within normal limits; not measurable during pause (0.40-second, constant interval shown)

Premature atrial contractions

Premature atrial contractions (PACs) usually result from an irritable focus in the atria that supersedes the sino-atrial node as the pacemaker for one or two beats. Although PACs commonly occur in normal hearts, they're also associated with coronary and valvular heart disease. In an inferior wall myocardial infarction (MI), PACs may indicate a concomitant right atrial infarct. In an anterior wall MI, PACs are an early sign of left-sided heart failure. They also may warn of a more severe atrial arrhythmia, such as atrial flutter or fibrillation.

Possible causes include digitalis toxicity, hyperthyroidism, elevated catecholamine levels, acute respiratory failure, and chronic obstructive pulmonary disease.

Intervention

Symptomatic patients may be treated with propranolol (Inderal) and disopyramide (Norpace).

Characteristics and interpretation

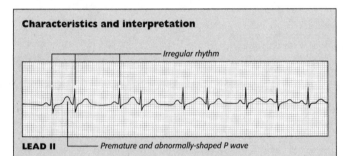

Irregular rhythm

LEAD II — *Premature and abnormally-shaped P wave*

Atrial rhythm: irregular (Incomplete compensatory pause follows PAC. Underlying rhythm may be regular.)
Ventricular rhythm: irregular (Incomplete compensatory pause follows PAC. Underlying rhythm may be regular.)
Atrial rate: varies with underlying rhythm (90 beats/minute shown)
Ventricular rate: varies with underlying rhythm (90 beats/minute shown)
P wave: premature and abnormally shaped; possibly lost in previous T wave (Varying configurations indicate multiform PACs.)

PR interval: usually normal but may be shortened or slightly prolonged, depending on the origin of ectopic focus (0.16-second, constant interval shown)
QRS complex: usually normal duration and configuration (0.08-second, constant duration shown)
T wave: usually normal configuration; may be distorted if the P wave is hidden in the previous T wave
QT interval: usually normal (0.36-second, constant interval shown)
Other: may occur in bigeminy or couplets

Atrial tachycardia

In atrial tachycardia, the atrial rhythm is ectopic and the atrial rate is rapid, shortening diastole. This results in a loss of atrial kick, reduced cardiac output, reduced coronary perfusion, and ischemic myocardial changes.

Although atrial tachycardia occurs in healthy patients, it's usually associated with high catecholamine levels, digitalis toxicity, myocardial infarction, cardiomyopathy, hyperthyroidism, hypertension, and valvular heart disease. Three types of atrial tachycardia exist: atrial tachycardia with block, multifocal atrial tachycardia, and paroxysmal atrial tachycardia.

Intervention

If the patient is symptomatic, prepare for immediate cardioversion. If the patient is stable, the doctor may perform carotid sinus massage (if no bruits are present) or order drug therapy, such as adenosine (Adenocard), verapamil (Calan), digoxin (Lanoxin), beta blockers, or diltiazem (Cardizem). If these measures fail, cardioversion may be necessary.

Characteristics and interpretation

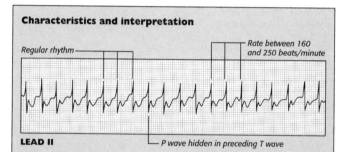

Regular rhythm

Rate between 160 and 250 beats/minute

LEAD II

P wave hidden in preceding T wave

Atrial rhythm: regular
Ventricular rhythm: regular
Atrial rate: three or more successive ectopic atrial beats at a rate of 160 to 250 beats/minute (210 beats/minute shown)
Ventricular rate: varies with atrioventricular conduction ratio (210 beats/minute shown)
P wave: 1:1 ratio with QRS complex, though often indiscernible because of rapid rate; may be hidden in previous ST segment or T wave
PR interval: may be unmeasurable if P wave can't be distinguished from preceding T wave (If P wave is present, PR interval is short when conduction through the AV node is 1:1. On this strip, the PR interval isn't discernible.)
QRS complex: usually normal unless aberrant intraventricular conduction is present (0.10-second duration shown)
T wave: may be normal or inverted if ischemia is present (inverted T waves shown)
QT interval: usually normal but may be shorter because of rapid rate (0.20-second interval shown)
Other: appearance of ST-segment and T-wave changes if tachyarrhythmia persists longer than 30 minutes

Atrial flutter

Characterized by an atrial rate of 300 beats/minute or more, atrial flutter results from multiple reentry circuits within the atrial tissue. Causes include conditions that enlarge atrial tissue and elevate atrial pressures. Atrial flutter is associated with myocardial infarction, increased catecholamine levels, hyperthyroidism, and digitalis toxicity. A ventricular rate of 300 beats/minute suggests the presence of an anomalous pathway.

If the patient's pulse rate is normal, he usually has no symptoms. If his pulse rate is high, he'll probably have signs and symptoms of decreased cardiac output, such as hypotension and syncope.

Intervention

The doctor may perform vagal stimulation to slow the ventricular response and demonstrate the presence of flutter waves. This intervention is contraindicated if a carotid bruit is present. If the patient is symptomatic, prepare for immediate cardioversion. Drugs that may be ordered to slow atrioventricular conduction include calcium channel blockers (diltiazem, verapamil) and beta-adrenergic blockers (esmolol, metoprolol). Digoxin may be ordered, but some experts question its use for urgent treatment. After the rate slows, if conversion to a normal rhythm hasn't occurred, procainamide (Pronestyl) or quinidine (Quinidex) may be ordered.

Characteristics and interpretation

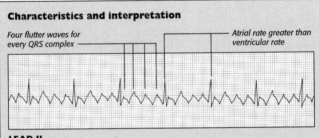

Four flutter waves for every QRS complex

Atrial rate greater than ventricular rate

LEAD II

Atrial rhythm: regular
Ventricular rhythm: may be regular or irregular, depending on the conduction ratio (regular rhythm shown)
Atrial rate: 300 to 350 beats/minute (300 beats/minute shown)
Ventricular rate: variable (70 beats/minute shown)
P wave: atrial activity seen as flutter waves, often with a saw-toothed appearance

PR interval: not measurable
QRS complex: usually normal but can be distorted by the underlying flutter waves (0.10-second, normal duration shown)
T wave: unidentifiable
QT interval: not measurable

Atrial fibrillation

Defined as chaotic, asynchronous electrical activity in the atrial tissue, atrial fibrillation results from impulses in many reentry pathways. These multiple and multidirectional impulses cause the atria to quiver instead of contract regularly.

With this arrhythmia, blood may pool in the left atrial appendage and form thrombi that can be ejected into the systemic circulation. An associated rapid ventricular rate can decrease cardiac output.

Possible causes include valvular disorders, hypertension, coronary artery disease, myocardial infarction, chronic lung disease, ischemia, thyroid disorders, and Wolff-Parkinson-White syndrome. The disorder may also result from high adrenergic tone secondary to physical exertion, sepsis or alcohol withdrawal, and the use of such drugs as aminophylline (Aminophyllin) and digitalis glycosides.

Intervention

If the patient is symptomatic, synchronized cardioversion should be used immediately. Vagal stimulation may be used to slow the ventricular response, but it won't convert the arrhythmia. Drugs that may be ordered to slow atrioventricular conduction include calcium channel blockers (diltiazem) and beta blockers (metoprolol). Digoxin may be ordered if the patient is stable. After the rate slows, if conversion to a normal sinus rhythm hasn't occurred, amiodarone (Cordarone), procainamide (Pronestyl), or quinidine (Quinidex) may be ordered. If atrial fibrillation is of several days' duration, anticoagulant therapy is recommended before pharmacologic or electrical conversion. If atrial fibrillation is of recent onset, ibutilide (Corvert) may be used to convert the rhythm.

Characteristics and interpretation

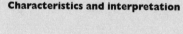

Coarse fibrillatory pattern

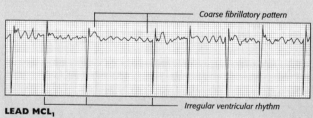

LEAD MCL₁

Irregular ventricular rhythm

Atrial rhythm: grossly irregular
Ventricular rhythm: grossly irregular
Atrial rate: greater than 400 beats/minute
Ventricular rate: 60 to 150 beats/minute, depending on treatment (80 beats/minute shown)
P wave: absent; appearance of erratic baseline fibrillatory waves (f waves) (When the f waves are pronounced, the arrhythmia is called coarse atrial fibrillation. When the f waves aren't pronounced, the arrhythmia is known as fine atrial fibrillation. On this strip, the f waves are pronounced.)
PR interval: indiscernible
QRS complex: duration usually within normal limits, with aberrant intraventricular conduction (0.08-second duration shown)
T wave: indiscernible
QT interval: not measurable

Junctional rhythm

Junctional rhythm occurs in the atrioventricular junctional tissue, producing retrograde depolarization of the atrial tissue and antegrade depolarization of the ventricular tissue. It results from conditions that depress sinoatrial node function, such as an inferior wall myocardial infarction (MI), digitalis toxicity, and vagal stimulation. The arrhythmia may also stem from an increased automaticity of the junctional tissue, which can be brought about by digitalis toxicity or ischemia associated with an inferior wall MI.

A junctional rhythm with a ventricular rate of 60 to 100 beats/minute is known as an accelerated junctional rhythm. If the ventricular rate exceeds 100 beats/minute, the arrhythmia is called junctional tachycardia.

Intervention

Treatment aims to identify and manage the arrhythmia's primary cause. If the patient is symptomatic, treatment may include atropine to increase the sinus or junctional rate. Or the doctor may insert a pacemaker to maintain an effective heart rate.

Characteristics and interpretation

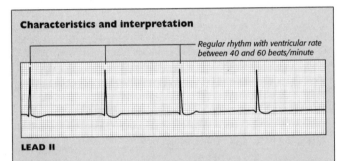

Regular rhythm with ventricular rate between 40 and 60 beats/minute

LEAD II

Atrial rhythm: regular
Ventricular rhythm: regular
Atrial rate: if discernible, 40 to 60 beats/minute (On this strip, the rate isn't discernible.)
Ventricular rate: 40 to 60 beats/minute (40 beats/minute shown)
P wave: usually inverted; may precede, follow, or fall within the QRS complex; may be absent (On this strip, the P wave is absent.)

PR interval: less than 0.12 second and constant if the P wave precedes the QRS complex; otherwise, not measurable (not measurable on this strip)
QRS complex: duration normal; configuration usually normal (0.08-second duration shown)
T wave: usually normal configuration
QT interval: usually normal (0.32-second duration shown)

Premature junctional contractions

In premature junctional contractions (PJCs), a junctional beat occurs before the next normal sinus beat. Ectopic beats, PJCs commonly result from increased automaticity in the bundle of His or the surrounding junctional tissue, which interrupts the underlying rhythm. The patient may complain of palpitations if PJCs are frequent.

PJCs most commonly result from digitalis toxicity. Other causes include ischemia associated with an inferior wall myocardial infarction, excessive caffeine ingestion, and excessive levels of amphetamines.

Intervention

In most cases, treatment is directed at the underlying cause.

Characteristics and interpretation

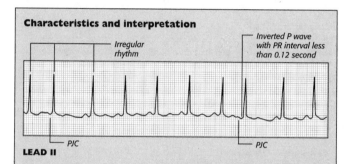

Atrial rhythm: irregular with PJC, but underlying rhythm may be regular
Ventricular rhythm: irregular with PJC, but underlying rhythm may be regular
Atrial rate: follows the underlying rhythm (100 beats/minute shown)
Ventricular rate: follows the underlying rhythm (100 beats/minute shown)
P wave: usually inverted; may precede, follow, or fall within the QRS complex; may be absent (shown preceding the QRS complex)

PR interval: less than 0.12 second on the PJC if P wave precedes the QRS complex; otherwise, not measurable (On this strip, the PR interval is 0.14 second and constant on the underlying rhythm and 0.06 second on the PJC.)
QRS complex: normal duration and configuration (0.06-second duration shown)
T wave: usually normal configuration
QT interval: usually within normal limits (0.30-second interval shown)

Premature ventricular contractions

Among the most common arrhythmias, premature ventricular contractions (PVCs) occur in both healthy and diseased hearts. These ectopic beats occur singly, in bigeminy, trigeminy, quadrageminy, or clusters.

PVCs may result from certain drugs, electrolyte imbalance, or stress.

When you detect PVCs, you must determine whether the pattern indicates danger. *Paired PVCs* can produce ventricular tachycardia because the second PVC usually meets refractory tissue. Three or more in a row is a run of ventricular tachycardia. *Multiform PVCs* look different from one another and may arise from different ventricular sites or be abnormally conducted. In *R-on-T phenomenon,* the PVC occurs so early

that it falls on the T wave of the preceding beat. Because the cells haven't fully depolarized, ventricular tachycardia or fibrillation can result.

The earlier the PVC, the shorter the diastolic filling time and the lower the stroke volume. Some patients complain of palpitations with frequent PVCs.

Intervention

If the PVCs are thought to result from a serious cardiac problem, lidocaine (Xylocaine)or other antiarrhythmics may be given to suppress ventricular irritability. When the PVCs are thought to result from a noncardiac problem, treatment aims at correcting the underlying cause — an acid-base or electrolyte imbalance, antiarrhythmic therapy, hypothermia, or high catecholamine levels.

Characteristics and interpretation

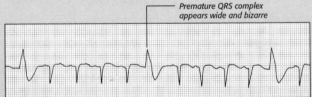

Premature QRS complex appears wide and bizarre

LEAD MCL₁

Atrial rhythm: irregular during PVC; underlying rhythm may be regular
Ventricular rhythm: irregular during PVC; underlying rhythm may be regular
Atrial rate: follows underlying rhythm (120 beats/minute shown)
Ventricular rate: follows underlying rhythm (120 beats/minute shown)
P wave: atrial activity independent of the PVC (If retrograde atrial depolarization exists, a retrograde P wave will distort the ST segment of the PVC. On this strip, no P wave appears before the PVC, but one occurs with each QRS complex.)
PR interval: determined by underlying rhythm; not associated with the PVC

(0.12-second, constant interval shown)
QRS complex: occurs earlier than expected; duration exceeds 0.12 second and complex has a bizarre configuration; may be normal in the underlying rhythm (On this strip, it's 0.08 second in the normal beats; it's bizarre and 0.12 second in the PVC.)
T wave: occurs in the direction opposite that of the QRS complex; normal in the underlying complexes
QT interval: not usually measured in the PVC but may be within normal limits in the underlying rhythm (On this strip, the QT interval is 0.28 second in the underlying rhythm.)

Ventricular tachycardia

The life-threatening arrhythmia ventricular tachycardia develops when three or more premature ventricular contractions occur in a row and the rate exceeds 100 beats/minute. It may result from enhanced automaticity or reentry within the Purkinje system. The rapid ventricular rate reduces ventricular filling time, and because atrial kick is lost, cardiac output drops. This puts the patient at risk for ventricular fibrillation.

Ventricular tachycardia usually results from acute myocardial infarction, coronary artery disease, valvular heart disease, heart failure, or cardiomyopathy. The arrhythmia can also stem from an electrolyte imbalance or from toxic levels of a drug such as a digitalis glycoside, procainamide (Pronestyl), or quinidine. You may detect two variations of this arrhythmia: R-on-T phenomenon and torsades de pointes.

Intervention

This rhythm often degenerates into ventricular fibrillation and cardiovascular collapse, requiring immediate cardiopulmonary resuscitation and defibrillation. If the patient is symptomatic, prepare for immediate cardioversion, followed by antiarrhythmic therapy. Lidocaine (Xylocaine) is usually administered immediately. If it proves ineffective, procainamide (Pronestyl) or bretylium (Bretylol) is used.

Characteristics and interpretation

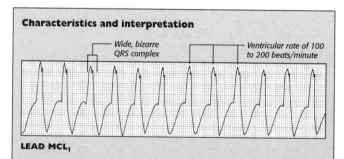

Wide, bizarre QRS complex

Ventricular rate of 100 to 200 beats/minute

LEAD MCL₁

Atrial rhythm: independent P waves possibly discernible with slower ventricular rates (On this strip, the P waves aren't visible.)
Ventricular rhythm: usually regular but may be slightly irregular (On this strip, it's regular.)
Atrial rate: can't be determined
Ventricular rate: usually 100 to 200 beats/minute (120 beats/minute shown)

P wave: usually absent; possibly obscured by the QRS complex; retrograde P waves possible presence
PR interval: not measurable
QRS complex: duration greater than 0.12 second; bizarre appearance, usually with increased amplitude (0.16 second-duration shown)
T wave: opposite the terminal forces of the QRS complex
QT interval: not measurable

Ventricular fibrillation

Defined as chaotic, asynchronous electrical activity within the ventricular tissue, ventricular fibrillation is a life-threatening arrhythmia that results in death if the rhythm isn't stopped immediately. Conditions leading to ventricular fibrillation include myocardial ischemia, hypokalemia, cocaine toxicity, hypoxia, hypothermia, severe acidosis, and severe alkalosis.

Patients with myocardial infarctions have the greatest risk of ventricular fibrillation during the initial 2 hours after the onset of chest pain. Those who experience ventricular fibrillation have a reduced risk of recurrence as healing progresses and scar tissue forms.

In ventricular fibrillation, a lack of cardiac output results in a loss of consciousness, pulselessness, and respiratory arrest. Initially, you may see coarse fibrillatory waves on the electrocardiogram strip. As the acidosis develops, the waves become fine and progress to asystole, unless defibrillation restores cardiac rhythm.

Intervention

Perform cardiopulmonary resuscitation until the patient can receive defibrillation. Administer epinephrine if initial defibrillation series is unsuccessful. Other drugs that may be used include lidocaine (Xylocaine), bretylium (Bretylol), and procainamide (Pronestyl). Magnesium sulfate may be used for torsades de pointes or refractory ventricular fibrillation.

Characteristics and interpretation

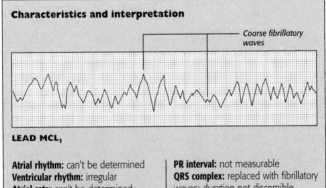

Coarse fibrillatory waves

LEAD MCL₁

Atrial rhythm: can't be determined
Ventricular rhythm: irregular
Atrial rate: can't be determined
Ventricular rate: can't be determined
P wave: indiscernible

PR interval: not measurable
QRS complex: replaced with fibrillatory waves; duration not discernible
T wave: can't be determined
QT interval: not measurable

Idioventricular rhythm

A life-threatening arrhythmia, id-ioventricular rhythm acts as a safety mechanism when all potential pace-makers above the ventricles fail to discharge or when a block prevents supraventricular impulses from reaching the ventricles.

The slow ventricular rate and loss of atrial kick associated with this life-threatening arrhythmia markedly re-duce cardiac output. In turn, this causes hypotension, confusion, verti-go, and syncope.

Intervention

Treatment aims to identify and man-age the primary problem that trig-gered this safety mechanism.

Atropine or dopamine (Intropin) may be given to increase the atrial rate. A pacemaker may also be insert-ed to increase the heart rate and thereby improve cardiac output.

Characteristics and interpretation

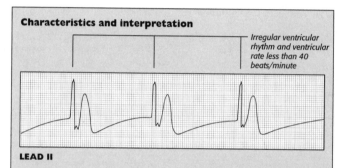

Irregular ventricular rhythm and ventricular rate less than 40 beats/minute

LEAD II

Atrial rhythm: can't be determined
Ventricular rhythm: usually regular, ex-cept with isolated escape beats (ir-regular rhythm shown)
Atrial rate: unable to be determined
Ventricular rate: less than 40 beats/minute (30 beats/minute shown)
P wave: absent
PR interval: usually not measurable

QRS complex: duration greater than 0.12 second; complex is wide and has a bizarre configuration (On this strip, the complex is 0.20 second and bizarre.)
T wave: directed opposite terminal forces of QRS complex
QT interval: usually greater than 0.44 second (0.46-second interval shown)

Accelerated idioventricular rhythm

When the pacemaker cells above the ventricles fail to generate an impulse or when a block prevents supraventricular impulses from reaching the ventricles, idioventricular rhythms result. When the rate of an idioventricular rhythm ranges from 40 to 100 beats/minute, it's considered accelerated idioventricular rhythm, denoting a rate greater than the inherent pacemaker.

In this life-threatening arrhythmia, the cells of the His-Purkinje system operate as pacemaker cells. The characteristic waveform results from an area of enhanced automaticity within the ventricles, which may be associated with myocardial infarction, digitalis toxicity, or metabolic imbalances. In addition, the arrhythmia commonly occurs during myo-cardial reperfusion after thrombolytic therapy.

The patient may or may not be symptomatic, depending on his heart rate and ability to compensate for the loss of the atrial kick. If symptomatic, he may experience signs and symptoms of decreased cardiac output, including hypotension, confusion, syncope, and blurred vision.

Intervention

An asymptomatic patient needs no treatment. For a symptomatic patient, treatment focuses on maintaining cardiac output and identifying the cause of the arrhythmia. The patient may require an atrial pacemaker to enhance cardiac output. Remember, this rhythm protects the heart from ventricular standstill and shouldn't be treated with lidocaine (Xylocaine) or other antiarrhythmic agents.

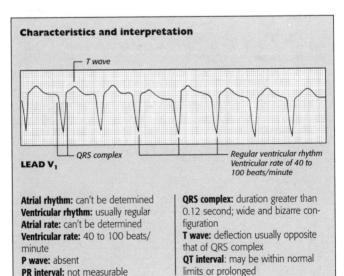

Characteristics and interpretation

T wave

QRS complex

LEAD V₁

Regular ventricular rhythm
Ventricular rate of 40 to
100 beats/minute

Atrial rhythm: can't be determined
Ventricular rhythm: usually regular
Atrial rate: can't be determined
Ventricular rate: 40 to 100 beats/minute
P wave: absent
PR interval: not measurable

QRS complex: duration greater than 0.12 second; wide and bizarre configuration
T wave: deflection usually opposite that of QRS complex
QT interval: may be within normal limits or prolonged

First-degree atrioventricular block

Defined as delayed conduction velocity through the atrioventricular (AV) node or His-Purkinje system, first-degree AV block is associated with an inferior wall myocardial infarction and the effects of digitalis glycosides or amiodarone (Cordarone). The arrhythmia is also associated with chronic degeneration of the conduction system.

Most patients with first-degree AV block are asymptomatic.

Intervention

Management of first-degree AV block includes identifying and treating the underlying cause as well as monitoring the patient for signs of progressive AV block.

Characteristics and interpretation

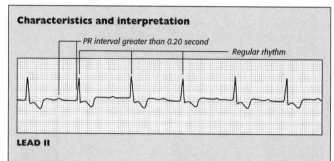

PR interval greater than 0.20 second

Regular rhythm

LEAD II

Atrial rhythm: regular
Ventricular rhythm: regular
Atrial rate: usually within normal limits (60 beats/minute shown)
Ventricular rate: usually within normal limits (60 beats/minute shown)
P wave: normal size and configuration (One P wave precedes each QRS complex.)

PR interval: greater than 0.20 second and constant (0.32-second duration shown)
QRS complex: usually normal duration and configuration (0.08-second duration and normal configuration shown)
T wave: normal size and configuration
QT interval: usually within normal limits (0.32-second interval shown)

Second-degree atrioventricular block, type I

In type I (Wenckebach or Mobitz I) second-degree atrioventricular (AV) block, diseased AV node tissues conduct impulses to the ventricles increasingly later, until one of the atrial impulses fails to be conducted or is blocked. Type I block most commonly occurs at the level of the AV node and is caused by an inferior wall myocardial infarction, vagal stimulation, or digitalis toxicity.

The arrhythmia usually doesn't cause symptoms. However, a patient may have signs and symptoms of decreased cardiac output, such as hypotension, confusion, and syncope. These effects occur especially if the patient's ventricular rate is slow.

Intervention

If the patient is asymptomatic, no intervention is required other than monitoring the electrocardiogram frequently to see if a more serious form of AV block develops.

If the patient is symptomatic, the doctor may order atropine to increase the rate and to stop the decremental conduction through the AV node. Occasionally, the doctor may insert a temporary pacemaker to maintain an effective cardiac output.

Characteristics and interpretation

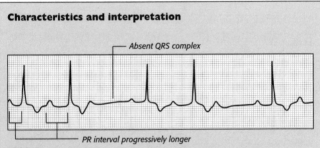

— Absent QRS complex

PR interval progressively longer

LEAD II

Atrial rhythm: regular
Ventricular rhythm: irregular
Atrial rate: determined by the underlying rhythm (80 beats/minute shown)
Ventricular rate: slower than the atrial rate (50 beats/minute shown)
P wave: normal size and configuration
PR interval: progressively prolonged with each beat until a P wave appears without a QRS complex

QRS complex: normal duration and configuration; periodically absent (0.08-second duration shown)
T wave: normal size and configuration
QT interval: usually within normal limits (0.46-second, constant interval shown)
Other: usually distinguished by a pattern of group beating, referred to as the footprints of Wenckebach

Second-degree atrioventricular block, type II

A life-threatening arrhythmia produced by a conduction disturbance in the His-Purkinje system, a type II (Mobitz II) second-degree atrioventricular (AV) block causes an intermittent absence of conduction. In type II block, two or more atrial impulses are conducted to the ventricles with constant PR intervals, when suddenly, without warning, the atrial impulse is blocked. This type of block occurs in an anterior wall myocardial infarction (MI), severe coronary artery disease, and chronic degeneration of the conduction system.

Intervention

If the patient is hypotensive, treatment aims at increasing his heart rate to improve cardiac output. Because the conduction block occurs in the His-Purkinje system, drugs that act directly on the myocardium usually prove more effective than those that increase the atrial rate. As a result, dopamine (Intropin) instead of atropine may be ordered to increase the ventricular rate.

If the patient has an anterior wall MI, the doctor will immediately insert a temporary pacemaker to prevent ventricular asystole. For long-term management, the patient usually needs a permanent pacemaker.

Characteristics and interpretation

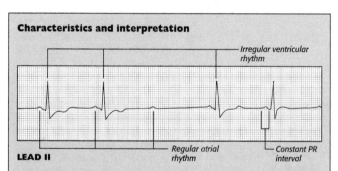

LEAD II

Atrial rhythm: regular
Ventricular rhythm: regular or irregular
Atrial rate: usually within normal limits (60 beats/minute shown)
Ventricular rate: may be within normal limits but less than the atrial rate (40 beats/minute shown)
P wave: normal size and configuration (Not all P waves are followed by a QRS complex.)
PR interval: constant and frequently within normal limits for all conducted beats

QRS complex: usually greater than 0.16 second because of the presence of a preexisting bundle-branch heart block (0.12-second complex shown)
T wave: usually normal size and configuration
QT interval: usually within normal limits (0.44-second interval shown)

Third-degree atrioventricular block

Also called complete heart block, life-threatening third-degree atrioventricular (AV) block occurs when all supraventricular impulses are prevented from reaching the ventricles. If this type of block originates at the AV node, a junctional escape rhythm occurs; if it originates below the AV node, an idioventricular escape rhythm occurs.

Third-degree AV block involving the AV node may result from an inferior wall myocardial infarction (MI)

or drug toxicity (digitalis glycosides, beta blockers, calcium channel blockers). Third-degree AV block below the AV node may result from an anterior wall MI or chronic degeneration of the conduction system.

Intervention

If cardiac output isn't adequate or the patient's condition is deteriorating, the doctor will order therapy to improve the ventricular rhythm. Initially, atropine may be ordered to increase the ventricular rate and improve cardiac output until a pacemaker is available.

Characteristics and interpretation

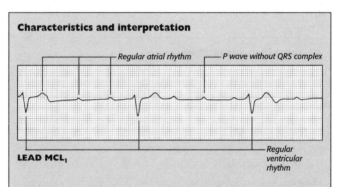

LEAD MCL₁

Atrial rhythm: usually regular
Ventricular rhythm: usually regular
Atrial rate: usually within normal limits (90 beats/minute shown)
Ventricular rate: slow (30 beats/minute shown)
P wave: normal size and configuration
PR interval: not measurable because the atria and ventricles beat independently of each other
QRS complex: determined by the site of the escape rhythm (With a junc-

tional escape rhythm, the duration and configuration are normal; with an idioventricular escape rhythm, the duration is greater than 0.12 second and the complex is distorted. In the complex shown, the duration is 0.16 second, the configuration is abnormal, and the complex is distorted.)
T wave: normal size and configuration
QT interval: may or may not be within normal limits (0.56-second interval shown)

12-lead ECGs

Basic components and principles

Whereas rhythm strips are used to detect arrhythmias, the 12-lead or standard ECG has a different purpose. The most common procedure for evaluating cardiac status, this diagnostic test helps identify various pathological conditions—most commonly, acute myocardial infarction.

The 12-lead ECG provides 12 views of the heart's electrical activity. (See *12 views of the heart.*) The 12 leads include:
• three bipolar limb leads (I, II, and III)
• three unipolar augmented limb leads (aV_R, aV_L, and aV_F)
• six unipolar precordial, or chest, leads (V_1, V_2, V_3, V_4, V_5, and V_6).

12 VIEWS OF THE HEART

The electrocardiogram's (ECG's) six limb leads view the heart from six different angles. This chart shows the direction of each lead relative to the wave of depolarization (shown in color) and lists the six views of the heart revealed by these leads.

Planes of heart	Leads	View of heart
	Standard limb leads (bipolar)	
	I	Lateral wall
	II	Inferior wall
	III	Inferior wall
	Augmented limb leads (unipolar)	
	aV_R	Provides no specific view
	aV_L	Lateral wall
	aV_F	Inferior wall
	Precordial, or chest, leads (unipolar)	
	V_1	Anteroseptal wall
	V_2	Anteroseptal wall
	V_3	Anterior and anteroseptal walls
	V_4	Anterior wall
	V_5	Anterolateral wall
	V_6	Anterolateral wall

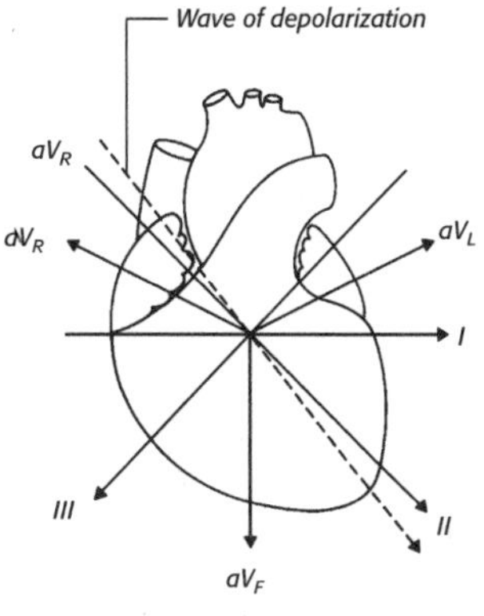

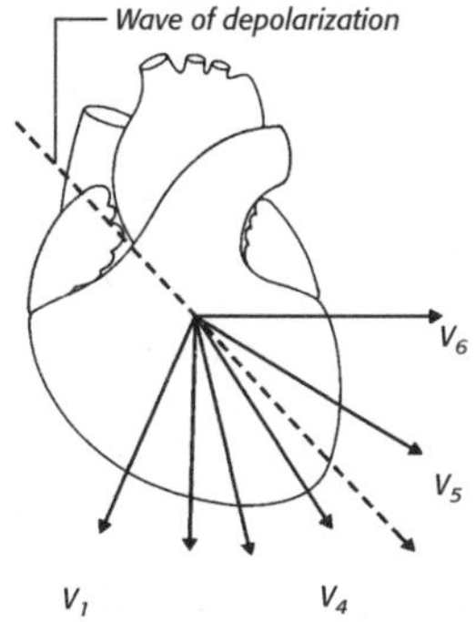

Wave of depolarization

aV_R dV_R aV_L I III II aV_F

Wave of depolarization

V_6 V_5 V_1 V_4

Leads

The six limb leads record electrical potential from the frontal plane, and the six precordial leads record electrical potential from the horizontal plane. Each waveform reflects the orientation of a lead to the wave of depolarization passing through the myocardium. Normally, this wave moves through the heart from right to left and from top to bottom.

Bipolar leads

These leads record the electrical potential difference between two points on the patient's body, where you place electrodes.
• Lead I goes from the right arm (−) to the left arm (+).
• Lead II goes from the right arm (−) to the left leg (+).
• Lead III goes from the left arm (−) to the left leg (+).

Because of the orientation of these leads to the wave of depolarization, the QRS complexes typically appear upright. In lead II, these complexes are usually the tallest because this lead parallels the wave of depolarization.

Unipolar leads

Unipolar leads (the augmented limb leads and the precordial leads) have only one electrode, which represents the positive pole. The negative pole is computed by the ECG. Lead aV_R typically records negative QRS complex deflections because the wave of depolarization moves away from it. In the aV_F lead, QRS complexes are positive; in the aV_L lead, they're biphasic.

Unipolar precordial leads V_1 and V_2 usually have a small R wave because the direction of ventricular activation is left to right initially. That's because conduction time is normally faster down the left bundle branch than it is down the right. But the wave of depolarization moves toward

the left ventricle and away from these leads, causing a low S wave.

In leads V_3 and V_4, the R and S waves may have the same amplitude, and you won't see a Q wave. In leads V_5 and V_6, the initial ventricular activation appears as a small Q wave; the following tall R wave represents the strong wave of depolarization moving toward the left ventricle. These leads record a small or absent S wave.

Determining electrical axis

As electrical impulses travel through the heart, they generate small electrical forces called *instant-to-instant vectors*. The mean of these vectors represents the direction and force of the wave of depolarization, also known as the heart's electrical axis.

In a healthy heart, the wave of depolarization originates in the sinoatrial node and travels through the atria and the atrioventricular node and on to the ventricles. So the normal movement is downward and to the left — the direction of a normal electrical axis.

In an unhealthy heart, the wave of depolarization (or the direction of the electrical axis) varies. That's because the direction of electrical activity swings away from areas of damage or necrosis.

A simple method to determine the direction of your patient's electrical axis is the quadrant method. Before you use this method, you need to understand the hexaxial reference system — a schematic view of the heart that uses the six limb leads.

As you know, these leads include the three standard limb leads (I, II, and III), which are bipolar, and the three augmented limb leads (aV_R, aV_L, and aV_F,), which are unipolar. Combined, these leads give a view of the wave of depolarization in the frontal plane, including the right, left, inferior, and superior portions of the heart.

Hexaxial reference system

The axes of the six limb leads also make up the hexaxial reference system, which divides the heart into six equal areas. To use the hexaxial reference system, picture in your mind the position of each lead: lead I connects the right arm (negative pole) with the left arm (positive pole); lead II connects the right arm (negative pole) with the left leg (positive pole); and lead III connects the left arm (negative pole) with the left leg (positive pole). The augmented limb leads have only one electrode, which represents the positive pole. As a result, lead aV_R goes from the heart toward the right arm (positive pole); aV_L goes from the heart toward the left arm (positive pole); and aV_F goes from the heart to the left leg (positive pole).

Now, take this mental picture one step further and draw an imaginary line to illustrate the axis of each lead. For example, for lead I, you'd draw a horizontal line between the right and left arms; for lead II, between the right arm and left leg; and so on. All the lines should intersect near the center, somewhere over the heart. If you draw a circle to represent the heart, you'd end up with a rough pie shape, with each wedge representing a portion of the heart monitored by each lead. (See *Understanding the hexaxial reference system.*)

This schematic representation of the heart allows you to plot your patient's electrical axis. If his axis falls in the right lower quadrant, between 0 degrees and +90 degrees, it's considered normal. An axis between +90 degrees and +180 degrees indicates right axis deviation; one between 0

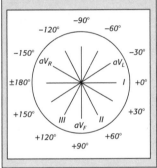
degrees and −90 degrees, left axis deviation; and one between −180 degrees and −90 degrees, extreme axis deviation (sometimes called the northwest axis). Some experts, however, feel that the portion from 0 degrees to −30 degrees has no clinical significance.

Quadrant method

A simple, rapid method for determining the heart's axis is the quadrant method, in which you observe the main deflection of the QRS complex in leads I and aV_F. The QRS complex serves as the traditional marker for

USING THE QUADRANT METHOD

This chart can help you quickly determine the direction of a patient's electrical axis, which is indicated by the gray arrow. First, observe the deflections of the QRS complexes in leads I and aV$_F$. Next, plot the deflections on the diagram (positive deflections are on the side that has positive degrees for that lead, and negative deflections are on the side that has negative degrees.) Then check the chart to determine if the patient's axis is normal or whether it has a left, right, or extreme deviation.

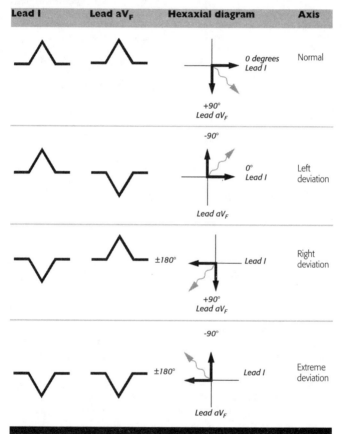

Lead I	Lead aV$_F$	Hexaxial diagram	Axis

determining the electrical axis because the ventricles produce the greatest amount of electrical force when they contract. Lead I indicates whether impulses are moving to the right or left; lead aV$_F$, whether they're moving up or down. (See *Using the quadrant method.*)

On the waveform for lead I, a positive main deflection of the QRS complex indicates that the electrical impulses are moving to the right, toward the positive pole of the lead, which is at the 0-degree position on the hexaxial reference system. Conversely, a negative deflection indicates that the impulses are moving to the left, toward the negative pole of the lead, which is at the ±180-degree position on the hexaxial reference system. On the waveform for lead aV_F, a positive deflection of the QRS complex indicates that the electrical impulses are traveling downward, toward the positive pole of the lead, which is at the +90-degree position of the hexaxial reference system. A negative deflection indicates that impulses are traveling upward, toward the negative pole of the lead, which is at the −90 degree position of the hexaxial reference system.

Plotting this information on the hexaxial reference system (with the horizontal axis representing lead I and the vertical axis representing lead aV_F) will reveal the patient's electrical axis. For example, if lead I shows a positive deflection of the QRS complex, darken the horizontal axis between the center of the hexaxial reference system and the 0-degree position. If lead aV_F also shows a positive deflection of the QRS complex, darken the vertical axis between the center of reference system and the +90-degree position. The quadrant between the two axes you've darkened indicates the patient's electrical axis. In this case, it's the left lower quadrant, which indicates a normal electrical axis.

Causes of axis deviation

Determining a patient's electrical axis can help confirm a diagnosis or narrow the range of clinical possibilities. Many factors influence the electrical axis, including the position of the heart within the chest, the size of the heart, the conduction pathways, and the force of electrical generation.

As you know, cardiac electrical activity swings away from areas of damage or necrosis. More specifically, electrical forces in the healthy portion of the heart take over for weak, or even absent, electrical forces in the damaged portion. For instance, after an inferior wall myocardial infarction, portions of the inferior wall can no longer conduct electricity. As a result, the major electrical vectors shift to the left, resulting in a left axis deviation.

Typically, the damaged portion of the heart is the last area to be depolarized. For example, in a left anterior hemiblock, the left anterior fascicle of the left bundle branch can no longer conduct electricity. Therefore, the portion normally served by the left bundle branch is the last portion of the heart to be depolarized. This shifts electrical forces to the left; consequently, the ECG shows left axis deviation.

An opposite shift occurs with right bundle-branch block. In this condition, the wave of impulse travels quickly down the normal left side but much more slowly down the damaged right side. This shifts the electrical forces to the right, causing a right axis deviation.

An axis shift also takes place when the right or left ventricle is being paced artificially. It likewise takes place when the ventricles are depolarizing abnormally, such as occurs in ventricular tachycardia. Both of these conditions can cause a left axis deviation or, occasionally, an extreme axis deviation.

Axis deviation may also result from ventricular hypertrophy. For example, an enlarged right ventricle generates greater electrical forces than normal and would consequently shift the electrical axis to the right. Wolff-Parkinson-White syndrome may produce a right, left, or extreme axis deviation, depending on which part of the ventricle is activated early.

Sometimes axis deviation may be a normal variation, as in infants and children, who normally experience right axis deviation. It may also stem from noncardiac causes. For example, if the heart is shifted in the chest cavity because of a high diaphragm from pregnancy, expect to find a left axis deviation. Also, if a patient's heart is situated on the right side of his chest instead of the left (a condition called dextrocardia), expect to find right axis deviation.

How to interpret a 12-lead ECG

You can use various methods to interpret a 12-lead ECG. Here's a logical, easy-to-follow, seven-step method that will help ensure that you're interpreting it accurately.

1. Find the lead markers and note the leads.

2. Note whether there are full or half standardization marks.

3. Using the four-quadrant method, observe the waveforms for leads I and aV_F, and determine the heart's axis. This can provide an early clue to a possible problem.

4. Note the R wave progression through the six precordial leads. Normally, in the precordial leads, the R wave (the first positive deflection of the QRS complex) appears progressively taller from lead V_1 to lead V_6. Conversely, the S wave (the negative deflection after an R wave) appears extremely deep in lead V_1 and becomes progressively smaller through lead V_6. (See *Normal findings.*)

5. Next, look at the T wave, which normally goes in the same direction as the QRS complex. If the main deflection of the QRS complex is positive, the T wave should be positive, too. If the main deflection of the QRS complex is negative, the T wave should be negative. The two exceptions to this are leads V_1 and V_2, in which a negative QRS complex with a positive T wave is normal.

If a T wave deflects in the opposite direction from the QRS complex, it's considered abnormal (except, as mentioned, in leads V_1 and V_2). Such a deflection is commonly referred to as an inverted T wave—a term that can be confusing when the QRS complex is negative and the T wave is actually positive. Keep in mind that in this case, inversion signifies that the T wave deflects in the direction opposite the QRS complex. It doesn't necessarily mean that the T wave is negative, as the word "inverted" suggests.

6. If you suspect myocardial infarction (MI), start with lead I and continue through to lead V_6, observing the waveforms for changes in ECG characteristics that can indicate acute MI, such as T-wave inversion, ST-segment elevation, and pathological Q waves. Note the leads in which you see such changes and describe the changes. When first learning to interpret the 12-lead ECG, ignore lead aV_R, because it won't provide clues to left ventricular infarction or injury.

7. Determine the site and extent of myocardial damage. To do so, use the chart *Locating myocardial damage,* on page 67 and follow these steps:

• Identify the leads recording pathological Q waves. Look at the second column of the chart for those leads. Then look at the first column to find the corresponding myocardial wall, where infarction has occurred. Keep in mind that this chart serves as a guideline only. Actual areas of infarction may overlap or be larger or smaller than listed.

• Identify the leads recording ST-segment elevation (or depression for reciprocal leads), and use the chart to locate the corresponding areas of myocardial injury.

• Identify the leads recording T-wave inversion, and locate the corresponding areas of ischemia.

NORMAL FINDINGS

LEAD I

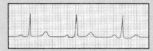

P wave: upright
Q wave: small or none
R wave: largest wave
S wave: none present, or smaller than R wave
T wave: upright
U wave: none present
ST segment: may vary from +1 to −0.5 mm

LEAD II

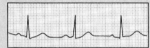

P wave: upright
Q wave: small or none
R wave: large (vertical heart)
S wave: none present, or smaller than R wave
T wave: upright
U wave: none present
ST segment: may vary from +1 to −0.5 mm

LEAD III

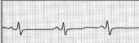

P wave: upright, diphasic, or inverted
Q wave: usually small or none (a Q wave must also be present in aV$_F$ to be considered diagnostic.)
R wave: none present to large wave
S wave: none present to large wave, indicating horizontal heart
T wave: upright, diphasic, or inverted
U wave: none present
ST segment: may vary from +1 to −0.5 mm

LEAD AV$_R$

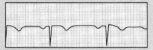

P wave: inverted
Q wave: none, small wave, or large wave present
R wave: none or small wave present
S wave: large wave (may be QS)
T wave: inverted
U wave: none present
ST segment: may vary from +1 to −0.5 mm

LEAD AV$_L$

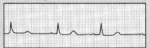

P wave: upright, diphasic, or inverted
Q wave: none, small wave, or large wave present (A Q wave must also be present in lead I or precordial leads to be considered diagnostic.)
R wave: none, small wave, or large wave present (A large wave indicates horizontal heart.)
S wave: none present to large wave (A large wave indicates vertical heart.)
T wave: upright, diphasic, or inverted
U wave: none present
ST segment: may vary from +1 to −0.5 mm

LEAD AV$_F$

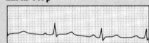

P wave: upright
Q wave: none, or small wave present
R wave: none, small wave, or large wave present (A large wave suggests vertical heart.)
S wave: none to large wave present (A large wave suggests horizontal heart.)
T wave: Upright, diphasic, or inverted
U wave: none present
ST segment: may vary from +1 to −0.5 mm *(continued)*

NORMAL FINDINGS *(continued)*

LEAD V₁

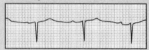

P wave: upright, diphasic, or inverted
Q wave: deep QS pattern may be present
R wave: none present or less than S wave
S wave: large (part of QS pattern)
T wave: usually inverted but may be upright and diphasic
U wave: none present
ST segment: may vary from 0 to +1 mm

LEAD V₂

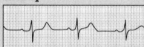

P wave: upright
Q wave: deep QS pattern may be present
R wave: none present or less than S wave (wave may become progressively larger)
S wave: large (part of QS pattern)
T wave: upright
U wave: upright, lower amplitude than T wave
ST segment: may vary from 0 to +1 mm

LEAD V₃

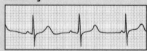

P wave: upright
Q wave: none or small wave present
R wave: less than, greater than, or equal to S wave (Wave may become progressively larger.)
S wave: large (greater than, less than, or equal to R wave)
T wave: upright
U wave: upright, lower amplitude than T wave
ST segment: may vary from 0 to +1 mm

LEAD V₄

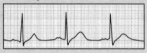

P wave: upright
Q wave: none or small wave present
R wave: progressively larger wave; R wave greater than S wave
S wave: progressively smaller (less than R wave)
T wave: upright
U wave: upright, lower amplitude than T wave
ST segment: may vary from +1 to −0.5 mm

LEAD V₅

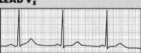

P wave: upright
Q wave: small
R wave: progressively larger but less than 26 mm
S wave. Progressively smaller; less than the S wave in V₄
T wave: upright
U wave: none present
ST segment: may vary from +1 to −0.5 mm

LEAD V₆

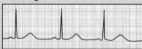

P wave: upright
Q wave: small
R wave: largest wave but less than 26 mm
S wave: smallest; less than the S wave in V₅
T wave: upright
U wave: none present
ST segment: may vary from +1 to −0.5 mm

LOCATING MYOCARDIAL DAMAGE

Wall affected	Leads	ECG changes	Artery involved	Reciprocal changes
Inferior (diaphragmatic)	II, III, aV$_F$	Q, ST, T	Right coronary artery (RCA)	I, aV$_L$ and, possibly, V$_4$ through V$_6$
Postero-lateral	I, aV$_L$, V$_5$, V$_6$	Q, ST, T	Circumflex, or branch of left anterior descending (LAD) artery	V$_1$, V$_2$, or II, III, and aV$_F$
Anterior	V$_1$, V$_2$, V$_3$, V$_4$, I, aV$_L$	Q, ST, T, loss of R-wave progression across precordial leads	Left coronary artery	II, III, aV$_F$
Posterior	V$_1$, V$_2$	None	RCA or circumflex, either of which supplies posterior descending artery (PDA)	R greater than S in V$_1$ and V$_2$, ST-segment depression, elevated T wave
Right ventricular	V$_4$, V$_5$, V$_6$	Q, ST, T	RCA	None
Anterolateral	I, aV$_L$, V$_4$, V$_5$, V$_6$	Q, ST, T	LAD and diagonal branches, circumflex and obtuse marginal branches	II, III, aV$_F$
Anteroseptal	V$_1$, V$_2$, V$_3$	Q, ST, T, loss of R wave in V$_1$	LAD	None
Ventricular	V$_{4R}$-V$_{6R}$	Q, ST, T	RCA	None

Acute myocardial infarction

An acute myocardial infarction (MI) can arise from any condition in which myocardial oxygen supply can't meet oxygen demand. Starved of oxygen, the myocardium suffers progressive ischemia, leading to injury and, eventually, to infarction.

In most cases, an acute MI involves the left ventricle, although it can also involve the right ventricle or the atria.

Typically, acute MIs are classified as either Q wave or non–Q wave.

In an acute transmural MI, the characteristic ECG changes result from the three I's (ischemia, injury, and infarction).

• Ischemia results from a temporary interruption of the myocardial blood supply. Its characteristic ECG change is T-wave inversion, a result of altered tissue repolarization. ST-segment depression also may occur.

ISCHEMIA

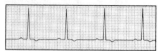

Ischemia produces T-wave inversion

• Injury to myocardial cells results from a prolonged interruption of blood flow. Its characteristic ECG change, ST-segment elevation, reflects altered depolarization. Usually, you'll consider an elevation greater than 0.1 mV significant.

INJURY

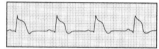

Injury produces ST-segment elevation

• Infarction results from an absence of blood flow to myocardial tissue, leading to necrosis. The ECG shows pathological Q waves, reflecting abnormal depolarization in damaged tissue or absent depolarization in scar tissue. The characteristic of a pathological Q wave is a duration of 0.04 second or an amplitude measuring at least one-third the height of the entire QRS complex.

INFARCTION

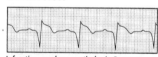

Infarction produces pathologic Q waves

Besides these three characteristic ECG changes, you may see reciprocal (or mirror image) changes. Reciprocal changes — most commonly, ST-segment depression or tall R waves — occur in the leads opposite those reflecting the area of ischemia, injury, or infarction.

Acute MI phases

To detect an acute MI, you'll look for ST-segment elevation first, followed by T-wave inversion and pathological Q waves.

Serial ECG recordings yield the best evidence of an MI. Normally, an acute MI progresses through the following phases.

Hyperacute phase

This phase begins a few hours after the onset of acute MI. You'll see ST-segment elevation and upright (usually peaked) T waves.

Fully evolved phase

This phase starts several hours after MI onset. You'll see deep T-wave inversion and pathological Q waves.

Resolution phase

This appears within a few weeks of acute MI. You'll see normal T waves.

Stabilized chronic phase

After the resolution phase, you'll see permanent pathological Q waves revealing an old infarction.

With an acute non–Q wave MI, you may see persistent ST-segment depression, T-wave inversion, or both. However, pathological Q waves may not appear. To differentiate an acute non–Q wave MI from myocardial ischemia, cardiac enzyme tests must be performed.

It's important to remember that for a true clinical diagnosis of an acute MI, a patient must have symptoms, ECG changes, and elevated cardiac enzyme levels. If the patient shows such signs and symptoms as chest pain, left arm pain, diaphoresis, and nausea, proceed as if he's had an acute MI until this possibility has been ruled out.

Right-sided ECG, Leads V₁ʀ to V₆ʀ

A right-sided ECG provides information about the extent of damage to

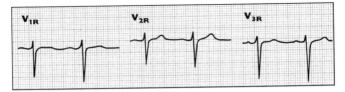

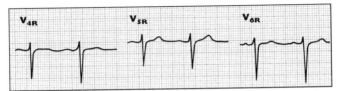

the right ventricle, especially during the first 12 hours of myocardial infarction. Right-sided ECG leads, placed over the right chest in similar but reversed positions from the left precordial leads, are called unipolar right-sided chest leads.

Placing electrodes

Right-sided ECG leads are precordial leads designated by the letter V, a number representing the electrode position, and the letter R, indicating right chest lead placement. Lead positions are:

• V_{1R}: fourth intercostal space, left sternal border
• V_{2R}: fourth intercostal space, right sternal border
• V_{3R}: midway between V_{1R} and V_{4R}, on a line joining these two locations
• V_{4R}: fifth intercostal space, right midclavicular line
• V_{5R}: fifth intercostal space, right anterior axillary line
• V_{6R}: fifth intercostal space, right midaxillary line.

Understanding polarity

The right-sided chest ECG leads measure the difference in electrical potential between a right chest electrode and a central terminal. The chest electrode used in each of the right V leads is positive. The negative electrode is obtained by adding together leads I, II, and III, whose algebraic sum equals zero.

Viewing the heart

Chest leads, whether on the left or the right chest, view the horizontal plane of the heart. The placement of left precordial leads gives a good picture of the electrical activity within the left ventricle. Because the right ventricle lies behind the left ventricle, the ability to evaluate right ventricular electrical activity when using only left precordial leads is limited. Right-sided ECG leads better visualize the right ventricular wall. This may be especially useful when evaluating a patient for a right ventricular myocardial infarction.

Leads V_{1R} and V_{2R} provide limited visualization of the right ventricle. Leads V_{3R} through V_{6R} are the most useful right ventricular leads. A decrease in the R wave with an increase in the S wave is normally seen from V_{1R} through V_{6R}, the reverse of the standard left precordial leads. V_{3R} to V_{6R} (particularly V_{4R}) are the most commonly used and the most helpful leads when looking for ECG changes indicating right ventricular ischemia and infarction.

Left bundle-branch block

In left bundle-branch block, a conduction delay or block occurs in both the left posterior and the left anterior fascicles of the left bundle. This delay or block disrupts the normal left-to-right direction of depolarization. As a result, normal septal Q waves are absent. Because of the block, the wave of depolarization must move down the right bundle first and then spread from right to left.

This arrhythmia may indicate underlying heart disease such as coronary artery disease. It carries a more serious prognosis than right bundle-branch block because of its close correlation with organic heart disease, and it requires a large lesion to block the thick, broad left bundle branch.

Intervention

When left bundle-branch block occurs along with an anterior wall myocardial infarction, it usually signals complete heart block, which requires insertion of a pacemaker.

Characteristics and interpretation

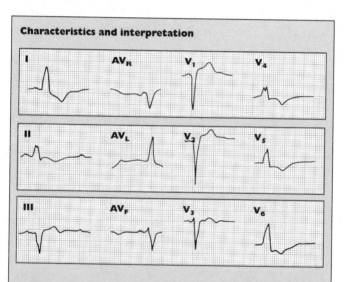

Rhythm: regular atrial and ventricular rhythms

Rate: atrial and ventricular rates within normal limits

P wave: normal size and configuration

PR interval: within normal limits

QRS complex: duration that varies from 0.10 to 0.12 second in incomplete left bundle-branch block (It's at least 0.12 second in complete block. Lead V_1 shows a wide, entirely negative rS complex [rarely a wide rS complex]. Leads I, aV_L, and V_6 show a wide, tall R wave without a Q or S wave.)

T wave: deflection opposite that of the QRS complex in most leads

QT interval: may be prolonged or within normal limits

Other: magnitude of changes paralleling the magnitude of the QRS complex aberration, with normal axis or left-axis deviation; delayed intrinsicoid deflection over the left ventricle (lead V_6)

Right bundle-branch block

In the conduction delay or block associated with right bundle-branch block, the initial left-to-right direction of depolarization isn't affected. The left ventricle depolarizes on time, so the intrinsicoid deflection in leads V_5 and V_6 (the left precordial leads) takes place on time as well. However, the right ventricle depolarizes late, causing a late intrinsicoid deflection in leads V_1 and V_2 (the right precordial leads). This late depolarization also causes the axis to deviate to the right.

Intervention

One potential complication of a myocardial infarction is a bundle-branch block. Some blocks require treatment with a temporary pacemaker. Others are monitored only to detect progression to a more complete block.

Characteristics and interpretation

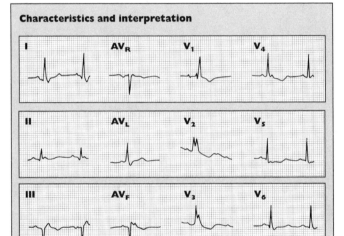

Rhythm: regular atrial and ventricular rhythms
Rate: atrial and ventricular rates within normal limits; P wave of normal size and configuration
PR interval: within normal limits
QRS complex: duration of at least 0.12 second in complete block and 0.10 to 0.12 second in incomplete block (In lead V_1, the QRS complex is wide and can appear in one of several patterns: an rSR I complex with a wide S and R I wave; an RS complex with a wide R wave; and a wide R wave with an M-shaped pattern. The complex is mainly positive, with the R wave occurring late. In leads I, aV_{L1} and V_6, a broad S wave can be seen.)
T wave: in most leads, deflection opposite that of the QRS deflection
QT interval: may be prolonged or within normal limits
Other: in the precordial leads, occurence of triphasic complexes because the right ventricle continues to depolarize after the left ventricle depolarizes, thereby producing a third phase of ventricular stimulation

Pericarditis

An inflammation of the pericardium, the fibroserous sac that envelops the heart, pericarditis can be acute or chronic. The acute form may be fibrinous or effusive, with a purulent serous or hemorrhagic exudate. Chronic constrictive pericarditis causes dense fibrous pericardial thickening. Regardless of the form, pericarditis can cause cardiac tamponade if fluid accumulates too quickly. It can also cause heart failure if constriction occurs.

In pericarditis, ECG changes occur in four stages. Stage 1 coincides with the onset of chest pain. Stage 2 begins within several days. Stage 3 starts several days after stage 2. Stage 4 occurs weeks later.

Intervention

Pericarditis is usually treated with aspirin or nonsteroidal anti-inflammatory drugs. A last resort is prednisone, quickly tapered over 3 days.

Characteristics and interpretation

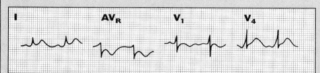

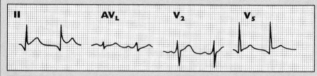

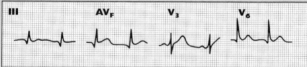

Rhythm: usually regular atrial and ventricular rhythms
Rate: atrial and ventricular rates usually within normal limits
P wave: normal size and configuration
PR interval: usually depressed in all leads except V_1 and aV_R, in which it may be elevated
QRS complex: within normal limits, but with a possible decrease in amplitude

ST segment: in stage 1, elevated 1 to 2 mm in a concave pattern in leads I, II, and III and the precordial leads
T wave: flattened in stage 2, inverted in stage 3 (lasting for weeks or months), and returning to normal in stage 4 (although sometimes becoming deeply inverted)
QT interval: within normal limits
Other: possible atrial fibrillation or tachycardia from sinoatrial node irritation

Digoxin: ECG effects

A potent digitalis glycoside, digoxin increases the force of myocardial contraction, decreases conduction velocity through the atrioventricular (AV) node to slow the heart rate, and prolongs the effective refractory period of the AV node by direct and sympatholytic effects on the sinoatrial node. Excess amounts of this drug can slow conduction through the AV node and cause irritable ectopic foci in the ventricles.

ECG changes only indicate that the patient is receiving a form of digoxin. If an arrhythmia develops, these ECG changes can help identify the cause of the arrhythmia as digitalis toxicity.

Virtually any type of arrhythmia can be caused by an excess of digoxin. The most common ones include premature ventricular contractions (especially bigeminy), paroxysmal atrial tachycardias with or without a block, second-degree heart block, and sinus arrest.

Interventions

Be alert for noncardiac symptoms of digoxin toxicity. Withhold digoxin for 1 to 2 days before performing electrical cardioversion.

Characteristics and interpretation

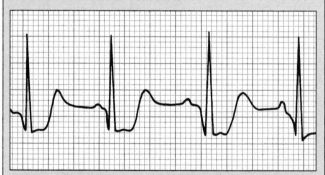

Rhythm: regular atrial and ventricular rhythms
Rate: atrial and ventricular rates are usually within normal limits, but bradycardia possible
P wave: decreased voltage; may be notched
PR interval: within normal limits or prolonged
QRS complex: within normal limits
ST segment: gradual sloping, causing ST-segment depression in the direction opposite that of the QRS deflection

T wave: may be flattened and inverted in a direction opposite that of the QRS deflection
Other: QT interval commonly shortened; ST sloping and depression and QT-segment interval shortening from digoxin use but not necessarily signs of digitalis toxicity; ST-segment depression and T-wave inversion in leads with negatively deflected QRS complexes, possibly indicating a need to reduce the digoxin dose

Quinidine: ECG effects

An antiarrhythmic drug that decreases sodium transport through cardiac tissues, quinidine slows conduction through the atrioventricular (AV) node. It also prolongs the effective refractory period and decreases automaticity.

Although ECG changes occur as a result of quinidine use, they aren't necessarily a sign of quinidine toxicity. At toxic levels, however, quinidine can cause sinoatrial and AV block and ventricular arrhythmias.

Interventions

Prolongation of the QT interval is a sign that the patient is predisposed to developing polymorphic ventricular tachycardia. Preventing ventricular tachyarrhythmias involves administering a digitalis glycoside for atrial tachyarrhythmias before quinidine.

Characteristics and interpretation

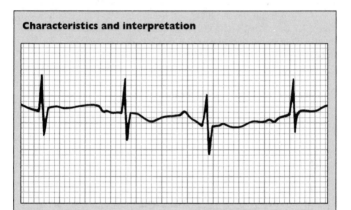

Rhythm: regular atrial and ventricular rhythms
Rate: atrial and ventricular rates within normal limits
P wave: may be widened and notched, especially in leads I and II
PR interval: within normal limits

QRS complex: widens slightly (Abnormal widening may be an early sign of developing quinidine toxicity.)
ST segment: often depressed
T wave: may be flattened or inverted
QT interval: may be prolonged
U wave: may be visible

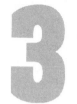

CHAPTER

3

Laboratory tests

Understanding the results in context

Common tests

Activated partial thromboplastin time

The activated partial thromboplastin time (APTT) is used to evaluate all the clotting factors of the intrinsic pathway except platelets by measuring the time required for formation of a fibrin clot after the addition of calcium and phospholipid emulsion to a plasma sample. An activator, such as kaolin, is used to shorten clotting time.

Purpose

• To aid preoperative screening for bleeding tendencies
• To screen for congenital coagulation deficiencies of the clotting factors
• To monitor heparin therapy

Reference values

Normally, a fibrin clot forms 21 to 35 seconds after addition of reagents. For a patient on anticoagulant therapy, ask the attending doctor to specify the reference values for the therapy being delivered.

Abnormal findings

Prolonged APTT may indicate a deficiency of certain plasma clotting factors, the presence of heparin, or the presence of fibrin split products, fibrinolysins, or circulating anticoagulants that act as antibodies to specific clotting factors.

Arterial blood gas analysis

Arterial blood gas (ABG) analysis is used to measure the partial pressures of oxygen (Pao_2) and carbon dioxide ($Paco_2$) and the pH of an arterial sample. Oxygen content (O_2CT), oxygen saturation (Sao_2), and bicarbonate (HCO_3^-) values are also measured. A blood sample for ABG analysis may be drawn by percutaneous arterial puncture or from an arterial line.

Purpose

• To evaluate gas exchange in the lungs
• To assess integrity of the ventilatory control system
• To determine the acid-base level of the blood
• To monitor respiratory therapy

Reference values

Normal ABG values fall within the following ranges:
• Pao_2: 75 to 100 mm Hg
• $Paco_2$: 35 to 45 mm Hg
• pH: 7.35 to 7.45
• O_2CT: 15% to 22%
• Sao_2: 95% to 100%
• HCO_3^-: 24 to 28 mEq/L.

Abnormal findings

A Pao_2 value below 50 mm Hg usually indicates hypoxia. A value between 50 and 75 mm Hg may indicate hypoxia, depending on the patient's age and the oxygen concentration he's receiving. After age 60, a patient's normal Pao_2 may fall below 75 mm Hg.

A $Paco_2$ above 45 mm Hg indicates hypoventilation or hypercapnia; below 35 mm Hg, hyperventilation or hypocapnia. The $Paco_2$ value can also signal a respiratory acid-base imbalance. A value above 45 mm Hg points to respiratory acidosis; below 35 mm Hg, respiratory alkalosis. (See *Recognizing acid-base disorders*.)

A pH greater than 7.42 indicates alkalosis. A pH less than 7.35 indicates acidosis.

RECOGNIZING ACID-BASE DISORDERS

This chart lists the arterial blood gas (ABG) values, possible causes, and clinical effects associated with acid-base disorders.

Disorders and ABG findings	Possible causes	Signs and symptoms
Respiratory acidosis (excess CO_2 retention) pH < 7.35 HCO_3^- > 28 mEq/L (if compensating) $Paco_2$ > 45 mm Hg	• Central nervous system depression from drugs, injury, or disease • Asphyxia • Hypoventilation due to pulmonary, cardiac, musculoskeletal, or neuromuscular disease	• Diaphoresis, headache, tachycardia, confusion, restlessness, apprehension
Respiratory alkalosis (excess CO_2 excretion) pH > 7.45 HCO_3^- < 24 mEq/L (if compensating) $Paco_2$ < 35 mm Hg	• Hyperventilation due to anxiety, pain, or improper ventilator settings • Respiratory stimulation caused by drugs, disease, hypoxia, fever, or high room temperature • Gram-negative bacteremia	• Rapid, deep breathing; paresthesia; light-headedness; twitching; anxiety; fear
Metabolic acidosis (HCO_3^- loss, acid retention) pH < 7.35 HCO_3^- < 24 mEq/L $Paco_2$ < 35 mm Hg (if compensating)	• HCO_3^- depletion due to renal disease, diarrhea, or small-bowel fistulas • Excessive production of organic acids due to hepatic disease, endocrine disorders (including diabetes mellitus), hypoxia, shock, and drug intoxication • Inadequate excretion of acids due to renal disease	• Rapid, deep breathing; fruity breath; fatigue; headache; lethargy; drowsiness; nausea; vomiting; coma (if severe)
Metabolic alkalosis (HCO_3^- retention, acid loss) pH > 7.45 HCO_3^- > 28 mEq/L $Paco_2$ > 45 mm Hg	• Loss of hydrochloric acid from prolonged vomiting or gastric suctioning • Loss of potassium due to increased renal excretion (as in diuretic therapy) or steroid overdose • Excessive alkali ingestion	• Slow, shallow breathing; hypertonic muscles, restlessness; twitching; confusion; irritability; apathy; tetany; seizures; coma (if severe)

A patient with a Pao_2 value between 60 and 100 mm Hg should have an Sao_2 value above 85%. If his Sao_2 value drops sharply, his Pao_2 value has probably fallen below 50 mm Hg.

An HCO_3^- value above 26 mEq/L points to metabolic, or kidney-related, alkalosis; below 22 mEq/L, metabolic acidosis.

Carcinoembryonic antigen

Carcinoembryonic antigen (CEA) is a protein normally found in embryonic entodermal epithelium and fetal GI tissue. Production of CEA stops before birth, but it may begin again later if a neoplasm develops. Because CEA levels are also raised by biliary obstruction, alcoholic hepatitis, chronic heavy smoking, and other conditions, this test can't be used as a general indicator of cancer. However, measurement of enzyme CEA levels by immunoassay is useful for staging and monitoring treatment of certain cancers.

Purpose

• To monitor the effectiveness of cancer therapy
• To assist in preoperative staging of colorectal cancers, assess adequacy of surgical resection, and test for recurrence of colorectal cancers

Reference values

Normal serum CEA values are less than 5 ng/ml.

Abnormal findings

If CEA levels are higher than normal before surgical resection, chemotherapy, or radiation therapy, their return to normal within 6 weeks suggest successful treatment. However, persistently elevated CEA levels suggest residual or recurrent tumor.

High CEA levels are characteristic in various malignant conditions, particularly endodermally derived neoplasms of the GI organs and the lungs, and in certain nonmalignant conditions, such as benign hepatic disease, hepatic cirrhosis, alcoholic pancreatitis, and inflammatory bowel disease.

Elevated CEA concentrations may also result from nonendodermal carcinomas, such as breast cancer and ovarian cancer.

Cerebrospinal fluid analysis

For qualitative analysis, cerebrospinal fluid (CSF) is most commonly obtained by lumbar puncture (usually between the third and fourth lumbar vertebrae) and, rarely, by cisternal or ventricular puncture. A CSF specimen may also be obtained during other neurologic tests, such as myelography.

Purpose

• To measure CSF pressure to help detect obstruction of CSF circulation
• To aid diagnosis of viral or bacterial meningitis, subarachnoid or intracranial hemorrhage, tumors, and brain abscesses
• To aid diagnosis of neurosyphilis and chronic central nervous system infections

Normal and abnormal findings

Normally, the CSF pressure is recorded and the appearance of the specimen is checked. Three tubes are collected routinely and sent to the laboratory for analysis of protein, sugar, and cells as well as for serologic testing, such as the Venereal Disease Research Laboratory (VDRL) test for neurosyphilis. A separate specimen is sent to the laboratory for culture and sensitivity testing. Electrolyte analysis and Gram stain may be ordered as supplementary tests. CSF electrolyte levels are of special interest in patients with abnormal serum electrolyte levels or CSF infection and in those receiving hyperosmolar agents.

For a summary of normal and abnormal findings in CSF analysis, see *Analysis of cerebrospinal fluid.*

ANALYSIS OF CEREBROSPINAL FLUID

Test	Normal	Abnormal	Implications
Pressure	50 to 180 mm H_2O	Increase	Increased intracranial pressure due to hemorrhage, tumor, or edema caused by trauma
		Decrease	Spinal subarachnoid obstruction above puncture site
Appearance	Clear, colorless	Cloudy	Infection (elevated white blood cell [WBC] count and protein levels, or many microorganisms)
		Xanthochromic or bloody	Subarachnoid, intracerebral, or intraventricular hemorrhage; spinal cord obstruction; traumatic tap (usually noted only in initial specimen)
		Brown, yellow, or orange	Elevated protein levels, red blood cell (RBC) breakdown (blood present for at least 3 days)
Protein	*Lumbar:* – neonates: 15 to 100 mg/dl – ages 3 months to 60 years: 15 to 45 mg/dl – over age 60: 15 to 60 mg/dl *Cisternal:* 15 to 25 mg/dl *Ventricular:* 15 to 16 mg/dl	Marked increase	Tumors, trauma, hemorrhage, diabetes mellitus, polyneuritis, blood in cerebrospinal fluid (CSF)
		Marked decrease	Rapid CSF production
Glucose	40 to 70 mg/dl (two-thirds of blood glucose level)	Increase	Systemic hyperglycemia
		Decrease	Systemic hypoglycemia, bacterial or fungal infection, meningitis, mumps, postsubarachnoid hemorrhage
Cell count	0 to 5 WBCs in adults; 0 to 30 WBCs in neonates	Increase RBCs	Active disease: meningitis, acute infection, onset of chronic illness, tumor, abscess, infarction, demyelinating disease (such as multiple sclerosis)
	No RBCs		Hemorrhage or traumatic tap

(continued)

Test	Normal	Abnormal	Implications
Venereal Disease Research Laboratory and other serologic tests	Nonreactive	Positive	Neurosyphilis
Chloride	118 to 132 mEq/L	Decrease	Infected meninges (as in tuberculosis or meningitis)
Gram stain	No organisms	Gram-positive or gram-negative organisms	Bacterial meningitis

ANALYSIS OF CEREBROSPINAL FLUID (continued)

Creatine kinase

Creatine kinase (CK) is an enzyme that catalyzes the creatine-creatinine metabolic pathway in muscle cells and brain tissue. Because of its intimate role in energy production, CK reflects normal tissue catabolism; increased serum levels indicate trauma to cells.

Fractionation and measurement of three distinct CK isoenzymes— CK-BB (CK_1), CK-MB (CK_2), and CK-MM (CK_3)—have replaced the use of total CK levels to accurately localize the site of increased tissue destruction. CK-BB is most often found in brain tissue. CK-MM and CK-MB are found primarily in skeletal and heart muscle.

Purpose

• To detect and diagnose acute myocardial infarction (MI) and reinfarction (CK-MB is primarily used)
• To evaluate possible causes of chest pain and to monitor the severity of myocardial ischemia after cardiac surgery, cardiac catheterization, and cardioversion (CK-MB is primarily used)
• To detect musculoskeletal disorders that are not neurogenic in origin, such as Duchenne muscular dystrophy (total CK is primarily used),

rhabdomyolysis, and early dermatomyositis

Reference values

Total CK values determined by ultraviolet or kinetic measurement range from 40 to 175 U/L for men and from 25 to 140 U/L for women. CK levels may be significantly higher in muscular people. Infants up to age 1 have levels two to four times higher than those in adults, possibly reflecting birth trauma and striated muscle development.

Normal ranges for isoenzyme levels are as follows: CK-BB, undetectable; CK-MB, undetectable to 7 U/L; CK-MM, 5 to 7 U/L.

Abnormal findings

CK-MM makes up 99% of total CK normally present in serum. Detectable CK-BB isoenzyme may indicate, but doesn't confirm, a diagnosis of brain tissue injury, widespread malignant tumors, severe shock, or renal failure.

CK-MB levels greater than 5% of total CK (or more than 10 U/L) indicate MI, especially if the lactate dehydrogenase isoenzyme ratio (LD_1/LD_2) is greater than 1 (flipped LD). In acute MI and after cardiac surgery, CK-MB begins to increase within 2 to 4 hours, peaks within 12 to 24 hours,

SERUM PROTEIN AND ISOENZYME LEVELS AFTER M.I.

Because they're released by damaged tissue, serum proteins and isoenzymes (catalytic proteins that vary in concentration in specific organs) can help identify the compromised organ and assess the extent of damage. The serum protein and isoenzyme determinations listed below are most significant in myocardial infarction (MI).

Isoenzymes
• Creatine kinase-MB (CK-MB): in the heart muscle and a small amount in skeletal muscle
• Lactate dehydrogenase 1 and 2 (LD_1, LD_2): in the heart, brain, kidneys, liver, skeletal muscles, and red blood cells (RBCs)

Proteins
Troponin-I and troponin-T (the cardiac contractile proteins) have greater sensitivity than CK-MB in detecting myocardial injury.

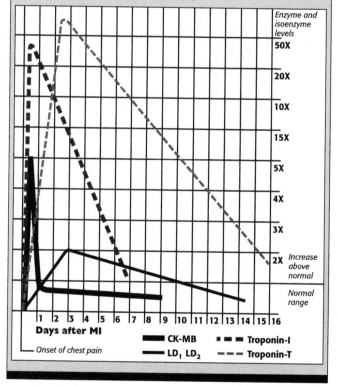

and usually returns to normal within 24 to 48 hours; persistent elevations and increasing levels indicate ongoing myocardial damage. Total CK follows roughly the same pattern but increases slightly later. CK-MB levels may not increase in heart failure or during angina pectoris not accompanied by myocardial cell necrosis. (See *Serum protein and isoenzyme levels after MI.*)

Serious skeletal muscle injury that occurs in certain muscular dystrophies, polymyositis, and severe myoglobinuria may produce a mild CK-MB increase because a small amount of this isoenzyme is present in some skeletal muscles.

Increasing CK-MM values follow skeletal muscle damage from trauma, such as surgery and I.M. injections, and from diseases, such as dermatomyositis and muscular dystrophy (values may be 50 to 100 times normal). A moderate increase in CK-MM levels develops in patients with hypothyroidism; sharp increases occur with muscle activity caused by agitation, such as during an acute psychotic episode.

Total CK levels may be increased in patients with severe hypokalemia, carbon monoxide poisoning, malignant hyperthermia, and alcoholic cardiomyopathy. They may also be increased after seizures and, occasionally, in patients who have suffered pulmonary or cerebral infarctions.

Creatinine clearance

An anhydride of creatine, creatinine is formed and excreted in constant amounts by an irreversible reaction and functions solely as the main end product of creatine. Creatinine production is proportional to total muscle mass and is relatively unaffected by urine volume or normal physical activity or diet.

An excellent diagnostic indicator of kidney function, the creatinine clearance test determines how efficiently the kidneys are clearing creatinine from the blood. The rate of clearance is expressed in terms of the volume of blood (in milliliters) that can be cleared of creatinine in 1 minute. Creatinine levels become abnormal when more than 50% of the nephrons have been damaged.

Purpose

• To assess kidney function (primarily glomerular filtration)
• To monitor progression of renal insufficiency

Reference values

Normal creatinine clearance varies with age; in males, it ranges from 55 to 146 ml/minute/1.73 m^2; in females, from 52 to 134 ml/minute/1.73 m^2. For older patients, creatinine clearance normally decreases by 6 ml/minute for each decade.

Abnormal findings

Low creatinine clearance may result from reduced renal blood flow (associated with shock or renal artery obstruction), acute tubular necrosis, acute or chronic glomerulonephritis, advanced bilateral chronic pyelonephritis, advanced bilateral renal lesions (which may occur in polycystic kidney disease, renal tuberculosis, and cancer), nephrosclerosis, heart failure, or severe dehydration.

High creatinine clearance rates generally have little diagnostic significance.

Erythrocyte sedimentation rate

The erythrocyte sedimentation rate (ESR) measures the degree of erythrocyte settling in a blood sample during a specified time period. The ESR is a sensitive but nonspecific test that is frequently the earliest indicator of disease when other chemical or physical signs are normal. The ESR commonly increases significantly in widespread inflammatory disorders; elevations may be prolonged in localized inflammation and malignant disease.

Purpose

• To monitor inflammatory or malignant disease
• To aid detection and diagnosis of occult disease, such as tuberculosis, tissue necrosis, and connective tissue disease

Reference values

Using the Westergren method, the ESR normally ranges from 0 to 10 mm/hour in children, 0 to 15 mm/hour in males, and 0 to 20 mm/hour in females. Rates gradually increase after age 50.

Abnormal findings

The ESR rises in pregnancy, anemia, acute or chronic inflammation, tuberculosis, paraproteinemias (especially multiple myeloma and Waldenström's macroglobulinemia), rheumatic fever, rheumatoid arthritis, and some malignant diseases.

Polycythemia, sickle cell anemia, hyperviscosity, and low plasma fibrinogen or globulin levels tend to depress the ESR.

Estrogen, serum

Estrogens (and progesterone) are secreted by the ovaries. They're responsible for the development of secondary female sexual characteristics and for normal menstruation; levels are usually undetectable in children. These hormones are secreted by ovarian follicular cells during the first half of the menstrual cycle and by the corpus luteum during the luteal phase and during pregnancy. In menopause, estrogen secretion drops to a constant, low level.

This radioimmunoassay measures serum levels of estradiol, estrone, and estriol (the only estrogens that appear in serum in measurable amounts) and has diagnostic significance in evaluating female gonadal dysfunction. Tests of hypothalamic-pituitary function may be required to confirm the diagnosis.

Purpose

• To determine sexual maturation and fertility
• To aid diagnosis of gonadal dysfunction, such as precocious or delayed puberty, menstrual disorders (especially amenorrhea), and infertility
• To determine fetal well-being
• To aid diagnosis of tumors known to secrete estrogen

Reference values

Normal serum estrogen levels for premenopausal women vary widely during the menstrual cycle, ranging from 30 to 400 pg/ml. The range for postmenopausal women is 0 to 30 pg/ml.

Serum estrogen levels in men range from 10 to 50 pg/ml. In children under age 6, the normal level of serum estrogen is less than 10 pg/ml.

Abnormal findings

Decreased estrogen levels may indicate primary hypogonadism, or ovarian failure, as in Turner's syndrome or ovarian agenesis; secondary hypogonadism, as in hypopituitarism; or menopause.

Abnormally high estrogen levels may occur with estrogen-producing tumors, in precocious puberty, and in severe hepatic disease, such as cirrhosis, that prevents clearance of plasma estrogens. High levels may also result from congenital adrenal hyperplasia (increased conversion of androgens to estrogen).

Glucose, fasting plasma

The fasting plasma glucose (or fasting blood sugar) test is used to measure plasma glucose levels after a 12- to 14-hour fast. This test is commonly used to screen for diabetes mellitus, in which absence or deficiency of insulin allows persistently high glucose levels.

Purpose

• To screen for diabetes mellitus
• To monitor drug or diet therapy in patients with diabetes mellitus

Reference values

The normal range for fasting plasma glucose varies according to the laboratory procedure. However, the American Diabetes Association's guidelines, revised in 1998, call for normal blood glucose levels of less than 126 mg/dl.

Abnormal findings

Confirmation of diabetes mellitus requires fasting plasma glucose levels of 126 mg/dl or more obtained on two or more occasions. In patients with borderline or transient elevated levels, a 2-hour postprandial plasma glucose test or oral glucose tolerance test may be performed to confirm diagnosis.

Increased fasting plasma glucose levels can also result from pancreatitis, recent acute illness (such as myocardial infarction), Cushing's syndrome, acromegaly, and pheochromocytoma. Hyperglycemia may also stem from hyperlipoproteinemia (especially type III, IV, or V), chronic hepatic disease, nephrotic syndrome, brain tumor, sepsis, or gastrectomy with dumping syndrome and is typical in eclampsia, anoxia, and seizure disorder.

Low plasma glucose levels can result from hyperinsulinism, insulinoma, von Gierke's disease, functional and reactive hypoglycemia, myxedema, adrenal insufficiency, congenital adrenal hyperplasia, hypopituitarism, malabsorption syndrome, and some cases of hepatic insufficiency.

Glucose, 2-hour postprandial plasma

Also called the 2-hour postprandial blood sugar test, the 2-hour postprandial plasma test is a valuable screening tool for detecting diabetes mellitus. It's performed when the patient demonstrates symptoms of diabetes (polydipsia and polyuria) or when results of the fasting plasma glucose test suggest diabetes.

Purpose

• To aid diagnosis of diabetes mellitus
• To monitor drug or diet therapy in patients with diabetes mellitus

Reference values

In a person who doesn't have diabetes, postprandial glucose values are 65 to 139 mg/dl by the glucose oxidase or hexokinase method; levels are slightly elevated in people over age 50. (See *Two-hour postprandial plasma glucose levels by age.*)

Abnormal findings

Two 2-hour postprandial blood glucose values of 200 mg/dl or above indicate diabetes mellitus. High levels may also occur with pancreatitis, Cushing's syndrome, acromegaly, and pheochromocytoma. Hyperglycemia may also be caused by hyperlipoproteinemia (especially type III, IV, or V), chronic hepatic disease, nephrotic

TWO-HOUR POSTPRANDIAL PLASMA GLUCOSE LEVELS BY AGE

The greatest difference in normal and diabetic insulin responses, and thus in plasma glucose concentration, occurs about 2 hours after a glucose challenge. Values of this test can fluctuate according to the patient's age. After age 50, for example, normal levels rise markedly and steadily, sometimes reaching 160 mg/dl or higher. In younger patients, glucose concentration over 145 mg/dl suggests incipient diabetes and requires further evaluation.

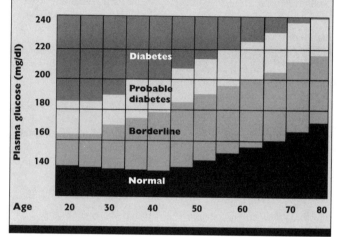

syndrome, brain tumor, sepsis, gastrectomy with dumping syndrome, eclampsia, anoxia, and seizure disorders.

Low glucose levels occur in hyperinsulinism, insulinoma, von Gierke's disease, functional and reactive hypoglycemia, myxedema, adrenal insufficiency, congenital adrenal hyperplasia, hypopituitarism, malabsorption syndrome, and some cases of hepatic insufficiency.

Glucose tolerance test, oral

The oral glucose tolerance test is the most sensitive method of evaluating borderline cases of diabetes mellitus. Plasma and urine glucose levels are monitored for 3 hours after ingestion of a challenge dose of glucose to assess insulin secretion and the body's ability to metabolize glucose.

The oral glucose tolerance test isn't generally used in patients with fasting plasma glucose values greater than 140 mg/dl or postprandial plasma glucose values greater than 200 mg/dl.

Purpose

• To confirm diabetes mellitus in selected patients
• To aid diagnosis of hypoglycemia and malabsorption syndrome (requires monitoring for an additional 2 to 3 hours to aid diagnosis, which is contraindicated when insulinoma is strongly suspected because prolonged fasting may lead to fainting and coma)

Reference values

Normal plasma glucose levels peak at 110 to 170 mg/dl within 30 minutes to 1 hour after administration of an oral glucose test dose and return to fasting levels or lower within 2 to 3 hours. Urine glucose tests remain negative throughout.

Abnormal findings

Decreased glucose tolerance, in which levels peak sharply before falling slowly to fasting levels, may confirm diabetes mellitus or may result from Cushing's disease, hemochromatosis, pheochromocytoma, or central nervous system lesions.

Increased glucose tolerance, in which levels may peak at less than normal, may indicate insulinoma, malabsorption syndrome, adrenocortical insufficiency (Addison's disease), hypothyroidism, or hypopituitarism.

Hemoglobin, glycosylated

Also called total fasting hemoglobin, the glycosylated hemoglobin test is a tool for monitoring diabetes therapy. Measurement of glycosylated hemoglobin levels provides information about the average blood glucose level during the preceding 2 to 3 months. This test requires only one venipuncture every 6 to 8 weeks and can, therefore, be used for evaluating long-term effectiveness of diabetes therapy.

Purpose

• To assess control of diabetes mellitus

Reference values

Glycosylated hemoglobin values are reported as a percentage of the total hemoglobin within an erythrocyte. Glycosylated hemoglobin accounts for 4% to 7%.

Abnormal findings

In diabetes, the patient has good control of blood glucose concentrations when the glycosylated hemoglobin value is less than 8%. A glycosylated hemoglobin value greater than 10% indicates poor control.

Hepatitis tests

This panel of tests confirms a diagnosis of hepatitis and identifies the causative type. (See *Hepatitis panel*.)

Human chorionic gonadotropin, serum

Human chorionic gonadotropin (hCG) is a glycoprotein hormone produced in the placenta. If conception occurs, a specific assay for hCG, commonly called the beta-subunit assay, may detect this hormone in the blood 9 days after ovulation. This interval coincides with the implantation of the fertilized ovum into the uterine wall. Although the precise function of hCG is unclear, it appears that hCG, with progesterone, maintains the corpus luteum during early pregnancy.

Production of hCG increases steadily during the first trimester, peaking around the 10th week of gestation. Levels then fall to less than 10% of first-trimester peak levels during the remainder of the pregnancy. About 2 weeks after delivery, the hormone may no longer be detectable.

This serum immunoassay, a quantitative analysis of hCG beta-subunit level, is more sensitive (and costlier) than the routine pregnancy test using a urine specimen.

HEPATITIS PANEL

These tests are performed on patients with symptoms of hepatitis. Positive results not only confirm a hepatitis diagnosis but differentiate the type and status of the infection as well.

Test	Purpose	Implication of positive result
Anti-HAV (antibody to hepatitis A virus [HAV] antigen; also called HAV-Ab)	• To rule out HAV infection • To determine immune status to HAV	• Indicates need for supportive care and education • Can test for anti-HAV immunoglobulin (Ig) M and anti-HAV IgG • Presence of IgG: indicates unlikely cause of current symptoms and immunity to HAV
Anti-HBc (IgG and IgM) (antibody to hepatitis B virus [HBV] core antigen)	• To differentiate acute from chronic HBV infection	• Is occasionally falsely positive • Must be interpreted in context of other tests • Indicates HBV infection as this marker doesn't appear after vaccination • If primarily anti-HBc IgM result: reveals acute hepatitis B (infected usually < 6 months) and needs follow-up • If primarily anti-HBc IgG result: reveals chronic hepatitis B and needs follow-up
Anti-HBeAg (antibody to hepatitis Be antigen)	• To select patients for interferon therapy • To select patients for liver transplantation	• If anti-HBeAg is present: indicates favorable prognosis because body has mounted a defensive attack against HBV • Usually appears 8 to 16 weeks after exposure to HBV antigen; indicates an immune response has occurred
Anti-HbsAg (antibody to hepatitis B surface antigen; also called anti-HBs)	• To check immune status to HBV	• Indicates immune response to HBV due to HBV infection, HBV immunoglobulin, or HBV vaccination • In acute infection, detectable after HbsAg disappears
Anti-HCV (antibody to hepatitis C virus [HCV]) enzyme-linked immunosorbent assay (ELISA)	• To aid differential diagnosis of HCV • To screen blood donors (ELISA-1 and ELISA-2: inexpensive, simple to perform, high sensitivity [ELISA-2 more sensitive])	• Does NOT indicate immunity • Appears 2 to 6 months after acute HCV infection, but may take up to 1 year • In the presence of elevated LFTs: diagnostic for hepatitis C and needs follow-up • Low specificity compared to RNA testing*

(continued)

HEPATITIS PANEL (continued)

Test	Purpose	Implication of positive result
Anti-HDV (antibody to hepatitis D virus [HDV])	• To detect antibodies to HDV ribonucleic acid (RNA) by polymerase chain reaction (HDV is a defective RNA virus that replicates efficiently only in the presence of HbsAg.)	• If positive for HDV: indicates poor prognosis • 50% of patients with fulminant HBV also have HDV
HBeAg (hepatitis Be antigen)	• To measure viral replication	• High levels: very infectious patient
HbsAg (also called hepatitis-associated antigen and Australia antigen)	• To screen blood donors and high risk populations • As part of prenatal testing • To establish differential diagnosis of viral hepatitis	• Needs follow-up • Elevation for > 6 months indicative of chronic hepatitis B infection
HBV deoxyribonucleic acid	• To measure viral presence (not antibodies) • To confirm HBV if HBV screen is positive result but liver function tests (LFTs) are normal	• Confirms HBV status and requires careful follow-up care
HCV RNA (also called enzyme immunoassay 2 [EIA-2], HCV RNA RT-PCR [reverse transcriptase-polymerase chain reaction])	• To measure viral presence (not antibodies) • To confirm hepatitis C virus (HCV) status (gold standard because it's the most sensitive, but it's expensive and requires technical skill) • To confirm HCV if HCV screen is positive but LFTs are normal	• Confirms HCV status and requires careful follow-up care

*A second-generation recombinant immunoblot assay (also called RIBA) is a commonly used supplemental assay, particularly in patients with normal alanine aminotransferase levels. The reactivity of antibodies toward each antigen band is reported as 1+ to 4+. If two or more bands react with an intensity of at least 1+, the result is indeterminate; however the bands c22-3 and c33c are strongly associated with HCV RNA and even an indeterminate result that includes one of them may indicate positive HCV infection.

Purpose

• To detect early pregnancy
• To determine adequacy of hormonal production in high-risk pregnancies (for example, habitual abortion)
• To aid diagnosis of trophoblastic tumors, such as hydatidiform moles and choriocarcinoma, and tumors that ectopically secrete hCG
• To monitor treatment for induction of ovulation and conception

Reference values

Normally, hCG levels are less than 4 IU/L. During pregnancy, hCG levels vary widely, depending partly on the number of days after the last normal menses.

Abnormal findings

Elevated hCG beta-subunit levels indicate pregnancy; significantly higher concentrations are present in a multiple pregnancy. Increased levels may also suggest hydatidiform mole, trophoblastic neoplasms of the placenta, and nontrophoblastic carcinomas that secrete hCG (including gastric, pancreatic, and ovarian adenocarcinomas). Low hCG beta-subunit levels can occur in ectopic pregnancy or pregnancy of less than 9 days. Beta-subunit levels can't differentiate between pregnancy and tumor recurrence because they're high in both conditions.

Human immunodeficiency virus

These tests detect antibodies, antigens, or ribonucleic acid caused by human immunodeficiency virus (HIV) in serum. HIV is the virus that causes acquired immunodeficiency syndrome (AIDS). Transmission occurs by direct exposure of a person's blood to body fluids containing the virus. The virus may be transmitted from one person to another through exchange of contaminated blood and blood products, during sexual intercourse with an infected partner, when I.V. drugs are shared, and from an infected mother to her child during pregnancy or breast-feeding.

Initial identification of HIV is usually achieved through enzyme-linked immunosorbent assay. Positive findings are confirmed by Western blot test and immunofluorescence. (See *HIV testing*, pages 90 and 91.)

Purpose

- To screen for HIV in high-risk patients
- To screen donated blood for HIV

Normal findings

Test results are normally negative. However, HIV-1 or HIV-2 antibodies may fall to undetectable levels in the final stages of AIDS. A positive result, indicating the presence of antibodies, necessitates further investigation.

 ALERT Immunocompromised patients may not produce these antibodies.

Abnormal findings

The test detects exposure to HIV-1 or HIV-2 1 to 6 months after infection occurs; antibody to p24 is commonly the first HIV-1 antibody detectable. However, the test doesn't identify patients who have been exposed to the virus but haven't yet made antibodies. Most patients with AIDS have antibodies to HIV. A positive test for the HIV antibody can't determine whether a patient harbors actively replicating virus or when the patient will manifest signs and symptoms of AIDS.

Many apparently healthy people have been exposed to HIV and have circulating antibodies. The test results for such people aren't false-positives.

International Normalized Ratio

The International Normalized Ratio (INR) system is viewed as the best means of standardizing measurement of prothrombin time to monitor oral anticoagulant therapy. It isn't used as a screening test for coagulopathies.

H.I.V. TESTING

Test and purpose	For low-risk people (retesting in few months for high-risk people)	Sensitivity and specificity
Enzyme-linked immunosorbent assay (ELISA) or enzyme immunoassay (EIA) HIV-1/HIV-2 *Screening test*	Positive result needs a confirmatory test. Negative result needs no follow-up.	99.9% when combined with Western blot test
P24 antigen ELISA *Screening test*	Requires confirmatory test for both negative and positive results.	Moderately low sensitivity; high specificity
Western blot *Confirmatory test*	Two or more bands indicates HIV. Absence of bands rules out HIV. Indeterminate result (1 band associated with HIV present) needs a retest in 1 month or a p24 or HIV ribonucleic acid (RNA) test.	99.9% when combined with ELISA/EIA test; 99.9 specificity
HIV RNA by RT-polymerase chain reaction (detects RNA after infection but before sero-conversion) *Aids prognosis determination*	Positive result rules in HIV. Negative result needs no follow-up.	98%; high specificity
HIV RNA by b deoxyribonucleic acid *Quantifies activity of antiviral agents*	Not for low risk population	90%; high specificity
Oral mucosal transudate *Screening test*	Positive result needs a confirmatory test. Negative result needs no follow-up.	As accurate as blood tests
CD4+ (indicates immune competence) *Aids treatment decisions*	CD4+ count < 200 gives a diagnosis of AIDS.	High sensitivity and high specificity for prognosis
Reactive rapid test (detects HIV-1 in 5 to 30 minutes) *Rapid-result screening test*	Positive result needs a confirmatory test. Negative result needs no follow-up.	99.9%; high specificity

Purpose

• To evaluate effectiveness of oral anticoagulant therapy

Reference values

Normal INR for patients receiving warfarin therapy is 2.0 to 3.0. For those with prosthetic heart valves, an INR of 2.5 to 3.5 is suggested.

Abnormal findings

An increased INR may indicate disseminated intravascular coagulation, cirrhosis, hepatitis, vitamin K deficiency, or salicylate intoxication lactic acid, an essential step in the metabolic processes that ultimately produce cellular energy. Because LD is present in almost all body tissues, cellular damage increases total serum LD, limiting the diagnostic usefulness of LD.

Five tissue-specific isoenzymes can be identified and measured: LD_1 and LD_2 appear primarily in the heart, red blood cells, and kidneys; LD_3 is found primarily in the lungs; and LD_4 and LD_5 are in the liver, skin, and the skeletal muscles.

Purpose

• To aid differential diagnosis of myocardial infarction (MI), pulmonary infarction, anemias, and hepatic disease
• To support creatine kinase (CK) isoenzyme test results in diagnosing MI, or to provide diagnosis when CK-MB samples are drawn too late to display increase
• To monitor patient response to some forms of chemotherapy

Reference values

Total LD levels normally range from 94 to 257 U/L in adults and from 108 to 540 U/L in children. Normal distribution is as follows:
• LD_1: 17.5% to 28.3% of total
• LD_2: 30.4% to 36.4% of total
• LD_3: 19.2% to 24.8% of total
• LD_4: 9.6% to 15.6% of total
• LD_5: 5.5% to 12.7% of total.

Abnormal findings

Because many common diseases increase total LD levels, isoenzyme electrophoresis is usually necessary for diagnosis. In some disorders, total LD levels may be within normal limits, but abnormal proportions of each isoenzyme indicate specific organ tissue damage. For instance, in acute MI, the LD_1/LD_2 isoenzyme ratio is

---

Seroconversion time

1 to 6 months

Often the first detectable level (<6 weeks)

1 to 6 months

1 to 6 months

1 to 6 months

1 to 6 months

Not applicable

1 to 6 months

or may be due to massive blood transfusion.

Lactate dehydrogenase

Lactate dehydrogenase (LD) catalyzes the reversible conversion of muscle

PERITONEAL FLUID ANALYSIS

Element	Normal value or finding
Gross appearance	Sterile, odorless, clear to pale yellow; scant amount (< 50 ml)
Red blood cells	None
White blood cells	< 300/µl (undiluted peritoneal fluid) or < 500/µl (lavage fluid)
Protein	< 4.1 g/dl
Glucose	70 to 100 mg/dl
Amylase	140 to 400 U/L
Ammonia	< 50 g/dl
Alkaline phosphatase	30 to 110 U/L
Cytology	No abnormal cells present
Bacteria	None
Fungi	None

typically greater than 1 within 12 to 48 hours after onset of symptoms (known as flipped LD).

Midzone fractions (LD_2, LD_3, LD_4) can be increased in granulocytic leukemia, lymphomas, and platelet disorders.

Peritoneal fluid analysis

Peritoneal fluid analysis assesses a specimen obtained by paracentesis. This procedure requires insertion of a trocar and cannula through the abdominal wall after the patient receives a local anesthetic. If the specimen is obtained for therapeutic purposes, the trocar may be connected to a drainage system. However, if only a small amount of fluid is obtained for diagnostic purposes, an 18G needle may be used in place of the trocar and cannula. In a four-quadrant tap, fluid is aspirated from each quadrant of the abdomen to verify abdominal trauma and confirm the need for surgery.

Purpose

- To determine the cause of ascites
- To detect abdominal trauma

Reference values

For normal peritoneal fluid values, see *Peritoneal fluid analysis*.

Abnormal findings

Milk-colored peritoneal fluid may result from chyle or lymph fluid escaping from a thoracic duct that is damaged or blocked by a malignant tumor, lymphoma, tuberculosis, parasitic infestation, adhesion, or hepatic cirrhosis; a pseudochylous condition may result from the presence of leukocytes or tumor cells. Differential diagnosis of true chylous ascites depends on the presence of elevated triglyceride levels (greater than

400 mg/dl) and microscopic fat globules.

Cloudy or turbid fluid may indicate peritonitis due to primary bacterial infection, ruptured bowel (after trauma), pancreatitis, strangulated or infarcted intestine, or appendicitis. Bloody fluid may result from a benign or malignant tumor, hemorrhagic pancreatitis, or a traumatic tap; however, if the fluid fails to clear on continued aspiration, traumatic tap isn't the cause. Bile-stained fluid may indicate a ruptured gallbladder, acute pancreatitis, or perforated intestine or duodenal ulcer.

A red blood cell count over 100/µl indicates neoplasm or tuberculosis; a count over 100,000/µl indicates intra-abdominal trauma. An elevated white blood cell count with more than 25% neutrophils occurs in 90% of patients with spontaneous bacterial peritonitis and in 50% of those with cirrhosis. A high percentage of lymphocytes suggest tuberculous peritonitis or chylous ascites. Numerous mesothelial cells indicate tuberculous peritonitis.

Protein levels rise above 3 g/dl in malignant conditions and above 4 g/dl in tuberculosis. Peritoneal fluid glucose levels fall below 60 mg/dl in 30% to 50% of patients with tuberculous peritonitis and peritoneal carcinomatosis.

Amylase levels rise in about 90% of patients with pancreatic trauma, pancreatic pseudocyst, or acute pancreatitis and may also rise in those with intestinal necrosis or strangulation.

Peritoneal alkaline phosphatase levels rise to more than twice the normal serum levels in about 90% of patients with ruptured or strangulated small intestine. Peritoneal ammonia levels also exceed twice the normal serum levels in ruptured or strangulated large and small intestines and in ruptured ulcer or appendix.

A protein ascitic fluid–serum ratio of 0.5 or greater may suggest a malignant condition, such as tuberculous or pancreatic ascites. The presence of this finding indicates a nonhepatic cause; its absence suggests uncomplicated hepatic disease. An albumin gradient between ascitic fluid and serum greater than 1 g/dl indicates chronic hepatic disease; a lesser value suggests a malignant condition.

Cytologic examination of peritoneal fluid accurately detects malignant cells. Microbiological examination can reveal coliforms, anaerobes, and enterococci, which can enter the peritoneum from a ruptured organ or from infections accompanying appendicitis, pancreatitis, tuberculosis, or ovarian disease. The presence of gram-positive cocci commonly indicate primary peritonitis; gram-negative organisms, secondary peritonitis. The presence of fungi may indicate histoplasmosis, candidiasis, or coccidioidomycosis.

Pleural fluid analysis

The pleura, a two-layer membrane that covers the lungs and lines the thoracic cavity, maintains a small amount of lubricating fluid between its layers to minimize friction during respiration. Increased fluid in this space may result from diseases such as cancer and tuberculosis or from blood or lymphatic disorders and can cause respiratory difficulty.

In pleural fluid aspiration (thoracentesis), the thoracic wall is punctured to obtain a specimen of pleural fluid for analysis or to relieve pulmonary compression and resultant respiratory distress.

Purpose

• To determine the cause and nature of pleural effusion

Reference values

Normally, the pleural cavity maintains negative pressure and contains less than 20 ml of serous fluid.

Abnormal findings

Pleural effusion results from the abnormal formation or reabsorption of pleural fluid. Certain characteristics classify pleural fluid as either a transudate (a low-protein fluid that has leaked from normal blood vessels) or an exudate (a protein-rich fluid that has leaked from blood vessels with increased permeability).

Pleural fluid may contain blood (hemothorax), chyle (chylothorax), or pus and necrotic tissue. Blood-tinged fluid may indicate a traumatic tap; if so, the fluid should clear as aspiration progresses.

Transudative effusion generally results from diminished colloidal pressure, increased negative pressure within the pleural cavity, ascites, systemic and pulmonary venous hypertension, heart failure, hepatic cirrhosis, and nephritis.

Exudative effusion results from disorders that increase pleural capillary permeability (possibly with changes in hydrostatic or colloid osmotic pressures), lymphatic drainage interference, infections, pulmonary infarctions, and neoplasms. Exudative effusion associated with depressed glucose levels, elevated lactate dehydrogenase (LD) isoenzyme levels, rheumatoid arthritis cells, and negative smears, cultures, and cytologic examination may indicate pleurisy associated with rheumatoid arthritis.

The most common pathogens that appear in culture studies of pleural fluid are *Mycobacterium tuberculosis, Staphylococcus aureus, Streptococcus pneumoniae* and other streptococci, *Haemophilus influenzae* and, in the case of a ruptured pulmonary abscess, anaerobes such as *Bacteroides.* Cultures are usually positive during the early stages of infection; however, antibiotic therapy may produce a negative culture despite a positive Gram stain and grossly purulent fluid. Empyema may result from complications of pneumonia, pulmonary abscess, perforation of the esophagus, or penetration from mediastinitis. A high percentage of neutrophils suggests septic inflammation; predominating lymphocytes suggest tuberculosis or fungal or viral effusions.

Serosanguineous fluid may indicate pleural extension of a malignant tumor. Elevated LD levels in a nonpurulent, nonhemolyzed, nonbloody effusion may also suggest a malignant condition. Pleural fluid glucose levels that are 30 to 40 mg/dl lower than blood glucose levels may indicate a malignant tumor, a bacterial infection, nonseptic inflammation, or metastasis. Increased amylase levels occur in pleural effusions associated with pancreatitis.

Prostate-specific antigen

Prostate-specific antigen (PSA) appears in normal, benign hyperplastic, and malignant prostatic tissue as well as in metastatic prostatic carcinoma. Serum PSA levels are used to monitor the spread or recurrence of prostate cancer and to evaluate the patient's response to treatment. This test isn't a suitable screening procedure for prostate cancer.

Purpose

• To monitor the course of prostate cancer and aid evaluation of treatment

Reference values

Normal serum values for PSA shouldn't exceed 2 ng/ml in males age 40 and younger and 4 ng/ml in men ages 41 to 61. In men over age 61, values shouldn't exceed 7 ng/ml.

Abnormal findings

About 80% of patients with prostate cancer have pretreatment PSA values greater than 4 ng/ml. However, PSA results alone don't confirm a diagnosis of prostate cancer. About 20% of patients with benign prostatic hyperplasia also have levels greater than 4 ng/ml. Further assessment and testing, including tissue biopsy, are needed to confirm cancer.

Prothrombin time

Prothrombin time (PT) measures the time required for a fibrin clot to form in a citrated plasma sample after addition of calcium ions and tissue thromboplastin (factor III).

Purpose

• To provide an overall evaluation of extrinsic coagulation factors V, VII, and X and of prothrombin and fibrinogen
• To monitor response to oral anticoagulant therapy

Reference values

Normally, PTs range from 10 to 13 seconds. Times vary, however, depending on the source of tissue thromboplastin and the type of sensing devices used to measure clot formation. In a patient receiving oral anticoagulants, PT is usually maintained between 2 and 2.5 times the normal control value.

Abnormal findings

Prolonged PT may indicate deficiencies in fibrinogen; prothrombin; factor V, VII, or X (specific assays can pinpoint such deficiencies); or vitamin K as well as hepatic disease. It may also result from ongoing oral anticoagulant therapy. Prolonged PT that exceeds 2.5 times the control is commonly associated with abnormal bleeding.

Thyroid-stimulating hormone

Thyroid-stimulating hormone (TSH), or thyrotropin, promotes increases in the size, number, and activity of thyroid cells and stimulates the release of triiodothyronine and thyroxine. These hormones affect total body metabolism and are essential for normal growth and development.

This test measures serum TSH levels by radioimmunoassay. It can detect primary hypothyroidism and determine whether the hypothyroidism results from thyroid gland failure or from pituitary or hypothalamic dysfunction. Normal serum TSH levels rule out primary hypothyroidism. This test may not distinguish between low-normal and subnormal levels, especially in secondary hypothyroidism.

Purpose

• To confirm or rule out primary hypothyroidism and distinguish it from secondary hypothyroidism

• To monitor drug therapy in patients with primary hypothyroidism

Reference values

Normal TSH values range from 0.3 to 5 mIU/L.

Abnormal findings

TSH levels may be slightly elevated in euthyroid patients with thyroid cancer. Extremely high levels suggest primary hypothyroidism or, possibly, endemic goiter.

Low or undetectable TSH levels may be normal but occasionally indicate secondary hypothyroidism (with inadequate secretion of TSH or thyrotropin-releasing hormone). Low TSH levels may also result from hyperthyroidism (Graves' disease) and thyroiditis; both disorders are marked by hypersecretion of thyroid hormones, which suppresses TSH release.

Thyroxine

Thyroxine (T_4) is an amine secreted by the thyroid gland in response to thyroid-stimulating hormone (TSH) and, indirectly, thyrotropin-releasing hormone. The rate of secretion is normally regulated by a complex system of negative and positive feedback mechanisms.

Only a fraction of T_4 (about 0.05%) circulates freely in the blood; the rest binds strongly to plasma proteins, primarily thyroxine-binding globulin (TBG). This minute fraction is responsible for the clinical effects of thyroid hormone. TBG binds so tenaciously that T_4 survives in the plasma for a relatively long time, with a half-life of about 6 days. This immunoassay should be interpreted in conjunction with the TBG level or as part of a free thyroxine index.

Purpose

• To evaluate thyroid function
• To aid diagnosis of hyperthyroidism and hypothyroidism
• To monitor response to antithyroid medication in hyperthyroidism or to thyroid replacement therapy in hypothyroidism

Reference values

Normally, total T_4 levels range from 5 to 12.5 μg/dl.

Abnormal findings

Abnormally elevated T_4 levels are consistent with primary and secondary hyperthyroidism, including excessive T_4 (levothyroxine) replacement therapy (factitious or iatrogenic hyperthyroidism). Subnormal levels suggest primary or secondary hypothyroidism or may be due to T_4 suppression by normal, elevated, or replacement levels of triiodothyronine (T_3). In doubtful cases of hypothyroidism, TSH measurement may be indicated.

Normal T_4 levels don't guarantee euthyroidism; for example, normal readings occur in T_3 thyrotoxicosis. Overt signs of hyperthyroidism require further testing.

Thyroxine and triiodothyronine (free)

These tests, often done simultaneously, measure serum levels of free thyroxine (FT_4) and free triiodothyronine (FT_3), the minute portions of T_4 and T_3 not bound to thyroxine-binding globulin (TBG) and other serum proteins. These unbound hormones are responsible for the thyroid's effects on cellular metabolism. Measurement of free hormone levels is the best indicator of thyroid function.

Because of disagreement as to whether FT_4 or FT_3 is the better indicator, laboratories commonly measure both. The disadvantages of these tests include a cumbersome and difficult laboratory method, inaccessibility, and cost. This test may be useful in the 5% of patients in whom the standard T_3 or T_4 tests fail to produce diagnostic results.

Purpose

• To measure the metabolically active form of the thyroid hormones
• To aid diagnosis of hyperthyroidism and hypothyroidism when TBG levels are abnormal

Reference values

Normal range for FT_4 is 0.7 to 2.0 ng/dl; for FT_3, 2.3 to 4.2 pmol/L. Values vary, depending on the laboratory.

Abnormal findings

Elevated FT_4 and FT_3 levels indicate hyperthyroidism, unless peripheral resistance to thyroid hormone is present. T_3 thryotoxicosis, a distinct form of hyperthyroidism, yields high FT_3 levels with normal or low FT_4 values. Low FT_4 levels usually indicate hypothyroidism, except in patients receiving replacement therapy with T_3. Patients receiving thyroid therapy may have varying levels of FT_4 and FT_3, depending on the preparation used and the time of sample blood collection.

Thyroxine-binding globulin

This test measures the serum level of thyroxine-binding globulin (TBG), the predominant protein carrier for circulating thyroxine (T_4).

Any condition that affects TBG levels and subsequent binding capacity also affects the amount of free T_4 (FT_4) in circulation. An underlying TBG abnormality renders tests for total triiodothyronine (T_3) and T_4 inaccurate but doesn't affect the accuracy of tests for free T_3 (FT_3) and FT_4.

Purpose

• To evaluate abnormal thyrometabolic states that don't correlate with thyroid hormone (T_3 or T_4) values (for example, a patient with overt signs of hypothyroidism and a low FT_4 level with a high total T_4 level due to a marked increase of TBG secondary to use of oral contraceptives)
• To identify TBG abnormalities

Reference values

Normal values vary by sex and age.

Males
• 1 to 6 years: 17 to 26 μg/ml
• 7 to 13 years: 15 to 24 μg/ml
• 14 to 18 years: 13 to 22 μg/ml
• 19 to 23 years: 11 to 20 μg/ml
• 24 years and older: 16 to 24 μg/ml

Females
• 1 to 6 years: 17 to 26 μg/ml
• 7 to 23 years: 15 to 26 μg/ml
• 24 years and older: 16 to 24 μg/ml

Abnormal findings

Elevated TBG levels may indicate hypothyroidism or congenital (genetic) excess, some forms of hepatic disease, or acute intermittent porphyria. TBG levels normally rise during pregnancy and are high in neonates. Suppressed levels may indicate hyperthyroidism or congenital deficiency and can occur in active acromegaly, nephrotic syndrome, and malnutrition associated with hypoproteinemia, acute illness, or surgical stress.

Patients with TBG abnormalities require additional testing, such as the serum FT_3 and serum T_4 tests, to evaluate thyroid function more precisely.

Triiodothyronine

This highly specific radioimmunoassay measures total (bound and free) serum content of triiodothyronine (T_3) to investigate clinical indications of thyroid dysfunction. Like thyroxine (T_4) secretion, T_3 secretion occurs in response to thyroid-stimulating hormone (TSH) and, secondarily, thyrotropin-releasing hormone.

Although T_3 is present in the bloodstream in minute quantities and is metabolically active for only a short time, its impact on body metabolism dominates that of T_4. Another significant difference between the two major thyroid hormones is that T_3 binds less firmly to thyroxine-binding globulin. Consequently, T_3 persists in the bloodstream for a short time; half disappears in about 1 day, whereas half of T_4 disappears in 6 days.

Purpose

• To aid diagnosis of T_3 thyrotoxicosis
• To aid diagnosis of hypothyroidism and hyperthyroidism
• To monitor clinical response to thyroid replacement therapy in hypothyroidism

Reference values

Serum T_3 levels vary by age:
• 1 to 14 years: 125 to 250 ng/dl
• 15 to 23 years: 100 to 220 ng/dl
• 24 years and older: 80 to 200 ng/dl.

Abnormal findings

Serum T_3 and serum T_4 levels usually rise and fall in tandem. However, in T_3 thyrotoxicosis, T_3 levels rise while total and free T_4 levels remain normal. T_3 thyrotoxicosis occurs in patients with Graves' disease, toxic adenoma, or toxic nodular goiter. T_3 levels also surpass T_4 levels in patients receiving thyroid replacement therapy containing more T_3 than T_4. In iodine-deficient areas, the thyroid may produce larger amounts of the more cellularly active T_3 than of T_4 in an effort to maintain the euthyroid state.

Generally, T_3 levels appear to be a more accurate diagnostic indicator of hyperthyroidism. Although both T_3 and T_4 levels are increased in about 90% of patients with hyperthyroidism, there's a disproportionate increase in T_3. In some patients with hypothyroidism, T_3 levels may fall within the normal range and not be diagnostically significant.

A rise in serum T_3 levels normally occurs during pregnancy. Low T_3 levels may appear in euthyroid patients with systemic illness (especially hepatic or renal disease), during severe acute illness, and after trauma or major surgery; in such patients, TSH levels are within normal limits. Low serum T_3 levels are found in some euthyroid patients with malnutrition.

Triiodothyronine uptake

The triiodothyronine (T_3) uptake test indirectly measures free thyroxine (FT_4) levels by demonstrating the availability of serum protein-binding sites for thyroxine (T_4). The results of T_3 uptake are frequently combined with a T_4 radioimmunoassay or T_4(D) (competitive protein-binding test) to determine the FT_4 index, a mathematical calculation that is thought to reflect FT_4 by correcting for thyroxine-binding globulin (TBG) abnormalities.

The T_3 uptake test has become less popular because rapid tests for T_3, T_4, and thyroid-stimulating hormone are readily available.

Purpose

• To aid diagnosis of hypothyroidism and hyperthyroidism when TBG levels are normal
• To aid diagnosis of primary disorders of TBG levels

Reference values

Normal T_3 uptake values are 25% to 35%.

Abnormal findings

A high T_3 uptake percentage in the presence of elevated T_4 levels indicates hyperthyroidism (implying few TBG free binding sites and high FT_4 levels). A low uptake percentage, together with low T_4 levels, indicates hypothyroidism (implying more TBG free binding sites and low FT_4 levels). Thus, in primary thyroid disease, T_4 and T_3 uptake vary in the same direction; availability of binding sites varies inversely.

Discordant variance in T_4 and T_3 uptake suggests abnormality of TBG. For example, a high T_3 uptake percentage and a low or normal FT_4 level suggest decreased TBG levels. Such decreased levels may result from protein loss (as in nephrotic syndrome), decreased production (due to androgen excess or genetic or idiopathic causes), or competition for T_4 binding sites by certain drugs (salicylates, phenylbutazone, and phenytoin). Conversely, a low T_3 uptake percentage and a high or normal FT_4 level suggest increased TBG levels. Such

increased levels may be due to exogenous or endogenous estrogen (pregnancy) or result from idiopathic causes. Thus, in primary disorders of TBG levels, measured T_4- and T_3-uptake change in the same direction.

Troponin-I and troponin-T

Troponin (cardiac troponin-I [cTnI]) is the contractile regulatory protein of striated muscle (slow-twitch and fast-twitch skeletal muscle and cardiac muscle). Cardiac muscle produces specific forms of troponin: cTnI and cardiac troponin-T (cTnT). They are released into the circulation after cellular necrosis.

Purpose

• To rule out myocardial infarction (MI) on initial presentation, especially when the patient didn't seek care immediately after onset of symptoms; highest sensitivity occurs after 10 hours

Reference values

For cTnI, positive results vary with the laboratory, from any detectable enzyme to greater than 1.5 ng/ml, in part due to several different tests available. For cTnT, levels greater than 0.5 ng/ml have high sensitivity in detecting acute MI.

Abnormal findings

The presence of cTnI indicates cellular necrosis.

The prolonged persistence of troponin gives it much greater sensitivity than creatine kinase-MB (CK-MB) for diagnosis of MI beyond the first 48 hours, and it replaces lactate dehydrogenase isoenzymes for the detection of infarction at these times. The troponins are more specific for MI than CK-MB with a decreased sensitivity early in the course of infarction (less than 5 hours) but with near perfect sensitivity and specificity later (more than 10 hours). Troponin appears in serum about 4 hours after onset of chest pain, peaks at 8 to 12 hours, and drops after 5 to 7 days.

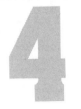

Common X-rays

Deciphering the images

Understanding an X-ray

When a radiologist assesses X-ray film, it's usually to find an answer to a particular problem or question. Examples include whether a chest tube or central line is positioned correctly, whether there is fluid in the lungs, and whether the bowel loops are distended.

Comparing an X-ray film with previous films is helpful, particularly when assessing progression of a clinical situation, such as pneumonia and pneumothorax. The patient's position when the film is taken should be noted. An anteroposterior (AP) versus a posteroanterior (PA) projection can change the apparent size of structures because of distance from the X-ray source. For instance, the heart may appear enlarged in an AP projection because it was closer to the X-ray tube (and farther from the film) when exposed.

A decubitus film may be a better projection for assessing fluid levels in the abdomen because the fluid is in a dependent position. Likewise, the quality and diagnostic usefulness of a portable film taken in a semi-upright position versus a full upright position are compromised because of fluid collecting in layers posteriorly and because the lungs aren't fully expanded. Often, the health care worker on the patient's unit decides whether the film is made in or out of the radiology department. Although it may be more convenient not to transport the patient, PA and lateral films taken in the radiology department ensure higher quality and greater diagnostic accuracy.

Differences in film quality, sharpness of detail, patient motion, lightness versus darkness of structures, and patient positioning can affect the diagnostic usefulness of an X-ray.

An X-ray should be considered a tool to aid the clinician in confirming a diagnosis or clinical finding. Wheezes or crackles in the lung bases heard on auscultation may be confirmed by the presence of fluid-filled, dense areas seen on a chest X-ray. But often an ordinary X-ray can't give the clinician all the information needed to make a diagnosis. In that case, the clinician may use another imaging modality to view anatomy or to identify a pathological process.

If you're present when X-rays are taken, take safety factors into account. (See *Factors in radiation protection*.)

FACTORS IN RADIATION PROTECTION

If you need to be with a patient or in the vicinity when X-rays are being taken, you need to be aware of your own safety as well as your patient's. These three factors affect your protection.

Time
Duration of exposure to the X-rays (Cutting exposure time by 50% cuts the dose by 50%.)

Distance
Distance from the source of the X-rays (Exposure decreases with distance, according to the inverse-square law; doubling the distance cuts exposure by 25%. A distance of 6′ is generally considered the minimum.)

Shielding
Protects against scatter radiation (Effective barriers include lead aprons, gloves, thyroid shields, leaded or photosensitive glass, walls, and fixed or movable partitions.)

X-rays of the torso

Normal chest X-ray

Bony and soft landmarks in this normal chest and upper abdomen X-ray stand out in this posteroanterior view.

Tracheal air shadow

Clavicles

Aortic notch

Ribs

Vertebrae

Lungs

Heart

Breasts

Diaphragm

Costophrenic angles

Liver

Stomach gas

Spleen

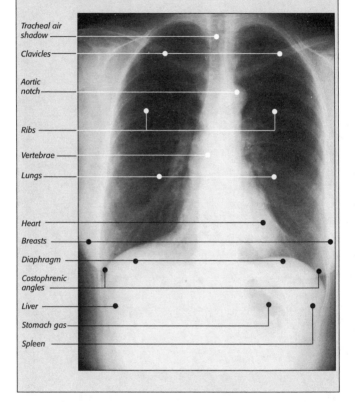

Foreign object in lung

The child in the X-rays on this page has inhaled an object that has lodged in the left bronchus. The anteroposterior chest X-ray taken during inspiration seems normal. An X-ray taken during expiration shows the effect of the foreign object. Trapped air has hyperinflated the left lung ➤. The mediastinum has shifted right ➤ and, compared to the inspiratory X-ray, the dark air-filled area on the left has become more lucent.

Inspiration

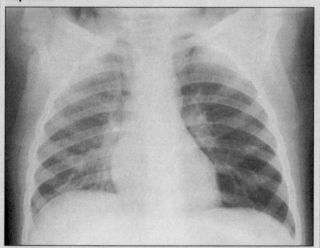

Expiration

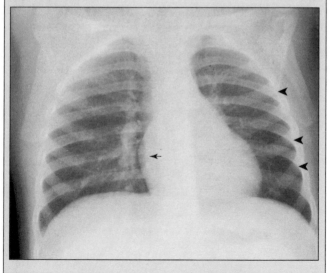

Heart valve replacement

This lateral chest X-ray taken after surgery to replace a defective heart valve shows the new valve in place ➤. It also shows a pleural effusion ➡.

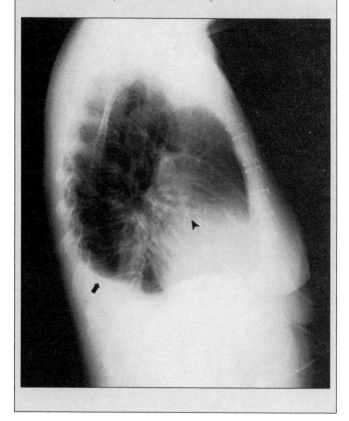

Lobar pneumonia

Typical signs of lobar pneumonia that involves the left lower lobe ➡ are apparent in this chest X-ray. Borders of the heart shadow and the left hemi-diaphragm are hidden (silhouette sign). Visible are mediastinal shift to the left, depressed left hilum, and atelectasis (indicated by the smaller left lung) ➤.

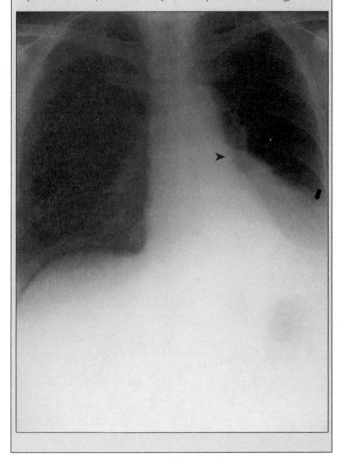

Lung cancer

In this chest X-ray, bronchogenic lung cancer shows up as a large mass ➡ with central cavitation ➤ in the right hilar area. Opacity of the right lower lobe indicates atelectasis caused by the tumor.

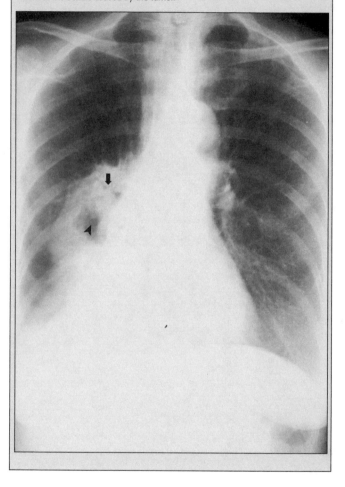

Pleural effusion

This posteroanterior chest X-ray of a patient with heart failure reveals pleural effusion. The right costophrenic angle is blunted by pleural fluid and the upper border of the pleural fluid ▷ is concave.

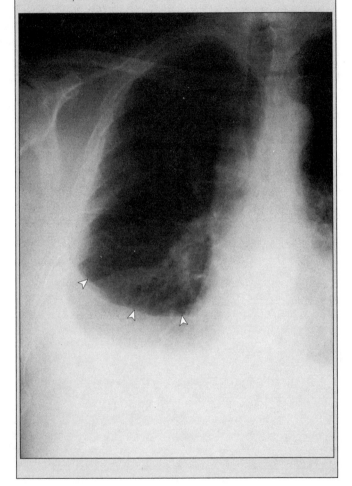

Pleural effusion with fluid in fissures

This lateral chest X-ray clearly demonstrates pleural fluid in the lung fissures ▷. These fissures, the spaces between the lung lobes, have been widened by the fluid.

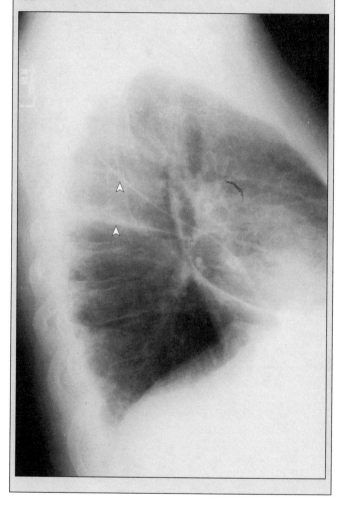

Pneumothorax with subcutaneous emphysema

This posteroanterior chest X-ray shows a pneumothorax as well as subcutaneous and mediastinal emphysema ⇒. Because the chest tube ⇒ has migrated outside the pleural space, the pneumothorax ▷ is larger than it was originally.

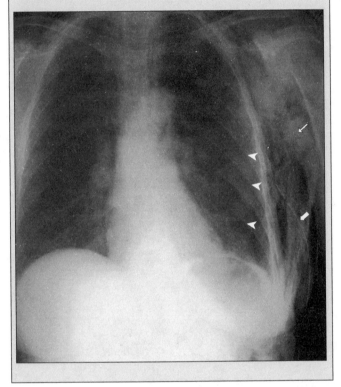

Pulmonary changes with asthma

The effects of asthma are apparent in this posteroanterior chest X-ray. The lungs
→ are hyperinflated, the heart ▷ small, and the diaphragm ⇨ depressed.

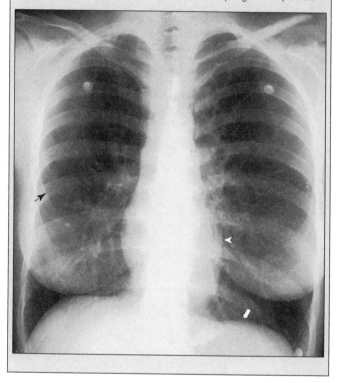

Rib fractures
This anteroposterior chest X-ray of a trauma patient shows lateral fractures of the fifth ➡ and sixth ➡ ribs on the left side. Displacement and associated fractures of the left clavicle ➤ and left scapula ➤ have created separation at the fracture sites.

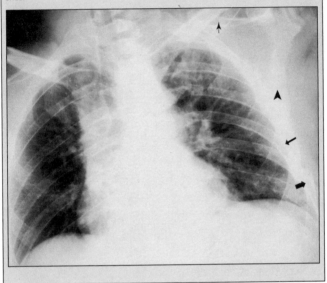

Other images

Bone tumor

A well-defined, eccentric, bubbly expansile tumor ▷ in the distal femoral diaphysis is clear in this plain X-ray.

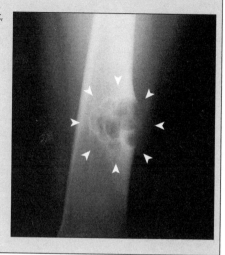

Leg fractures

This anteroposterior X-ray of the left leg and ankle shows the results of trauma. Visible are an oblique, comminuted fracture of the tibia ➤ and lateral displacement of distal parts as well as a comminuted avulsion-type fracture of the medial malleolus ➡.

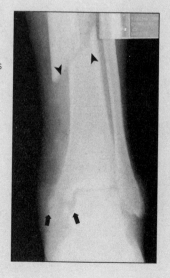

Osteoarthritis of the knee

This plain X-ray of a right knee shows narrowing of the medial joint space ➤ and mild osteophyte formation ▷.

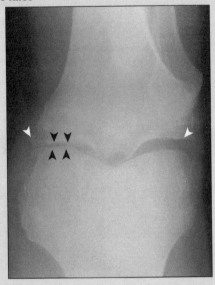

Rheumatoid arthritis of the hand

This plain X-ray of the left hand shows classic signs of advanced rheumatoid arthritis. Periarticular soft tissue swelling ⇢ is evident as are many erosions involving the distal ulna, carpals, metacarpals, and phalanges ▷. Joint spaces are narrowed. In addition, periarticular osteoporosis encircles the metacarpal and phalangeal joints ✳.

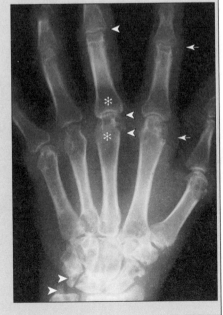

Rotator cuff tear and meniscal tear

The shoulder shown in this magnetic resonance imaging (MRI) scan (top), clearly has a torn right rotator cuff ▷. In the sagittal MRI image (bottom), an oblique tear ➤ is evident in the posterior horn of the medial meniscus.

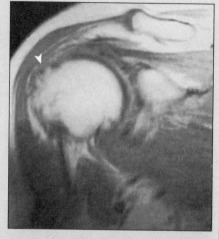

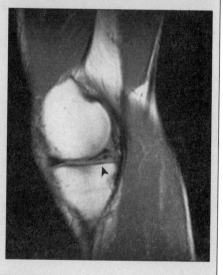

Small-bowel obstruction

In this plain abdominal X-ray, dilated, gas-filled bowel loops ▷ and a lack of colon gas indicate an obstruction of the small bowel.

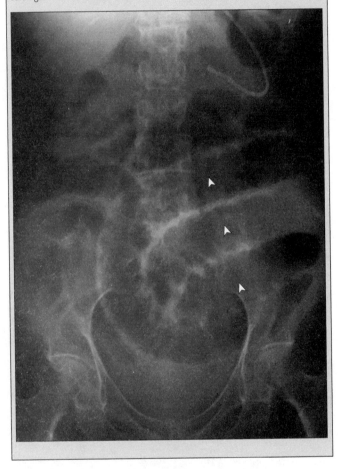

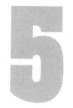

CHAPTER

Dermatologic disorders

Managing common skin problems

Selected skin problems

Introduction

More than half of all patients with skin problems receive treatment in a primary care setting, and this number is expected to increase. Because it's impossible to be familiar with the thousands of skin disorders and lesions, it's important to know when to refer or consult. In addition, it takes specialized training to differentiate which treatment plan will be most effective for a specific malignant lesion. This chapter explores some commonly seen lesions, how to manage them, and when to refer or consult.

Acne vulgaris

ICD-9-CM 706.1

An androgenically stimulated, inflammatory disease of the sebaceous follicles, acne vulgaris primarily affects adolescents, although lesions can appear as early as age 8. Although acne strikes boys more commonly and more severely, it usually occurs in girls at an earlier age and tends to last longer, sometimes into adulthood. Manifested as comedones, papules, pustules, and cysts, it can cause scarring. The prognosis is good with treatment.

Contagion

This condition isn't contagious.

Causes

The cause of acne is multifactorial but isn't caused by any dietary factor. An overproduction of androgen or an increased response by the sebaceous glands can lead to acne. Also, hyper-sensitivity to *Propionibacterium acnes* and its metabolic byproducts can cause acne. It results from a complex interaction between androgen and bacteria in the hair follicles.

 SPECIAL POPULATIONS
Acne vulgaris can occur in all adolescents, but incidence and severity are lower in people of African and Asian descent. Acne rosacea is more common in people of European and especially Celtic descent.

Predisposing factors include heredity; adolescence; male sex; oral contraceptive use (many females experience an acne flare-up during their first few menses after starting or discontinuing oral contraceptives); androgen stimulation; certain drugs, including corticosteroids, corticotropin, androgens, bromides, trimethadione, phenytoin, isoniazid, lithium, and halothane; cobalt irradiation; and hyperalimentation.

Other precipitating factors include exposure to heavy oils, greases, or tars; trauma or rubbing from tight clothing; oily cosmetics; emotional stress; and a hot, humid climate. Also, check the patient's drug history because certain medications, such as oral contraceptives, may cause an acne flare-up.

More is known about the pathogenesis of acne. Androgens stimulate sebaceous gland growth and production of sebum, which is secreted into dilated hair follicles that contain bacteria. The bacteria, usually *P. acnes* and *Staphylococcus epidermidis* — which are normal skin flora — secrete lipase. This enzyme interacts with sebum to produce free fatty acids, which provoke inflammation. Also, the hair follicles produce more keratin, which joins with the sebum to form a plug in the dilated follicle.

Clinical presentation

The appearance of characteristic acne lesions, especially in an adolescent patient, confirms the presence of acne vulgaris. The acne plug may appear as a closed comedone, or whitehead (if it doesn't protrude from the follicle and is covered by the epidermis), or as an open comedone, or blackhead (if it does protrude and isn't covered by the epidermis). The black coloration is caused by oxidation of tyrosine to melanin in the hair follicle.

Rupture or leakage of an enlarged plug into the dermis produces inflammation and characteristic acne pustules, papules or, in severe forms, acne cysts or abscesses. Chronic, recurring lesions produce acne scars.

Differential diagnosis

Conditions to consider before diagnosing acne vulgaris include folliculitis, rosacea, perioral dermatitis, steroid-induced acne, pseudofolliculitis barbae, staphylococcal infection (which may cause folliculitis or abscess), molluscum contagiosum, and ruptured inclusion cyst.

Diagnostic tests
• This condition is commonly diagnosed solely by clinical presentation.
• Consider ordering metabolite tests and testosterone levels when acne starts in a previously unaffected adult.

Management

• Be aware that acne can cause psychological problems, including depression and withdrawal from social situations. Pay special attention to the patient's perception of his physical appearance, and offer emotional support.

Drugs
• Frequently, acne is treated topically with benzoyl peroxide, a powerful antibacterial, alone or in combination with a keratin stabilizer (tretinoin) or another antiacne drug (such as azelaic acid).
• Systemic therapy consists primarily of antibiotics, usually metronidazole or tetracycline, used for their anti-inflammatory action. Usual doses are given but frequency is decreased to twice daily rather than four times a day. When the condition improves, a lower daily dosage is used for long-term maintenance.

 SPECIAL POPULATIONS Tetracycline is contraindicated during pregnancy because it discolors the teeth of the fetus. Erythromycin may be substituted for these patients.
• Exacerbation of pustules or abscesses during topical or systemic therapy requires a culture to identify a possible secondary bacterial infection.
• Oral isotretinoin combats acne by inhibiting sebaceous gland function and keratinization. Because of its severe adverse effects, the 16- to 20-week course of isotretinoin is limited to those with severe papulopustular or cystic acne that doesn't respond to conventional therapy (See *Tips on choosing a corticosteroid regimen*, page 120.)
• Though females may benefit from administration of estrogens to inhibit androgen activity, the high doses required present a risk of severe adverse effects. Improvement rarely occurs before 2 to 4 months, and exacerbations may follow estrogen discontinuation.

Referral or consultation

 COLLABORATION Consult with a dermatologist for cases that are severe or non-responsive after 12 weeks of

TIPS ON CHOOSING A CORTICOSTEROID REGIMEN

• Ointments enhance penetration, creams contain 50% water, and lotions and gels contain even more water. Water promotes evaporation, thus less medication is absorbed.
• Potency equals amount of skin penetration.
• Make directions relevant to the patient (for example, "squeeze out a pea-sized amount").
• Start with a higher potency and progress within 2 weeks (when possible) to a lower potency drug. Or, start with a moderate potency (for older and thin skin) but make it clear that you anticipate a slower response.
• Referral or consultation is indicated before using systemic corticosteroids, high-potency corticosteroids, or occlusive dressings to increase steroid absorption. These regimens increase the potential for adverse local and systemic effects.
• Adrenal axis suppression is uncommon but possible; local reactions usually resolve when the drug is stopped. Thinning of the skin and striae are usually permanent.

treatment or if considering isotretinoin (Accutane).

Follow-up

Two or three visits in a 12-week period are needed to evaluate treatment and adjust it according to the patient's response. Try to quantify skin eruptions to allow a more accurate evaluation of therapy. Advise monthly visits until an adequate response is obtained.

These visits can serve a second purpose in a population that doesn't frequently visit the primary care provider — to address high-risk behaviors like drugs, unprotected sex, and reckless or impaired driving.

Complications

Severe, confluent, inflammatory acne (acne conglobata); facial scarring; and resulting psychological effects may occur.

Patient teaching

• Try to identify predisposing factors that can be eliminated or modified.
• Emphasize that acne isn't caused or exacerbated by too much or too little sex, masturbation, dirty skin, or various foods.
• Explain the causes of acne to the patient and family. Make sure they understand that the prescribed treatment is more likely to improve acne than a strict diet and continual scrubbing with soap and water. Provide written instructions regarding treatment.
• Advise the patient to avoid exposure to sunlight or to use a sunscreen. If the prescribed regimen includes tretinoin and benzoyl peroxide, tell the patient to avoid skin irritation by using one preparation in the morning and the other at night.
• Instruct the patient to take tetracycline on an empty stomach and to avoid taking it with antacids or milk, which inhibit drug absorption.
• Tell the patient who is taking isotretinoin to avoid vitamin A supplements, which can worsen adverse effects. Also discuss how to deal with the dry skin and mucous membranes that usually occur during treatment.

 SPECIAL POPULATIONS Warn the female patient of child-bearing age about the severe risk of teratogenicity with isotretonoin. In addition to signing a special permission form, she'll need monthly measurement of lipid levels and liver function as well as monthly pregnancy tests.

• Inform the patient that acne takes a long time — sometimes years — for complete resolution. Encourage continued local skin care even after acne clears. Explain the adverse effects of all drugs.

Resources

American Academy of Dermatology (patient education materials): 708-330-0230; *www.aad.org/ P_Frameset.html* (Then select Patient Education Materials; Spanish versions are available.)

Anogenital pruritus

ICD-9-CM perianal 698.0, genital 698.1 (545)

An intense local itching of the vulva, scrotum, perineal skin, or anus, anogenital pruritus can exist with an underlying low-grade pruritus.

 SPECIAL POPULATIONS This disorder is most common in middle-aged white men.

Contagion

This condition isn't contagious.

Causes

Anogenital pruritus usually results from a combination of poor anal hygiene, obesity, excessive sweating, and pilonidal cysts. Another common cause is hemorrhoids.

Clinical presentation

Skin appearance reflects the primary disorder, secondary changes from scratching or rubbing, or both. Onset may be sudden or gradual. When the itch-scratch cycle starts, it's hard to break. Itching and rubbing episodes can be intense and interfere with daily activities, even with an underlying low-grade pruritus. It's worse at night; patients may scratch during sleep, to the point of drawing blood. Most people present after the itch-scratch cycle is well established and over-the-counter medications have failed. Many of these preparations exacerbate the process by irritating the damaged skin or keeping the area too moist. Even when treated appropriately, anogenital pruritus has a high relapse rate and should be considered a chronic disease.

Differential diagnosis

Anogenital pruritus can be idiopathic or result from an inflammatory process (such as contact dermatitis and psoriasis), an infestation (such as scabies, lice, and pinworms), a mechanical factor (such as irritation from rectal mucus and fecal material, hemorrhoids, and anal fissures), or a neoplasm.

Males with extensive pruritus and erythematous nodules of the scrotal area should be evaluated for scabies. If the patient doesn't respond to treatment, evaluate more thoroughly for an infectious cause by using a magnifying glass to look for burrows and nits.

Diagnostic tests

The condition is diagnosed by history and physical examination.

Management

• Maintain fastidious anal hygiene. Keep the area dry.
• Use hemorrhoid management when indicated.
• Counsel weight loss as appropriate.

Nonprescription medications

• Clean affected skin areas with cleansing pads (such as witch hazel and glycerin [Tucks]) or mild soap and water, especially after defecation.
• If the skin is dry or cracked, apply a topical emollient, such as petroleum jelly, after the patient defecates and at bedtime.
• Keep moist skin areas dry with absorbent powder.
• Control itching with a topical anesthetic, such as pramoxine hydrochloride (Caladryl Clear lotion and Itch-X gel and spray), applied up to every 4 hours.
• If fissures or erosions occur, apply compresses soaked in Burow's solution (aluminum sulfate and calcium acetate in water) for 10 to 15 minutes two or three times daily.

Prescription drugs

• Apply nonfluorinated topical steroids (hydrocortisone 1% or 2.5%) twice daily for 1 week after symptoms resolve; resume at first signs of itching.
• Use hydrocortisone and iodine creams (Vytone, Vioform-Hydrocortone) for anti-inflammatory, antibacterial, and antifungal properties. Iodine may stain or induce a contact allergy.
• Apply topical anesthetic (1% to 2.5% hydrocortisone plus pramoxine, Pramosone, PrameGel) two to three times daily.
• Use systemic antihistamines (hydroxyzine, doxepin) at bedtime for antihistamine and sedative effects.

Referral or consultation

 COLLABORATION Consult with a dermatologist for nonresponsiveness. Anticipate biopsy to rule out an underlying neoplasm.

Patient teaching

• Tell the patient to avoid topical antihistamines because of the high incidence of contact dermatitis.
• Help him identify and avoid potential trigger factors.
• Tell the patient to use air conditioning and wear loose cotton clothing and boxer shorts to reduce the retention of sweat.
• Tell the patient to avoid prolonged sitting, particularly on vinyl or leather.
• Advise him to avoid hot water; a warm sitz bath decreases pain and spasm in the anal canal.
• Tell him to avoid excessive washing and to use mild soap without fragrance or a nonsoap skin cleanser with a soft cotton cloth.
• Encourage the patient to drink six to eight glasses of water daily and to eat more fiber and fresh fruit or use bulk laxatives.
• Caution him to avoid spicy and irritating foods (caffeine, beer, tomatoes, pickles, curries).
• Instruct the patient to clean well after defecation and urination, dry thoroughly, and avoid using colored or scented toilet paper if possible.
• Tell the female patient to use unscented tampons and to avoid scented sanitary pads and panty liners.
• Teach the patient to use relaxation techniques, such as meditation and self-hypnosis.

 ALERT Tell the patient to call the primary care provider and report persistent, changing, worsening, anxiety-producing, or specific signs and symptoms, including:
– bright red rectal bleeding that doesn't stop within 1 hour
– black, tarry, or maroon-colored stools
– severe, unrelenting rectal or pelvic pain
– no relief within 3 days.

Basal cell carcinoma

ICD-9-CM facial 173.3; scalp or neck 173.4; trunk 173.5; upper limb 173.6; lower limb 173.7

A slow-growing, destructive skin tumor, basal cell carcinoma usually occurs in people over age 40.

 SPECIAL POPULATIONS Basal cell carcinoma is more prevalent in blond, fair-skinned men and is the most common malignant tumor affecting whites.

Contagion

This condition isn't contagious.

Causes

Prolonged sun exposure is the most common cause of basal cell carcinoma. Other possible causes include arsenic ingestion, radiation exposure, burns, immunosuppression and, rarely, vaccinations.

Although the pathogenesis of basal cell carcinoma is uncertain, some experts now hypothesize that it originates when, under certain conditions, undifferentiated basal cells become neoplastic instead of differentiating into sweat glands, sebum, and hair.

Clinical presentation

Four types of basal cell carcinoma occur:
• *Nodular,* which presents as shiny translucent lesions
• *Ulcerative,* which is often covered with a dry crust and appears as an ulcerated nodule
• *Rodent ulcerative,* which has an elevated skin border or rolled appearance. These lesions occur most often on the face, particularly the forehead, eyelid margins, and nasolabial folds. Telangiectatic vessels cross the surface, and the lesions are occasionally pigmented. As the lesions enlarge, their centers become depressed and their borders become firm and elevated. Ulceration and local invasion eventually occur. Rodent ulcers rarely metastasize; however, if untreated, they can spread to vital areas and become infected. If they invade large blood vessels, they can cause massive hemorrhage.
• *Sclerosing basal cell carcinomas (morphea-like)* are waxy, sclerotic, yellow to white plaques with indistinct borders. Occurring on the trunk, sclerosing basal cell carcinomas often look like small patches of scleroderma. They commonly appear as multiple erythematous lesions with occasional pearly papules at the periphery and typically have variegated pigmentation.

Basal cell carcinomas are usually detected on examination with good lighting, a hand lens, and careful palpation.

Differential diagnosis

Other possible diagnoses include sebaceous hyperplasia, intradermal nevi, actinic keratosis, benign mole, hyperpigmentation, and molluscum contagiosum.

Diagnostic tests

Biopsy and histologic study confirm the diagnosis by showing basal cells extending into the dermis.

Management

• In all physical examinations, look for unusual nevi or other skin lesions.

 COLLABORATION If melanoma is suspected, the lesion should never be curetted, shaved, or electrodesiccated. Refer all suspicious lesions to a dermatologist, not just for identification but also for determination of the most effective treatment plan. When a biopsy is taken, it maximizes the clinician's experience to make detailed notes in order to correlate the clinical presentation with the biopsy outcome.

• Depending on the size, location, and depth of the lesion, expected treatment may include curettage and electrodesiccation, chemotherapy, surgical excision, irradiation, or chemosurgery.

• Curettage and electrodesiccation offer good cosmetic results for small lesions.

• Topical fluorouracil is often used for superficial lesions. This medication produces marked local irritation or inflammation in the involved tissue but no systemic effects.

• Moh's surgery is a microscopically controlled surgical excision that carefully removes recurrent lesions until a tumor-free plane is achieved. After removal of large lesions, skin grafting may be required.

 SPECIAL POPULATIONS
Irradiation is used if the tumor location requires it and for elderly or debilitated patients who might not withstand surgery. It may cause disfigurement.

• Cryotherapy with liquid nitrogen freezes and kills the cells.

• Chemosurgery is often necessary for persistent or recurrent lesions. It consists of periodic applications of a fixative paste (such as zinc chloride) and subsequent removal of fixed pathologic tissue. Treatment continues until tumor removal is complete.

Referral or consultation

Consult a dermatologist for suspicious lesions and for biopsy.

Follow-up

Visits are needed monthly for 3 months, then every 3 months for 9 months, and then every 6 months for 5 years. After that, an annual visit is required.

Complications

Recurrences and new lesions usually occur within 5 years. Scarring is possible, but metastasis is rare.

Patient teaching

• Most skin cancers are curable, particularly if caught in early stages. Discuss diagnosis and treatment options. Warn the patient that it's common to have recurrences or new lesions within 5 years.

• Instruct the patient to eat frequent, small meals that are high in protein. Suggest eggnog, pureed foods, and liquid protein supplements if the lesion has invaded the oral cavity and caused eating problems.

• Stress the importance of routinely examining the skin, becoming familiar with the body, and focusing on moles and new lesions to detect changes early.

• Tell the patient that to prevent disease recurrence, he needs to avoid excessive sun exposure, use a strong sunscreen or sunshade, and wear a wide-brimmed hat to protect the face and back of the neck and long-sleeved shirts to protect his skin from damage by ultraviolet rays.

• Advise the patient to relieve local inflammation from topical fluorouracil with cool compresses or corticosteroid ointment.

• Instruct the patient with noduloulcerative basal cell carcinoma to wash his face gently when ulcerations and crusting occur; scrubbing too vigorously may cause bleeding.

• To help prevent malignant melanoma, stress the detrimental effects of overexposure to solar radiation, especially to fair-skinned, blonde, blue-eyed patients. Recommend that all patients use a sunscreen.

WARNING SIGNS OF LESIONS

Use this mnemonic device to help evaluate basal cell carcinoma or epithelioma.

A symmetrical
B leeding
C olor variegated within lesion
D iameter greater than 6 mm (pencil eraser)
E dges irregular
F eeling (sensitive to touch, burning, itching)
G rowing in height or diameter

ALERT Tell the patient to call the primary care provider and report persistent, changing, worsening, anxiety-producing, or specific signs and symptoms, including lesions that fit the mnemonic ABCDEFG. (See *Warning signs of lesions*.)

Resources

• Skin Cancer Foundation: 800-SKIN-490
• American Cancer Society: 800-ACS-2345
• Cancer Information Service: 800-4-CANCER
• Cancer Care: 800-813-HOPE
For patients, caregivers, and providers:
Association of Cancer Online Resources: *www.acor.org*

Contact dermatitis

ICD-9-CM 692.9

Contact dermatitis is a general term describing inflammatory skin reactions after contact with specific antigens. It's the most common skin disease attributed to the workplace and is the cause of a considerable portion of disability in industry. Contact dermatitis can be divided into two categories: nonallergic and allergic. Nonallergic dermatitis (for example, reaction to poison ivy) is caused by chemical irritation and tends to develop more rapidly. Reaction depends on the concentration of the irritant. Conversely, allergic dermatitis (for example, reaction to a specific brand of soap) is caused by an antigen (also called an allergen) that evokes a cell-mediated hypersensitivity reaction only in people who are sensitized to it. The reaction occurs even with small amounts of exposure, takes longer to appear, and occurs after each exposure. (See *Types of dermatitis,* pages 126 to 129.)

Contagion

This condition isn't contagious.

Causes

Contact dermatitis is a delayed hypersensitivity reaction and appears several hours to a week (and rarely even longer) after exposure to the antigen. The time delay is caused by the *cell-mediated immune cascade*. When immunoglobulin G or immunoglobulin M reacts with antigens as part of the body's immune response, complement factors are activated that move through the epidermis to the lymph nodes to stimulate T-cell proliferation. From the lymph nodes, T cells move by way of the bloodstream to tissues and then to the dermal layers to produce the dermatitis. Consequently, chronic skin irritation usually continues even after exposure to the allergen has ended or after the ir-

(Text continues on page 128.)

TYPES OF DERMATITIS

Type	Causes	Signs and symptoms
Exfoliative dermatitis Severe, chronic noninfectious inflammation characterized by redness and widespread erythema and scaling	• Preexisting lesions progressing to exfoliative stage, such as in contact dermatitis, drug reaction, lymphoma, leukemia, or atopic dermatitis • May be idiopathic	• Generalized dermatitis, with acute loss of stratum corneum, and erythema and scaling • Sensation of tight skin • Hair loss • Possibly fever, sensitivity to cold, shivering, gynecomastia, and lymphadenopathy
Hand or foot dermatitis Noninfectious disease characterized by inflammatory eruptions on the hands or feet	• Usually unknown but may result from progressive contact dermatitis • Excessive skin dryness often a contributing factor	• Redness and scaling of the palms or soles • May produce painful fissures • Some cases present with blisters (dyshidrotic eczema)
Localized neurodermatitis (lichen simplex chronicus, essential pruritus)		
Noninfectious superficial inflammation characterized by itching and papular eruptions that appear on thickened, hyperpigmented skin	• Chronic scratching or rubbing of a primary lesion or insect bite or other skin irritation • May be psychogenic	• Intense, sometimes continual scratching • Thick, sharp-bordered, possibly dry, scaly lesions with raised papules and accentuated skin lines (lichenification) • Usually affects easily reached areas, such as ankles, lower legs, anogenital area, back of neck, and ears • One or a few lesions may be present; asymmetrical distribution
Nummular dermatitis Noninfectious subacute disease characterized by inflammation of coin-shaped, scaling, or vesicular patches; usually quite pruritic	• Possibly precipitated by stress, skin dryness, irritants, or scratching	• Round, nummular (coin-shaped), red lesions, usually on arms and legs, with distinct borders of crusts and scales • Possibly oozing and severe itching • Summertime remissions common, with wintertime recurrence

Diagnosis	Treatment and interventions
• Diagnosis requires identification of the underlying cause.	• Hospitalization, with protective isolation and hygienic measures to prevent secondary bacterial infection • Open wet dressings with colloidal baths • Bland lotions over topical corticosteroids • Maintenance of constant environmental temperature to prevent chilling or overheating • Careful monitoring of renal and cardiac status • Systemic antibiotics and steroids
• Patient history and physical findings (distribution of eruption on palms and soles) confirm diagnosis.	• Antibiotics for secondary infection • Avoidance of excessive hand washing and drying and of accumulation of soaps and detergents under rings • Use of emollients with topical corticosteroids
• Physical findings confirm diagnosis.	• Scratching must stop; then lesions will disappear in about 2 weeks • Fixed dressings or Unna's boot (zinc gelatin dressing providing continuous pressure to affected areas) to cover affected areas • Topical corticosteroids under occlusive dressing or by intralesional injection • Antihistamines and open wet dressings • Emollients • Patient informed about underlying cause
• Physical findings and patient history confirm nummular dermatitis. • Diagnosis must rule out fungal infections, atopic or contact dermatitis, and psoriasis.	• Elimination of known irritants • Measures to relieve dry skin: increased humidification, limited frequency of baths, use of bland soap and bath oils, and application of emollients • Application of wet dressings in acute phase • Topical corticosteroids (occlusive dressing or intralesional injection) for persistent lesions • Tar preparations and antihistamines to control itching • Antibiotics for secondary infection

(continued)

TYPES OF DERMATITIS (continued)

Type	Causes	Signs and symptoms
Seborrheic dermatitis Noninfectious subacute skin disease that affects the scalp, face and, occasionally, other areas; characterized by lesions covered with yellow or brownish gray scales	• Unknown; stress and neurologic conditions may be predisposing factors; related to the yeast *Pityrosporum ovale*	• Eruptions in areas with many sebaceous glands (usually scalp, face, chest, axillae, and groin) and in skin folds • Itching, redness, and inflammation of affected areas; lesions may appear greasy; fissures may occur • Indistinct, occasionally yellowish, scaly patches from excess stratum corneum (dandruff may be a mild seborrheic dermatitis)
Stasis dermatitis Noninfectious condition characterized by eczema of the legs with edema, hyperpigmentation, and persistent inflammation	• Secondary to peripheral vascular diseases affecting legs, such as recurrent thrombophlebitis and resultant chronic venous insufficiency	• Varicosities and edema common, but obvious vascular insufficiency not always present • Usually affects the lower leg, just above internal malleolus, or sites of trauma or irritation • Early signs: dusky red deposits of hemosiderin in skin, with itching and dimpling of subcutaneous tissue • Later signs: edema, redness, and scaling of large areas of legs • Possibly fissures, crusts, and ulcers

ritation has been systemically controlled. In addition, because of the cell-mediated pathway, all skin becomes hypersensitive to the antigen.

Clinical presentation

The acute stage can occur over a few days and is characterized by well-demarcated, erythematous, edematous lesions that may be superimposed on other lesions, with skin erosions. Crusting and oozing may be present as well as pruritus.

Subacute cases present with mildly erythematous lesions, with small, dry scaling or exfoliation and, occasionally, small, firm papules.

Chronic dermatitis can last for months or years. It also has a mildly erythematous base, but thickening, scaling, excoriations, and fissuring predominate. Skin that is thinner or has more contact with the irritant is more strongly affected. Constitutional symptoms (such as fever) may occur in severe cases of acute dermatitis.

Common secondary conditions associated with contact dermatitis include viral, fungal, or bacterial infections and ocular disorders, probably due to scratching.

Diagnosis	Treatment and interventions
• Patient history and physical findings, especially distribution of lesions in sebaceous gland areas, confirm seborrheic dermatitis. • Diagnosis must rule out psoriasis.	• Removal of scales with frequent washing and shampooing with selenium sulfide suspension (most effective), zinc pyrithione, or tar and salicylic acid shampoo • Application of fluorinated corticosteroids to nonhairy areas
• Diagnosis requires positive history of venous insufficiency and physical findings such as varicosities.	• Measures to prevent venous stasis: avoidance of prolonged sitting or standing, use of support stockings, weight reduction in obesity, and leg elevation • Corrective surgery for underlying cause • After ulcer develops: rest periods with legs elevated; open wet dressings; Unna's boot; and antibiotics for secondary infection after wound culture

Differential diagnosis

Diagnosis is based on clinical impression. Other possible diagnoses include herpes simplex, bullous pemphigoid, photoallergy, scabies, tinea, or another type of dermatitis.

Typical distribution of skin lesions rules out other inflammatory skin lesions, such as diaper rash (lesions confined to the diapered area), seborrheic dermatitis (no pigmentation changes or lichenification occurs in chronic lesions), or atopic dermatitis (antecubital, groin, facial areas).

Diagnostic test
• The diagnosis is based on physical examination and patient history.
• A *skin patch test* confirms identity of the allergen.

Management

• Effective treatment of contact dermatitis consists of eliminating allergens and avoiding irritants. Local and systemic measures aim to relieve itching and inflammation.
• Large vesicles may be drained. However, to reduce the chance of infection, their tops shouldn't be removed.

SPECIAL POPULATIONS
Remember that coping with disfigurement is extremely difficult, especially for children and adolescents. Be careful not to show anxiety or revulsion when touching the lesions during examination. Help the patient accept his altered body image, and encourage him to verbalize his feelings.

• Although the patient can help clear lichenified skin by applying occlusive dressings (such as plastic film), this should be done only after consulting with a dermatologist because the dressing increases the potency of the corticosteroid cream.

Drugs

• Combination of zinc oxide, talc, menthol, and phenol reduces dryness and is protective.

• A high-potency corticosteroid ointment(fluocinonide, triamcinolone) may be applied thinly twice daily until lesions are controlled, especially after bathing, to alleviate inflammation. Avoid using corticosteroids (particularly high-potency types) on thin-skinned areas (face, skin folds) because they thin the skin over time.

• Calamine can alleviate pruritus.

• Systemic corticosteroids should be used only during extreme exacerbations and after consultation or referral with a dermatologist.

SPECIAL POPULATIONS In infants and children, use hydrocortisone ointment 2.5% (1% for face and intertriginous areas).

• Antibiotics (erythromycin) are used for secondary infections.

Referral or consultation

COLLABORATION For severe, refractory, or complex cases and before using systemic corticosteroids, refer to a primary care doctor or dermatologist.

Refer to a psychologist or psychiatrist as needed for counseling due to altered body image, particularly in adolescents and children.

Follow-up

Although the clinical picture may vary, generally follow up in 1 week to assess response. If nonresponsive to treatment, seek consultation. Two weeks after resolution of symptoms, consider patch testing to determine causative agent.

Complications

Generalized dermatitis and secondary bacterial infections may occur.

Patient teaching

• Instruct the patient to avoid contact with known allergens; if the patient develops a chronic problem of unknown cause, advise keeping a symptom diary to try to identify allergens.

• Advise the patient to set up an individual schedule and plan for daily skin care.

• Advise the patient to bathe in plain water. (He may have to limit bathing, according to the severity of the lesions.) Tell him to bathe with a non-fatty soap and tepid water (96° F [35.6° C]) but to avoid using any soap when lesions are acutely inflamed.

• For acute pruritus, tell the patient that taking an extra warm bath or shower (usually most helpful before bedtime) opens pores and allows cell-mediated factors to wash out, causing increased itching for up to 10 minutes, but this is followed by relief that can last about 8 hours. Not recommended more than once daily and for those with dry skin.

• Soaking in cool water with Burow's solution, Aveeno, or baking soda is helpful. A cool compress or ice cube can provide local relief.

• Caution the patient to avoid extended periods in a hot environment because that will exacerbate symptoms

• Advise the patient to shampoo frequently (no more than once daily) and apply corticosteroid solution to the scalp afterward

• As indicated, recommend hypoallergenic cosmetics, decreased use of milder deodorants, and use of mild detergents without fragrance. Check for the words "hypoallergenic" and "dye and perfume free."

• Daytime drowsiness is possible with the use of antihistamines to relieve itching. This may interfere with sleep. Advise the patient to use alternate methods for inducing natural sleep, such as drinking a glass of warm milk, to help prevent overuse of sedatives.

• Between steroid doses, applying a moisturizing cream can help retain lubricant in the skin, particularly if applied during and after a tub bath.

• Instruct the patient to keep fingernails short to limit excoriation and secondary infections caused by scratching.

• Advise the patient that irritants, such as detergents and wool, exacerbate dermatitis.

ALERT Tell the patient to call the primary care provider and report persistent, changing, worsening, anxiety-producing, or specific signs and symptoms, including:

– signs of infection (redness, edema, drainage, especially if cloudy, thick, or colored), fever (greater than 102.5° F [39.1° C]), and large, painful open areas

– itching or rash nonresponsive to management plan after 3 days

– signs of serious allergic reaction: lesions appear around or in eyes and mouth.

• Instruct the patient to call emergency medical services for difficulty breathing, shortness of breath, wheezing, swelling of tongue or throat, abdominal or chest pain, confusion, or loss of consciousness.

Resources

• American Academy of Allergy, Asthma & Immunology: 800-822-2762; *www.aaaai.org/public*

• Asthma and Allergy Foundation of America: 800-7-ASTHMA

• American Academy of Dermatology (patient-teaching materials): 708-330-0230; *www.aad.org*

Eczema

ICD-9-CM Atopic dermatitis (acute, allergic, chronic, erythematous, fissum, occupational, rubrum, squamous) 692.9, atopic 691.8, external ear 380.22, flexural 691.8, gouty 274.89, infantile (acute or chronic) 690.12

Eczema is defined as "the itch that rashes." Scratching causes weeping and skin infection that crusts over, progressing to thick, roughened skin. This condition can flare up intermittently throughout a person's lifetime.

 SPECIAL POPULATIONS Ninety percent of people afflicted with eczema have the characteristic rash by age 5.

Contagion

This condition isn't contagious.

Causes

The skin is unable to retain adequate water, and the dryness causes itching. Constant scratching leads to a vicious cycle: itch-scratch-rash-itch. Eczema is chronic and has a strong genetic component. More than two-thirds of patients have a personal or family history of asthma, eczema, hay fever, or other allergies. Increasing prevalence is thought to be due to increased exposure to allergens, a decline in breast-feeding, and heightened parental and clinician awareness.

Clinical presentation

Pruritus is the hallmark symptom of eczema. Scratching can cause weeping, infected skin, and crusting. When acute, lesions are poorly defined erythematous and edematous papules and plaques with tiny vesicles, exudation, crusting, and excoriation. Chronic lesions are lichenified, hyperpigmented, and thickened, with fissured skin folds. Presentation generally differs by age: in infants, it affects the face; in children, the antecubital and popliteal fossae; in adults, it's more generalized and often more severe.

Differential diagnosis

Conditions to consider include photosensitivity, contact dermatitis, scabies, seborrheic dermatitis, psoriasis, nummular eczema, dermatophytosis, and early-stage mycosis fungoides.

Diagnostic tests
• Diagnosis is made on clinical grounds.
• *Bacterial culture* is indicated because almost 90% of patients are secondarily colonized.
• *Viral culture* rules out herpes simplex virus in crusted lesions.
• *Radioallergosorbent testing* is rarely helpful.

Management
Drugs
• Topical corticosteroids decrease erythema, inflammation, and pruritus

and are the most commonly used agents. Adverse effects include adrenal suppression with chronic use, permanent thinning of the skin, and striae formation
• Menthol and camphor lotions (Sarna) help control itching.
• Topical anesthetics such as pramoxine alone or with hydrocortisone (Aveeno Anti-Itch, PrameGel, Epifoam) may be used for itching. Avoid benzocaine because of allergic reactions.
• Nonsedating (histamine-1) antihistamines (loratadine [Claritin] or cetirizine [Zyrtec]) are good for daytime itch.
• Sedating antihistamines (hydroxyzine or doxepin) can be used daily at bedtime.
• Topical antibacterials are used for excoriations and crusted areas. Avoid neomycin-containing topicals because of sensitization.
• Topical and oral antibiotics are used for secondary infections. Consider them for widespread excoriations and malodorous or yellow crusting areas. Cyclic administration of erythromycin (5 days every 2 weeks) can combat staphylococcal colonization.
• Oral antipruritics are of modest benefit, and topical antihistamines are rarely helpful. Particularly avoid diphenhydramine because of allergic reactions.
• Systemic corticosteroids help acute flares, but recurrence after discontinuation is common.
• Ultraviolet B and psoralen plus ultraviolet A may be useful in refractory disease after age 10.
• Acyclovir (I.V. or by mouth) is used for secondary infection by herpes simplex. Eczema herpeticum requires immediate treatment; it has a punched-out appearance and occurs in grouped and disseminated crusted erosions. Daily acyclovir for suppressive therapy may be needed.

Referral or consultation

 COLLABORATION Consult a dermatologist for refractory lesions, disease complicated by herpes simplex infection, or when allergic contact dermatitis is suspected. Refer or consult before using occlusive dressings with corticosteroids, systemic corticosteroids, or cyclosporine. Refer to an allergist or immunologist in cases with congenital immunodeficiency or significant respiratory atopy or when an environmental allergen is suspected.

Complications

Skin infections, usually caused by *Staphylococcus aureus*, may develop. Excessive use of corticosteroids on skin folds or the face can cause striae and skin atrophy. Systemic effects can accompany topical use of high-potency corticosteroids over large areas, particularly with occlusive dressings.

Patient teaching

Preventive measures

• Advise the patient to wear loose-fitting soft fabrics and to minimize skin irritants (clothes made of coarse fabric, harsh soaps, prolonged hot baths or showers).

• Instruct the patient to minimize drying of the skin and loss of epithelium, which lowers defenses and increases risk of infection. Tell him he should avoid bathing more than once per day; take lukewarm baths or showers and use moisturizing soaps (Dove, Aveeno Oilated Bath) or colloidal oatmeal (Aveeno); use soap to wash body folds, but on other parts of the body use only as needed; and pat dry and apply moisturizer (hydrated petroleum moisture creams) while skin is damp. Advise him to avoid ointments because they clog pores and increase itching

• Teach the patient to decrease stress because exacerbations are associated with emotional stress.

• Advise the patient to try not to scratch or rub. If he must do so, advise using pads of fingers, not nails.

 SPECIAL POPULATIONS Tell patents that children's nails should be trimmed to minimize damage from scratching.

• Tell the patient that wet-work activities (such as dishwashing) should be done while wearing white cotton gloves under rubber gloves. Contact with chlorine (in swimming pools as well as when cleaning) should be avoided.

 ALERT Tell the patient to call the primary care provider and report persistent, changing, worsening, anxiety-producing, or specific signs and symptoms, including:
– signs of infection (increased redness of lesions, swelling, cloudy or odorous drainage, and temperature above 102° F [38.8° C]
– itching unrelieved by management plan
– if rash not much improved after 1 week of management.

Resources

American Academy of Dermatology (patient education materials), 708-330-0230; *www.aad.org*

Fungal infections

ICD-9-CM Tinea corporis 110.5, pedis 110.4, capitis/barbae 110.0, unguium 110.1, cruris 110.3

Also called tinea, ringworm, or dermatophytosis, fungal infections can affect the scalp (tinea capitis), body (tinea corporis), nails (tinea unguium), feet (tinea pedis), groin (tinea cruris), and bearded skin (tinea barbae).

Tinea infections are quite prevalent in the United States and are usually more common in males than in females. With effective treatment, the cure rate is high, although about 20% of people with infected feet or nails develop chronic conditions.

Contagion

This infection is contagious. Transmission can occur directly (through contact with infected lesions) or indirectly (through contact with contaminated articles, such as shoes, towels, and shower stalls). Some infections come from contact with animals or soil.

Incubation period: 10 to 14 days.
Isolation: Avoid direct contact.
Communicable period: In humans, as long as lesions are present; on fomites (objects contaminated with causative organisms), extended time.

Causes

Tinea infections (except for tinea versicolor, which is caused by overgrowth of normal skin flora and isn't transmittable) result from infection with dermatophytes (fungi) of the genera *Trichophyton, Microsporum,* and *Epidermophyton*.

Clinical presentation

Lesions vary in appearance and duration with the type of infection.
• *Tinea capitis,* which mainly affects children, is characterized by round erythematous patches on the scalp, causing hair loss with scaling. In some children, a hypersensitivity reaction develops, leading to boggy, inflamed, often pus-filled lesions (kerions).
• *Tinea corporis* produces flat lesions on the skin at any site except the scalp, bearded skin, groin, palms, or soles. The lesions may be dry and scaly or moist and crusty; as they enlarge, their centers heal, causing the classic ring-shaped appearance.
• *Tinea unguium* (onychomycosis) infection typically starts at the tip of one or more toenails (fingernail infection is less common) and produces gradual thickening, discoloration, and crumbling of the nail, with accumulation of subungual debris. Eventually, the nail may be destroyed completely.
• *Tinea pedis* causes scaling and blisters between the toes. Severe infection may result in inflammation, with severe itching and pain on walking. A dry, squamous inflammation may affect the entire sole.
• *Tinea cruris* (jock itch) produces red, raised, sharply defined, itchy lesions in the groin that may extend to the buttocks, inner thighs, and the external genitalia. Warm weather and tight clothing encourage fungus growth.
• *Tinea barbae* is an uncommon infection that affects the bearded facial area of men.
• *Tinea versicolor,* also called pityriasis versicolor, is a chronic, asymptomatic, hypopigmented, scaling, macular rash with sharp margins. It's caused by opportunistic overgrowth of a lipophilic yeast that is normally present on the skin. High-risk factors include high humidity, excessive sebum production, and application of grease or corticosteroids for extended periods.

Differential diagnosis

Other conditions to consider when diagnosing a fungal infection are vitiligo, other types of dermatitis (seborrheic, atopic, contact), psoriasis, alopecia areata, and pityriasis alba.

Diagnostic tests

• Microscopic examination of lesion scrapings prepared in potassium hydroxide solution usually confirms tinea infection, detecting arthrospores within hair shafts.

• Other diagnostic procedures include Wood's light examination (which is useful in only 10% of cases of tinea capitis and further identifies the dermatophyte but doesn't affect treatment) and culture of the infecting organism.

Management

Drugs

• Tinea infections usually respond to topical antifungals, such as clotrimazole (Lotrimin), twice daily for 3 to 6 weeks. However, topical therapy is ineffective for tinea capitis; griseofulvin is the treatment of choice.

• Oral griseofulvin (250 to 500 mg twice daily for 1 to 3 months) is especially effective in tinea infections of the skin and hair but requires baseline complete blood count (CBC) and liver function tests (LFTs).

• Pulse therapy with oral terbinafine (250 mg) daily for 3 months or itraconazole (200 mg) by mouth twice per day for 1 week, repeated monthly for 3 to 6 months for fingernails and 8 to 12 months for toenails, depending on extent of infection is helpful in nail infections. Remember, the effect will continue after treatment because the drug is absorbed into the nail, and as the nail slowly grows out, the drug will continue to kill fungus.

• Other antifungals include naftifine, ciclopirox olamine, tolnaftate, ketoconazole (baseline CBC and LFTs required), plus numerous others. Topical treatments should continue for 2 weeks after lesions resolve.

• Tinea versicolor responds to selenium sulfide (2.5%) shampoo. The shampoo is applied to affected sites daily for 1 week, allowed to remain for 15 minutes, and then rinsed out.

• Supportive measures include open wet dressings, removal of scabs and scales, and application of keratolytics, such as salicylic acid, to soften and remove hyperkeratotic lesions of the heels or soles.

• For tinea corporis, use abdominal pads between skin folds for the patient with excessive abdominal girth; change pads frequently. Check daily for excoriated, newly denuded areas of skin. If the involved area is moist, apply open wet dressings two or three times daily to decrease inflammation and help remove scales.

Referral or consultation

Refer to or consult with a primary care doctor or dermatologist if the patient is nonresponsive in weeks.

Follow-up

Evaluate the patient's response to the drug every 2 weeks and then monthly for the duration of treatment (for nail involvement). If prescribing griseofulvin or ketoconazole, monitor with CBC and LFTs every 3 months.

Complications

Permanent scarring and hair loss are possible if marked inflammation occurs.

Patient teaching

 SPECIAL POPULATIONS
For tinea corporis or tinea capitis, remind parents to check with the school or day-care facility for its policy on tinea. Many children may attend with some restrictions, such as no swimming, gym, or activities likely to lead to close physical contact. Restrictions for younger children may be more

strict because of their inability to avoid intimate contact.

• For all tinea infections except those of the hair and nails, first line therapy is topical. Advise the patient to watch for sensitivity reactions and secondary bacterial infections. Tell him to continue topical treatments for 2 weeks after lesions are completely gone.

• Advise the patient to use good hand-washing technique. To prevent spreading the infection to others, advise washing towels, bedclothes, and combs frequently in hot water and to avoid sharing them. Suggest that family members be checked (particularly for tinea capitis).

• For tinea unguium, advise the patient to keep nails short and straight and to gently remove debris from under the nails with an emery board.

• For tinea pedis, encourage the patient to expose his feet to air whenever possible and to wear sandals or leather shoes and clean cotton socks. Instruct the patient to wash the feet twice daily and, after drying them thoroughly, to apply the antifungal cream followed by antifungal powder to absorb perspiration and prevent excoriation.

• For tinea cruris, instruct the patient to dry the affected area thoroughly after bathing and to evenly apply antifungal powder after applying the topical antifungal agent. Advise wearing loose-fitting clothing, which should be changed frequently and washed in hot water.

• For tinea barbae, suggest that the patient let his beard grow. (Whiskers should be trimmed with scissors, not a razor.) If the patient insists that he must shave, advise him to use an electric razor instead of a blade.

ALERT Tell the patient to call the primary care provider and report persistent, changing, worsening, anxiety-producing, or specific signs and symptoms, including:
– no improvement after 1 week of management plan (1 month for nails)
– lesions spread to the scalp or nails
– lesions appear infected (fever, increased redness, swelling, cloudy or colored drainage).

Resources
www.healthanswers.com (Enter "tinea" in the search box and then select from listed options.)

Herpes simplex

ICD-9-CM Herpes simplex 054.73, conjunctiva simplex 054.43, genital 054.10, whitlow 054.6

Herpes simplex is a recurring viral infection. Herpes Type 1 (HSV-1) may affect the mucous membranes, oropharynx, conjunctiva, and skin and most commonly produces cold sores and fever blisters. It also may infect the genital area.

Herpes Type 2 (HSV-2) primarily affects the genital area but may involve the anus, buttocks, and legs.

The usual course of primary infection is 2 weeks; recurrences are less severe with less viral shedding. However, the infection may disseminate, causing encephalitis or pneumonia.

 SPECIAL POPULATIONS Eighty-five percent of adults worldwide test positive for HSV-1, which is much more common than HSV-2. In the United States, HSV-2 is present in about 1 in 4 adults and is commonly found in patients with human immunodeficiency virus.

Primary herpesvirus hominis (HVH) is the leading cause of gingivostomatitis in children ages 1 to 3 and causes the most common nonepidemic encephalitis. It's the second most common viral infection in pregnant women and vertical transmission may cause spontaneous abortion.

Contagion

This infection is contagious. It's spread by skin-skin, mucosa-skin contact.

HSV-1 is spread in oral and respiratory secretions and can also be sexually transmitted.

HSV-2 is usually spread by sexual contact but is also vertically transmitted.

Incubation period: 2 to 12 days.
Communicable period: During viral shedding. This is generally 1 week after mouth lesions resolve, up to 12 days after genital lesions resolve in primary infection, and up to 7 days after genital lesions resolve in recurrences. However, reactivations may be asymptomatic and consist of viral shedding only.
Isolation: Avoid contact with infants under 4 months, people who are immunosuppressed, and children with eczema.

Causes

Most HVH infections are subclinical. The remainder produce localized lesions and systemic reactions. After the first infection, a patient is a carrier susceptible to reactivation, which may be provoked by physical or emotional stress. However, in recurrences, the patient usually has no constitutional symptoms.

Saliva, feces, urine, skin lesions, and purulent eye exudate are potential sources of infection.

Clinical presentation

Perioral (most common site), clustered, uniform vesicles on erythema-

tous base, which crust over before resolving.

Primary infection
- Prodrome of local pain, tender lymphadenopathy, headache, generalized ache, fevers
- Located on mucous membranes
- Clustered, often umbilicated vesicles on an erythematous base
- Lesions erode, forming moist erosions or yellowish crusts that last 2 to 4 weeks
- Virus travels to dorsal root ganglia and enters latent stage

Recurrent infection
- Reduced severity and duration but still infectious
- Prodrome of constitutional symptoms less common
- Dome-shaped lesions open and crust in 2 to 4 days
- Yellowish crust sheds in 8 days

 SPECIAL POPULATIONS In neonates, HVH symptoms usually appear 1 or 2 weeks after birth. They range from localized skin lesions to a disseminated infection of such organs as the liver, lungs, and brain. Ninety percent of infants with disseminated disease die. Herpetic stomatitis may lead to severe dehydration in children.

Vesicles may form on any part of the oral mucosa, especially the tongue, gingiva, and cheeks, and is usually HSV-1. In generalized infection, vesicles occur with submaxillary lymphadenopathy. Other symptoms include increased salivation, halitosis, anorexia, and temperature of up to 105° F (40.6° C).

Genital herpes usually affects adolescents and young adults and most often is HSV-2. Typically painful, the initial attack produces fluid-filled vesicles that ulcerate and heal in 1 to 3 weeks. Fever, regional lyphadenopathy, and dysuria may also occur.

Herpetic keratoconjunctivitis is usually unilateral, causing local symptoms: conjunctivitis, regional adenopathy, blepharitis, and vesicles on the lid. Other ocular symptoms may be excessive lacrimation, edema, chemosis, photophobia, and purulent exudate. Uveitis may cause permanent vision loss.

Differential diagnosis

Diagnosed by clinical appearance.
• Impetigo crusts and exudate are straw-colored.
• Aphthous stomatitis exhibits gray, shallow erosions with a ring of hyperemia on the anterior mouth and lips.
• Hand-foot-and-mouth disease presents with lesions on distal extremities.
• Herpes zoster appears on unilateral dermatome.
• Syphilitic chancre is a painless ulcer.
• Herpangina appears on the posterior buccal mucosa (soft palate, oropharynx) but not the anterior gums and on lips; Stevens-Johnson syndrome is suspected if the person recently started on a new medication.
• Herpetic whitlow, a primary finger infection, commonly affects health care workers. First the finger tingles or itches and then it becomes inflamed with neuralgia. Herpetic whitlow may also present with satellite vesicles, fever, chills, malaise, and a red streak up the arm.

Diagnostic tests

• *Tzanck smear* shows multinucleated giant cells (herpes zoster has identical findings).
• *HSV culture* takes from 2 to 6 days to get results.
• *Herpes antibody titers* don't differentiate HSV-1 from HSV-2.
• Screen for other sexually transmitted diseases with primary genital herpes.

Management

• Counseling is needed because the patient usually feels "dirty" or as if she has done something wrong to "deserve" this incurable disease.

Drugs

• Early lesions: remove the top of the lesion and apply Campho-Phenique
• Systemic antivirals (valacyclovir, famciclovir)
• Analgesic-antipyretic for fever and pain (acetaminophen, aspirin, ibuprofen)
• Local anesthetic (viscous lidocaine) for the pain of gingivostomatitis, enabling the patient to eat and preventing dehydration
• Drying agents (calamine lotion) to make labial lesions less painful
• Ophthalmic: acyclovir, vidarabine plus referral
• Optional daily suppressive therapy for patients with more than six recurrences each year (After 1 year, discontinue drug and reevaluate.)

Referral or consultation

Consult with a doctor for extensive lesions.

 COLLABORATION Consult an ophthalmologist for eye involvement.

Complications

Encephalitis, pneumonia, aseptic meningitis, viremia, or ocular involvement may occur.

 SPECIAL POPULATIONS In infants, systemic complications are severe, with a 90% mortality rate.

Patient teaching

• Advise the patient with central nervous system infection alone that there is no need for isolation.

- Teach the patient to apply intermittent cool, moist dressings with Domeboro or Burow's solution.
- Explain that this disease isn't curable and recurrence rates vary widely.
- Antivirals won't cure the disease but shorten its duration; advise the patient to seek treatment at the first sign of recurrence.
- Tell the patient to apply analgesic spray (Americaine) to the genital area, to use a hair dryer on a low setting on the area after showering, and to keep the area dry.
- Tell the patient that painful urination can be eased by pouring a cup of warm water over the genitals while urinating.
- Tell patients to monitor children over age 3 months for signs and symptoms of dehydration: less than three voids in 24 hours, cotton mouth, tenting skin, no tears when crying.
- For oral pain, advise the patient to use a soft toothbrush, eat a soft diet, and drink plenty of clear liquids. Avoid citrus fruits and salty or spicy foods.
- Tell him to rinse with warm water after meals.
- For mouthwash, advise saline (¼ tsp salt in 8 oz of warm water).
- To prevent spread, avoid immunocompromised people; teach about safer sex (herpes can be transmitted even when no lesions are present); explain condom benefits and limitations; teach avoidance of sexual contact during active periods; wash hands frequently.

ALERT Tell the patient to call the primary care provider and report persistent, changing, worsening, anxiety-producing, or specific signs and symptoms, including:
- worsening of sores
- high fever non-responsive to antipyretics
- signs of dehydration (less than three voids in 24 hours; dark, foul-smelling urine; skin tenting; crying without tearing)
- severe mouth pain
- patient is difficult to awaken or complains of stiff neck.

Resources
- Herpes Resource Center: 800-230-6039
- National Herpes Hotline: 919-361-8488
- National STD Hotline: 800-227-8922
- For teens: *www.plannedparenthood.org/* or *www.teenwire.com/index.asp*
- Sexual assault information: *www.cs.utk.edu/~bartley/saInfoPage.html*

Herpes zoster

ICD-9-CM Herpes zoster 053.9, eye zoster 053.29

Also called shingles, herpes zoster is an acute unilateral and segmental inflammation of the dorsal root ganglia. The virus continues to multiply in the ganglia, destroys the host neuron, and spreads down the sensory nerves to the skin.

Although herpes zoster is less contagious than varicella zoster (V-Z), contact with the vesicle fluid can cause chickenpox in V-Z–negative people. Shingles usually occurs in those older than 50 and seldom recurs. It may be activated by emotional or physical stress, immunocompromise, or immunosuppressive therapy. It produces localized vesicular skin lesions confined to a dermatome and severe neuralgia. Occasionally, postherpetic neuralgia (PHN) may persist for months or years.

SPECIAL POPULATIONS
Whites are four times more likely to develop herpes zoster than blacks. After age 80, the risk of developing zoster is as high as 30% during a person's remaining lifetime. In patients with human immunodeficiency virus infection, the annual incidence of zoster is 3%.

Contagion

This condition is contagious. It doesn't cause shingles but may cause chickenpox (V-Z) if the patient isn't immune. Herpes zoster is much less infectious than V-Z. Transmission is by contact with fluid from the vesicles, which can also become airborne. Vertical transmission is possible.
Incubation period: 2 to 3 weeks.
Communicable period: Infectious for up to 5 days before rash appears until 7 days after lesions first appeared but up to 21 days after rash appears in an immunocompromised person.
Isolation: Make sure lesions are covered (as with a shirt) when in public. Avoid immunocompromised and pregnant people for 7 or 21 days after lesions appeared (depending on the patient's immunocompetence).

Causes

This condition is caused by infection with the herpesvirus varicella-zoster, a local reactivation of latent varicella infection.

Clinical presentation

Prodrome: itching, burning, stabbing pain; usually involving one dermatome more common on the trunk.

Eruptions

• Red clustered lesions of varied size become edematous vesicles on an erythematous base, filled with cloudy fluid; they continue to appear for 7 days.
• About 10 days after they appear, the vesicles dry and form scabs. Compared to V-Z, they are unilateral, more deeply seated, more closely aggregated, and restricted to the area supplied by the dorsal root ganglia that contains the reactivated V-Z.

Postherpetic neuralgia

• Risk increases with age, may last, and can be severe.

Differential diagnosis

Diagnosis is made by patient history and physical examination.

Diagnostic tests

Rarely indicated.
• *Viral culture* is an expensive test but shows varicella isolate.
• *Tzanck smear* shows multinucleated giant cells but doesn't differentiate from herpes simplex.
• Staining antibodies from vesicular fluid and identification under fluorescent light differentiate herpes zoster from localized herpes simplex.

Management

Drugs

• Analgesic and antipyretics: acetaminophen, aspirin, nonsteroidal anti-inflammatory drugs
• Systemic antivirals (valacyclovir, famciclovir, or I.V. acyclovir) appear to prevent disseminated, life-threatening disease in immunocompromised patients and those with encephalitis or pneumonitis
• Systemic antivirals (acyclovir) for a week to reduce illness severity
• Topical antibacterial (Bactroban) for open lesions
• Systemic antibiotics for bacterial superinfection (erythromycin)
  For PHN, consider the following four treatments:

- Narcotic analgesia (codeine): as needed
- Topical analgesic (capsaicin cream): deletes pain impulse transmitter substance P and prevents its resynthesis
- 5% lidocaine patch (Lidoderm): extended-release topical analgesic
- Tricyclic antidepressant (amitriptyline): for neurogenic pain.

 ALERT A long-term study is in progress in patients over age 65 to prove efficacy of primary prevention with varicella vaccine (VZV), particularly for immunocompromised people. VZV has an established 80% prevention rate for varicella zoster. When varicella zoster rash develops, patients average 50 lesions instead of 400.

Referral or consultation

Consult with a doctor if the patient is immunocompromised.

 ALERT Refer the patient to an ophthalmologist for lesions affecting the eyes.

Follow-up

Follow up in 2 weeks to verify resolution and check for PHN.

Complications

Complications of herpes zoster include PHN, ocular involvement, corneal ulceration, meningoencephalitis, cutaneous dissemination, superinfection of lesions, hepatitis, pneumonitis, peripheral motor weakness, segmental myelitis, cranial nerve syndromes, and Guillain-Barré syndrome.

Patient teaching

- Advise the patient to get adequate rest during the acute phase.
- Teach the patient to apply drying agent (calamine lotion) liberally to lesions.

- Teach him to apply Burow's solution for widespread lesions.
- For itch relief, suggest that the patient soak in a tepid water bath with ½ cup baking soda.
- Instruct the patient to avoid scratching the lesions and to trim fingernails to decrease superinfection from scratching.
- Tell the patient to wash his hands frequently and to wash lesions gently with antibacterial soap and warm water without rubbing or scrubbing.
- Tell the patient to apply a cold compress if vesicles rupture.
- Tell the patient that the rash usually resolves in 2 to 3 weeks.
- If the patient believes he has been in proximity to an immunocompromised person, he should notify the person.
- To minimize PHN, teach the patient not to delay analgesics because the pain is severe. Teach that antidepressant drugs are used for their effect on nerve endings, not as antidepressants
- Repeatedly reassure the patient that herpetic pain will eventually subside but may take months to years.

 ALERT Tell the patient to call the primary care provider and report persistent, changing, worsening, anxiety-producing, or specific signs and symptoms, including:
– visual changes and pain
– signs of infection or if scabs change from soft brown to soft golden yellow
– development of cough
– temperature above 101° F (38.3° C).

Hives

ICD-9-CM Urticaria 708.9, hereditary 277.6, allergic 708.0, due to cold/heat 708.2, idiopathic/nonal-

lergic 708.1, larynx 995.1, recur-
rent periodic 708.8 (480)

Also called urticaria, hives are raised skin lesions secondary to edema of the superficial dermis. Angioedema describes deeper swellings with poorly defined borders that are slightly painful or pruritic. Angioedema often involves eyelids, lips, tongue, genitalia, hands, and feet.

Contagion

This condition isn't contagious.

Causes

Usually immunoglobulin E (IgE)–mediated, hives are caused by numerous factors, both immunologic and non-immunologic, that result in edema. The most common causes are food and medications. Other causes are hard to identify absolutely but include physical agents (such as heat, pressure, and light), infection, insect bites, and idiopathic processes.

Clinical presentation

Transient wheals (irregular borders, bright to light pink, some with central clearing) with larger edematous areas appear and are frequently pruritic. Each lesion resolves in less than 24 hours. Angioedema involves subcutaneous tissue as well as the dermis.

Diagnosis is made by checking the history for possible causes and by physical examination. For acute episodes, screening laboratory tests and a radioallergosorbent test (RAST) are of little value. For lack of expected response to antihistamines, reevaluate the diagnosis.

Differential diagnosis

It is important to quickly differentiate a severe allergic reaction that may be life-threatening from one that isn't. Most commonly, insect bites and adverse drug reactions can cause this reaction. Other conditions to consider include contact dermatitis, vasculitis, lupus, lymphoma, and mononucleosis.

Diagnostic tests

• For chronic urticaria, consider a hepatitis test panel (see chapter 4.)
• *RAST* identifies IgE antibodies (for allergies)
• *Erythrocyte sedimentation rate* may indicate necrotizing vasculitis if elevation is persistent.
• *Complete blood count* reveals high eosinophils in a patient with a fever and suggests angioedema-urticaria-eosinophilia syndrome. It may detect transient eosinophilia from reaction to foods, parasites, and drugs.

Management

Drugs

• Avoidance of known allergens is the first step but is rarely successful.
• Antihistamine therapy with histamine-1 (H_1) antagonists is the therapy of choice. Hydroxyzine is the best sedating drug; it should be given continuously and should be pushed to the limit of tolerance.
• Nonsedating H_1 antagonists can be used if sedation isn't desired.
• Doxepin, a tricyclic antidepressant, has both H_1- and H_2- antagonist effects and is a potent antihistamine.
• Epinephrine (subcutaneous form) is indicated for severe acute episodes. Clinical effects last a few hours, so this is an adjunct to an antihistamine. This emergency medication should be carried at all times. Ask to see it at each visit to reinforce behavior and check for expiration of medication.
• Corticosteroids (prednisone) are reserved for refractory or unresponsive cases.

• Many patients won't have a detectable cause for chronic urticaria or angioedema. In this case, it's important to offer support and medication, combined with realistic expectations.

Referral or consultation

Consult with a dermatologist for any patient with acute angioedema if symptoms aren't relieved with antihistamines and for patients with chronic urticaria lasting more than 6 weeks. Anticipate these therapies: nifedipine, nonsteroidal anti-inflammatory drugs, danazol, colchicine, dapsone, sulfasalazine, cyclosporine, androgens, ultraviolet light, and plasmapheresis.

Complications

Severe systemic allergic reaction, respiratory distress, or respiratory collapse may occur.

Patient teaching

• Give the patient a thorough explanation of the disorder so he can control the frequency and severity of symptomatic episodes by adjusting his lifestyle.
• Patients with severe allergies should carry an emergency anaphylaxis kit such as Epi-Pen. Advise the patient to wear medical identification jewelry if he has a history of anaphylaxis.
• Teach the patient to eliminate triggers if known.
• Suggest baking soda (½ cup per tub) or Aveeno baths with cool water to relieve itching. For temporary relief, suggest cool showers and compresses to temporarily relieve itching.
• In cold-induced urticaria, warn the patient that vascular collapse is possible if he jumps into a cool pool.
• If food allergies are strongly suspected, teach the patient about an elimination diet. The patient eats basically rice and chicken for several days; after hives have resolved, foods are reintroduced one at a time.
• Tell the patients with ultraviolet B–induced solar urticaria that sun avoidance and the use of sunscreens may be adequate. However, sunscreens may be insufficient for those sensitive to ultraviolet A and visible light. Some patients with solar urticaria improve by gradually increasing their exposure to natural or artificial light

ALERT Tell the patient to call the primary care provider and report persistent, changing, worsening, anxiety-producing, or specific signs and symptoms, including:
—symptoms that aren't mostly gone within 24 hours of following management plan
—signs of infection (increased redness of lesions, swelling, cloudy or odorous drainage, temperature above 102° F [38.8°])
—hives that develop shortly after beginning a new medication
• Warn the patient to call emergency medical services for a severe reaction (shortness of breath, difficulty swallowing, wheezing, swelling of tongue or throat, severe abdominal or chest pain, cold sweats, pallor, or strong feelings of impending doom).

Lice

ICD-9-CM Pediculosis infestation 132.9, corporis 132.1, capitis 132.0, eyelid 373.6, more than one site 132.3, pubic 132.2

The presence of lice means a cutaneous parasitic infestation with lice and eggs. Head lice (*Pediculus humanus capitis*), body lice (*P. humanus corporis*), and pubic or crab lice (*Phthirus pubis*) are tiny (less than 2 mm) parasitic insects that suck blood from the skin. Female lice live for approximately 1 month and deposit up to 10 eggs per day on the host. Eggs (nits) hatch in 7 to 10 days and are mature at 2 weeks. Capitis and corporis are more likely in children; pubis, in young adults.

Contagion

This condition is highly contagious. Lice are spread by personal contact. Fomites are commonly implicated in the transmission of body lice; culprits include infested clothing, combs, brushes, bedding, and upholstered chairs. Overcrowding increases transmission. Fever of the host encourages lice to migrate to new host.

Incubation period: Eggs hatch in 7 to 10 days.

Communicable period: Until insecticide is applied to skin. On fomites: lice can survive 10 days away from a host before starving to death; eggs survive less than 2 weeks.

Isolation: Contact isolation for 24 hours after insecticide is applied; fomites, 3 weeks.

 COLLABORATION School or day-care staff should be notified if evidence of lice is found on children.

Clinical presentation

All lice cause intense itching. The nits, or clusters of louse eggs, are seen as tiny grayish white or honey-colored ovals glued to hair shafts. Body lice are difficult to find because they burrow under the skin. A secondary excoriation or infection may be caused by scratching.

Differential diagnosis

Rule out scabies and other mites that cause cutaneous reactions in humans. Dandruff, hair lacquer, and hair gel droplets may be mistaken for head lice. The diagnosis is made on clinical grounds. No testing is indicated.

Management

• Pubic lice have a 90% sexual transmission rate. About one-third of these patients have another sexually transmitted disease.
• Eyelash lice on a child may indicate sexual abuse and must be evaluated.

Drugs

• Permethrin (Nix) is used as a one-time treatment.
• Pyrethrins and lindane aren't totally ovicidal; thus it's often necessary to retreat in 7 to 14 days because of the 7- to 10-day incubation period.
• Antibiotics (usually erythromycin or dicloxacillin) can be used in treatment of secondary infection.
• Over-the-counter preparations such as calamine lotion, hydrocortisone cream, and topical antihistamines, can be used to control itching.

Referral or consultation

Consult with a primary care doctor or dermatologist if the patient is unresponsive to treatment.

Follow-up

Follow up as needed for persistent or recurring symptoms.

Complications

Secondary skin infection due to scratching and disruption of skin barrier may occur.

Patient teaching

• Teach the patient that poor hygiene isn't a risk factor in acquiring pediculosis.
• Advise the patient that the dead nits remain in the scalp or pubic hair af-

ter treatment with shampoo or lotion. Nits are best removed with a very fine comb (a nit comb is included in the RID package). Tell the patient that removal is eased by soaking the hair in a solution of equal parts water and white vinegar and wrapping wet hair and scalp in a towel for 15 minutes.
• Instruct the patient that all family members and close contacts should be treated concomitantly to prevent recurrence or reinfection.

SPECIAL POPULATIONS Tell parents to keep children's fingernails short to minimize damage from scratching.
• Teach the patient that linens, clothing, and close contact items (like bed decorations) must be washed in hot water (140° F [60° C]) or dry-cleaned; carpets and rugs should be well vacuumed and the bags disposed of immediately; brushes and combs should be soaked in rubbing alcohol for 1 hour; and anything that can't be cleaned in this manner (hats, upholstery, stuffed animals) should be put in a sealed plastic bag and set aside for 3 weeks (2 week incubation period, 1 week starvation period).
• Tell the patient to remove eyelash lice by applying petroleum jelly (Vaseline) to lashes (eyelid margins) twice daily for 8 days, followed by removal of nits.
• Warn the patient that persistent itching may be caused by too-frequent use of pediculicide.

ALERT Tell the patient to call the primary care provider and report persistent, changing, worsening, anxiety-producing, or specific signs and symptoms, including:
– signs of infection (redness of lesions, edema, drainage from sites, temperature above 101° F [38.3° C])
– itching that isn't relieved within 3 days.

Resources
Helpful information regarding lice and myths regarding management of lice: *www.headlice.org/special/mission.html*

Lyme disease

ICD-9-CM 088.81

A multisystemic disorder, Lyme disease is caused by the spirochete *Borrelia burgdorferi,* which is carried by the minute tick *Ixodes dammini* or another tick in the Ixodidae family. It often begins in the summer with the classic skin lesion called erythema migrans (EM). Weeks or months later, cardiac or neurologic abnormalities sometimes develop, possibly followed by arthritis.

Initially, Lyme disease was identified in a group of children in Lyme, Connecticut. Now Lyme disease is known to occur primarily in three parts of the United States:
• Northeast – Massachusetts to Maryland
• Midwest – Wisconsin and Minnesota
• West – California and Oregon.

Although Lyme disease is endemic to these areas, cases have been reported in 43 states and 20 other countries, including Germany, Switzerland, France, and Australia.

Contagion

This condition isn't contagious. It's transmitted by ticks only. (Animal studies show a tick must be attached for 24 hours to transmit; this may also be true for humans.)
Incubation period: 3 to 32 days.
Communicable period: None.
Isolation: None.

Causes

Lyme disease occurs when a tick injects spirochete-laden saliva into the bloodstream or deposits fecal matter on the skin. After incubating for 3 to 32 days, the spirochetes migrate out to the skin, causing EM. They then disseminate to other skin sites or organs by way of the bloodstream or lymph system. The spirochetes' life cycle isn't completely clear: they may survive for years in the joints or they may trigger an inflammatory response in the host and then die.

Clinical presentation

Typically, Lyme disease has three stages.

Stage I

EM heralds stage I with a red macule or papule, often at the site of a tick bite. This lesion often feels hot and itchy and may grow to more than 20″ (50 cm) in diameter. Within a few days, more lesions may erupt along with a malar rash, conjunctivitis, or diffuse urticaria. In 3 to 4 weeks, lesions are replaced by small, red blotches, which persist for several more weeks.

Malaise and fatigue are constant, but other findings (headache, fever, chills, myalgias, and regional lymphadenopathy) are intermittent. Less common effects are meningeal irritation, mild encephalopathy, migrating musculoskeletal pain, and hepatitis. A persistent sore throat and dry cough may appear several days before EM.

Stage 2

Weeks to months later, the second stage begins with neurologic abnormalities—fluctuating meningoencephalitis with peripheral and cranial neuropathy—that usually resolve after days or months. Facial palsy is especially noticeable. Cardiac abnormalities, such as a brief, fluctuating atrioventricular heart block, may also develop.

Stage 3

Characterized by arthritis, stage 3 begins weeks or years later. Migrating musculoskeletal pain leads to frank arthritis with marked swelling, especially in the large joints. Recurrent attacks may precede chronic arthritis with severe cartilage and bone erosion.

Differential diagnosis

Because isolation of *B. burgdorferi* is unusual in humans and because indirect immunofluorescent antibody tests are marginally sensitive, diagnosis often rests on the characteristic EM lesion and related clinical findings, especially in endemic areas. This is important because early treatment is most beneficial in preventing long-term sequelae.

Conditions to consider when making the diagnosis for constitutional symptoms include viral syndromes, rheumatoid arthritis, tularemia, lupus, Bell's palsy, Reiter's syndrome, encephalitis, Rocky Mountain spotted fever, and rheumatic fever. When classifying the lesion, consider tinea corporis, herald patch of pityriasis rosea, insect bite, cellulitis, urticaria, erythema multiforme, drug eruption, syphilis, and cutaneous lymphomas.

Diagnostic tests

• *Enzyme-linked immunosorbent assay* may be positive for immunoglobulin G and M. *B. burgdorferi* antibodies; however, false negatives can arise in first-stage infection or in late stages where patients received early antibiotic treatment. False positives have been seen with Rocky Mountain spotted fever, syphilis, lupus, and rheumatoid arthritis.

• Cerebrospinal fluid and synovial fluid analyses can be cultured for *B. burgdorferi*.
• Blood culture or skin biopsy has less than a 40% detection rate for *B. burgdorferi* spirochetes and must be placed on Kelly's medium.
• *Complete blood count* and *erythrocyte sedimentation rate (ESR)* may detect mild anemia, an elevated ESR and leukocyte count, and elevated aspartate aminotransferase levels, all supporting the diagnosis.

The PreVue *B. burgdorferi* antibody detection assay can be performed and read in 1 hour. Positive results must be confirmed by the Western blot test.

Management

Urgent

Stage 2 and stage 3 Lyme disease may require inpatient care, determined by the clinical picture. Treatment involves either high-dose penicillin (penicillin G) or third-generation cephalosporins (ceftriaxone, cefotaxime) for 2 to 4 weeks I.V.

General

• Take a detailed patient history, asking about travel to endemic areas and exposure to ticks.
• Check for drug allergies, and check for adverse effects when starting an antibiotic the patient hasn't been exposed to before.
• Primary prevention is available for patients over age 15 through a vaccine. Research is still in progress.

SPECIAL POPULATIONS
Education regarding avoidance and detection is paramount to preventing infection, particularly for children.

B. burgdorferi can cross the placenta; therefore pregnant patients with active infection require parenteral antibiotics.

Drugs

• A 14- to 21-day course of oral tetracycline (doxycycline) is the treatment of choice for adults. Beta-lactamase-inhibiting penicillins (amoxicillin) and second-generation cephalosporins (cefuroxime) are alternates. Oral amoxicillin is usually prescribed for children. When given in the early stages, these drugs can minimize later complications.
• A short course of corticosteroids (prednisone) may be helpful.
• For patients at heightened risk in endemic areas, there is a new vaccine, recombinant OspA (Lymerix), a series of three injections that is approved for people over age 15. Long-term efficacy and safety aren't yet established.

Referral or consultation

Consult with a doctor, especially for disease stages 2 and 3 or severe manifestations. Refer the patient to a physical therapist for arthritis to increase range of motion and strengthening.

SPECIAL POPULATIONS
Consult with an obstetrician if the patient is pregnant. Expect no treatment if the patient is asymptomatic. For early disease, drugs are administered by mouth; for later stages, the parenteral route is used.

Follow-up

Follow-up is determined by clinical presentation. Reevaluate mild cases at the end of oral treatment. Stages 2 and 3 require careful monitoring over months to years. At each visit, focus on the patient's neurologic system; check for signs of increased intracranial pressure and cranial nerve involvement, such as ptosis, strabismus, and diplopia; also check for cardiac abnormalities, such as arrhythmias and heart block.

Complications

The disease may lead to recurrent synovitis, tendinitis, bursitis, chronic neurologic symptoms, peripheral neuropathies, and chronic Lyme disease (arthritis, meningitis, and carditis).

Patient teaching

• Emphasize the importance of range-of-motion and strengthening exercises, and the avoidance of overexertion.

Preventive measures

• Stress that prevention of Lyme disease is possible by early detection and prompt removal of ticks (removal within 24 hours may preclude transmission of spirochete).
• *B.burgdorferi* is carried by deer ticks, but despite the name, the ticks occur on mice and vegetation as well as on deer. They are about the size of the period at the end of this sentence. Teach the patient to try to walk in the center of paths to avoid brushing against vegetation, to cover all skin with bright-colored clothes so that ticks are seen easily, and to tuck pants inside boots or socks.
• Advise the patient to use insect repellents containing N,N-diethyl-m-toluamide (DEET) on clothing and exposed skin surfaces sparingly but as often as every 2 hours (follow product instructions). Permethrin can also be used as a repellent on clothing. To minimize skin irritation and systemic absorption, tell the patient to cover the skin with cloth and the cloth with repellent. Advise him to examine his skin carefully after outdoor activities, especially around vegetation, and to wash repellent off when inside.

ALERT Tell the patient to call the primary care provider and report persistent, changing, worsening, anxiety-producing, or specific signs and symptoms, including:
—inability to remove whole tick (including head)
—whole tick removed, but duration of presence unknown or more than 18 hours
—development of an expanding circular lesion (bull's-eye appearance of red border with clear center); flulike symptoms, rash, or headaches 3 to 32 days after known or possible tickbite; high fever; paralysis of any part of the body; palpitations; pain and swelling of more than one joint.

Resources

• Lyme Borreliosis Foundation: 203-871-2900.
• Arthritis Foundation: 800-283-7300
For all: *www.drreddy; www.cdc.gov*

Psoriasis

ICD-9-CM 696.1

Psoriasis is a chronic, recurrent disease marked by epidermal proliferation. Its lesions, which appear as sharply demarcated papules and plaques covered with silver scales or as erythematous pustules, vary widely in severity and distribution.

 SPECIAL POPULATIONS
Psoriasis affects about 2% of the population in the United States, and incidence is higher among whites than other races. Incidence is low in West Africans, Japanese, Inuits, and Native Americans.

Although this disorder commonly presents in young adults, it may strike at any age, including infancy. Recurring partial remissions and exacerbations characterize psoriasis. Flare-ups are often related to specific systemic and environmental factors but may be unpredictable; they can usually be controlled with therapy. The disease is more common in colder areas.

Contagion

This condition isn't contagious.

Causes

The tendency to develop psoriasis is genetically determined. Researchers have discovered a significantly higher-than-normal incidence of certain human leukocyte antigens in families with psoriasis, suggesting a possible immune disorder. This theory is supported by the presence of many T cells in psoriatic lesions and successful treatment with cyclosporine. Another theory is that psoriasis results from a genetic error of mitotic control. Onset of the disease is also influenced by environmental factors.

Trauma can trigger the isomorphic effect (Koebner's phenomenon) in which lesions develop at sites of injury. Rubbing and scratching stimulate the proliferative process. Infections, especially those resulting from beta-hemolytic streptococci, may cause a flare-up of guttate (drop-shaped) lesions. Other contributing factors include pregnancy, endocrine changes, climate (cold weather tends to exacerbate psoriasis), and emotional stress.

Generally, a skin cell takes 14 days to move from the basal layer to the stratum corneum, where after 14 days of normal wear and tear, it's sloughed off. The life cycle of a normal skin cell is 28 days, compared with only 4 days for a psoriatic skin cell. This markedly shortened cycle doesn't allow time for the cell to mature. Consequently, the stratum corneum becomes thick and flaky, producing the cardinal manifestations of psoriasis.

Clinical presentation

The most common complaint of the patient with psoriasis is itching and occasional pain from dry, cracked, encrusted lesions.

Plaques

Psoriatic lesions are erythematous and usually form well-defined plaques, sometimes covering large areas of the body. Such lesions most commonly appear on the scalp, chest, elbows, knees, back, and buttocks. The plaques consist of characteristic silver scales that either flake off easily or can thicken, covering the lesion. Removal of psoriatic scales frequently produces fine bleeding points (Auspitz sign). Occasionally, small guttate lesions appear, either alone or with plaques; these lesions are typically thin and erythematous with few scales.

Widespread shedding of scales is common in exfoliative or erythrodermic psoriasis and may also develop in chronic psoriasis.

In about 25% of patients, psoriasis spreads to the fingernails, producing small indentations and yellow or brown discolorations. In severe cases, the accumulation of thick, crumbly debris under the nail causes it to separate from the nail bed.

Pustular psoriasis

Rarely, psoriasis becomes pustular, taking one of two forms. In localized pustular (Barber) psoriasis, pustules appear on the palms and soles and remain sterile until opened. In generalized pustular (Von Zumbusch) psoriasis, which often occurs with fever, leukocytosis, and malaise, groups of pustules coalesce to form lakes of pus on red skin. These pustules also remain sterile until opened and commonly involve the tongue and oral mucosa.

Arthritic symptoms

Some patients with psoriasis develop arthritic symptoms, usually in one or more joints of the fingers or toes or sometimes in the sacroiliac joints, which may progress to spondylitis. Such patients may complain of morning stiffness. Joint symptoms show no consistent linkage to the course of the cutaneous manifestations of psoriasis; they demonstrate remissions and exacerbations similar to those of rheumatoid arthritis.

Differential diagnosis

Conditions to consider when making the diagnosis include dermatitis (seborrheic, nummular, atopic, or hand), eczema, candidiasis, tinea, pityriasis, syphilis, Reiter's disease, pustular eruptions, drug eruptions (such as beta blockers, gold, methyldopa), lichen planus, and cancer. The distribution and shape of lesions commonly confirm the diagnosis, with some consideration of patient history.

Diagnostic tests

• *Skin biopsy* on microscopic examination may detect thickened stratum corneum, epidermal hyperplasia, and minimal inflammation.
• *Serum uric acid levels, leukocytes,* and *sedimentation rates* may be elevated because of accelerated nucleic acid degradation, but indications of gout are absent.
• *HLA-Cw6, B-13, and B-w57* may be present in early-onset psoriasis.
• *Rheumatoid factor* isn't present.
• *Complete blood count with differential* may indicate anemia and vitamin B_{12}, folate, and iron deficiencies.

Management

 ALERT Severe and unstable forms like acute pustular psoriasis (Von Zumbusch's) and acute erythroderma require emergency inpatient treatment. Symptoms include frightened appearance, tachycardia, tachypnea, fever that may be high, and burning erythema preceding clusters of tiny pustules that become confluent, forming "lakes" of pus. Treatment includes bed rest, isolation, fluid replacement, and repeated blood cultures for early diagnosis and treatment of secondary infection. Medication options include I.V. antibiotics, retinoids, methotrexate, and psoralen plus ultraviolet–A (PUVA) when tolerated.

• Appropriate treatment depends on the type of psoriasis, the extent of the disease, the patient's response to it, and what effect the disease has on the patient's lifestyle. No permanent cure exists, and all methods of treatment are palliative.
• Be aware that psoriasis can cause psychological problems, including depression and withdrawal from social situations. Pay special attention to the patient's perception of his physical appearance, and offer emotional support.
• To remove psoriatic scales, the patient must apply an occlusive ointment, such as petroleum jelly, salicylic acid preparations, or preparations containing urea. These medications soften the scales, which can then be removed by scrubbing them carefully with a soft brush while bathing.

UVB exposure or solar radiation

Methods to retard rapid cell production include exposure to ultraviolet B (UVB) or natural sunlight to the point of minimal erythema.

A thin layer of petroleum jelly may be applied before UVB exposure (the most common treatment for generalized psoriasis). Exposure time can increase gradually. Outpatient or day treatment with UVB avoids long hospitalizations and prolongs remission.

Drugs
• A potent fluorinated steroid ointment (betamethasone valerate or fluocinolone acetonide) works well except on the face and intertriginous areas. These ointments are applied twice daily, preferably after bathing to facilitate absorption, and with overnight use of occlusive dressings, such as plastic wrap, plastic gloves and booties, a vinyl exercise suit, or corticosteroid-impregnated tape (Cordran tape), under direct medical or nursing supervision. Switching products prevents tachyphylaxis.
• Limit high-potency topical steroids to 2 weeks, avoid occlusive dressings, and taper applications to prevent rebound.
• Small (less than 4.1 cm), stubborn plaques may require intralesional steroid injections (2 to 5 mg/ml triamcinolone acetonide). Injection is intradermal, not subcutaneous (requires pressure to inject, otherwise needle is in subcutaneous tissue).

SPECIAL POPULATIONS
Hypopigmentation at the site can result from steroid injection and is more apparent in darker-pigmented patients.
• Anthralin, combined with a paste mixture, may be used for well-defined plaques but must not be applied to unaffected areas because it causes injury and stains normal skin. Apply petroleum jelly around the affected skin before applying anthralin. Often used concurrently with steroids, anthralin is applied at night and steroids during the day
• Topical vitamin D analogue (calcipotriene) is slower acting (2 months) than steroids but does last. Apply to less than 40% of body surface (not to facial area) and less than 100 g/week.

Goeckerman, Ingram, and PUVA
In a patient with severe chronic psoriasis, the Goeckerman regimen, which combines tar baths and UVB treatments, may help achieve remission and clear the skin in 3 to 5 weeks. The Ingram technique is a variation of this treatment, using anthralin instead of tar. PUVA therapy combines administration of psoralens with exposure to high-intensity UVA.

Other treatments
• Low-dose antihistamines, oatmeal baths, emollients, and open wet dressings may help relieve pruritus. Aspirin and local heat help alleviate the pain of psoriatic arthritis; severe cases may require nonsteroidal anti-inflammatory drugs.
• Therapy for psoriasis of the scalp consists of a tar shampoo followed by application of a steroid lotion. No effective treatment exists for psoriasis of the nails.
• An immunosuppressant (cyclosporine or tacrolimus) is indicated as short-term treatment for recalcitrant psoriases.
• As a last resort, a cytotoxin (usually methotrexate) may help severe, refractory psoriasis.

SPECIAL POPULATIONS
Isotretinoin (Accutane), a retinoid acid derivative, is effective in treating extensive cases of psoriasis. Warn the female patient of child-bearing age about the severe risk of teratogenicity. In addition to signing a special permission form, she'll need monthly measurements of lipid levels and liver function as well as monthly pregnancy tests.
• Many common drugs can exacerbate psoriasis. Monitor hepatic and renal function when using cytotoxic drugs.

Referral or consultation

 COLLABORATION Refer the patient to a dermatologist who specializes in UV therapy for patients with extensive disease. Also refer the patient to a dermatologist before using systemic steroids, before using occlusive dressings with high-potency topical steroids, and for scalp or perineal involvement.

Consult with a doctor for nonresponsiveness to treatment within 2 months, extensive disease, psoriatic arthritis, or inflammatory disease.

Consult with a psychologist or psychiatrist for counseling and coping mechanisms.

Follow-up

Follow up with a monthly focus on examination of skin, effectiveness of treatment, evaluation of psychological health, and adverse drug effects. Monitor for adverse reactions, especially allergic reactions to anthralin, atrophy and acne from steroids, and burning, itching, nausea, and squamous cell carcinomas from PUVA.

Evaluate the patient on methotrexate pretreatment weekly and then monthly for red blood cell, white blood cell, and platelet counts; aspartate aminotransferase; and albumin because cytotoxins may cause hepatic or bone marrow toxicity.

Liver biopsies may be done to assess the effects of methotrexate (pretreatment, after 3 months, and then with every cumulative methotrexate dose of 1.5 g; usually about every 2 years).

Complications

Secondary infection, pustular psoriasis, exfoliative erythrodermatitis, psychological distress, continuous chronic flare-ups, rebound after stopping corticosteroids, thinning of skin, striae, immunocompromise, hypopigmentation, and tachyphylaxis from topical corticosteroids may occur.

Patient teaching

• Teach correct application of prescribed ointments, creams, and lotions. A steroid cream, for example, should be applied in a thin film and rubbed gently into the skin until the cream disappears,
• Instruct the patient to apply all topical medications, especially those containing anthralin and tar, with a downward motion to avoid rubbing them into the follicles. He must wear gloves because anthralin stains and injures the skin. After application, the patient may dust himself with powder to prevent anthralin from rubbing off on his clothes,
• Warn the patient never to put an occlusive dressing over anthralin. Suggest the use of mineral oil and then soap and water to remove anthralin.
• Caution the patient to avoid scrubbing his skin vigorously, to prevent Koebner's phenomenon (appearance of isomorphic lesions).If a medication has been applied to the scales to soften them, suggest that the patient use a soft brush to remove them.
• Caution the patient receiving PUVA therapy to stay out of the sun on the day of treatment and to protect his eyes with sunglasses that screen UVA for 24 hours after treatment. Tell him to wear goggles during exposure to this light.
• Assure the patient that psoriasis isn't contagious and, although exacerbations and remissions occur, they're controllable with treatment. However, there is no cure.
• Because stressful situations tend to exacerbate psoriasis, help the patient learn to cope with these situations.
• Explain the relation between psoriasis and arthritis, but point out that

psoriasis causes no other systemic disturbances.

• Warn the patient to avoid alcoholic beverages, stimulating drugs, indomethacin, lithium, angiotensin-converting enzyme inhibitors, beta blockers, some antibiotics, salicylates or nonsteroidal anti-inflammatory drugs, amiodarone, morphine, procaine, potassium iodide, and antimalarials.

ALERT Tell the patient to call the primary care provider and report persistent, changing, worsening, anxiety-producing, or specific signs and symptoms, including:

– symptoms of acute erythroderma (frightened appearance, racing heartbeat, rapid breathing or shortness of breath, fever that may be high, burning erythema preceding clusters of tiny pustules that run together, forming "lakes" of pus)

– depression

– flare-up

– signs of infection (increasing redness, cloudy or colored drainage, large open areas, swelling).

• Make sure the patient understands his prescribed therapy; provide written instructions to avoid confusion.

Resources

National Psoriasis Foundation : 800-723-9166; *76135.2746@compuserve.com www.healthanswers.com* (Enter "psoriasis" in the search box.)

Scabies

ICD-9-CM 133.0

Scabies is a parasitic skin infection by a mite (*Sarcoptes scabiei*) that causes intense itching. A secondary eczematous dermatitis (classic itch causes scratching, which exacerbates itching, which increases scratching) usually occurs.

Contagion

This contagious skin infestation usually spreads by skin-to-skin contact but also by clothing or bedding. It's usually spread by sexual contact, contact with mite-infested sheets in institutionalized individuals, and close contact (frequently among children under age 6). It's transmitted rarely by fomites because the mite survives only 4 days apart from the host.

Incubation: No symptoms in primary infection for 2 to 6 weeks. Because of prior sensitization, recurrent infestations cause symptoms in 1 to 4 days.

Communicable period: Until after effective application of insecticide. On fomites: 10 days (time for eggs to hatch and mites to starve).

Isolation: Exclude from school or work for 24 hours after effective treatment (5% of infestations require a second treatment after 1 week to eliminate scabies).

 COLLABORATION School or day-care staff should be notified.

Clinical presentation

Generalized itching, mostly at night when mites feed, is almost always present. Lesions, burrows, vesicles, and nodules may occur in the web spaces of fingers and toes, on the wrists and axillae, and in the groin or buttock areas.

 SPECIAL POPULATIONS In elderly people, scabies may be found on the back, and skin may appear to be simply excoriated. Patients with human immunodeficiency virus infection may present with "crusted" scabies that look like psoriasis.

Differential diagnosis

Generalized pruritus with no apparent cause may respond to treatment for scabies. Consider atopic dermatitis, dermatitis herpetiformis, insect bites, pityriasis rosea, prurigo, seborrheic dermatitis, and secondary syphilis.

Diagnostic tests
• Magnifying lens examination may detect a dark point at the end of the burrow (the mite). Place a drop of mineral oil over a lesion and scrape and examine under microscope for mites, eggs, egg casings, and feces. Scraping from under fingernails may be positive.
• If burrows aren't visible, apply ink to an area of rash and then wipe off with alcohol. Burrows become more distinct as the ink gets under the skin.

Management

• It's usually necessary to treat close family and contacts (within the past month).
• If treatment is unsuccessful after 2 applications 1 week apart, consider poor application technique or another diagnosis.

Drugs
• Scabicides (permethrin or crotamiton creams or lotions) are left on 8 to 12 hours (follow product instructions), washed off, and repeated after 1 week if indicated.
• Another scabicide (lindane) may be used; however, some lindane resistant scabies have been reported. This drug shouldn't be used after a bath or by those with extensive dermatitis because of extensive absorption and increased risk of seizures. Lindane can also cause aplastic anemia.
• Antihistamines are used for symptomatic relief of itching only.

• Mupirocin ointment or systemic antimicrobials are used for secondary bacterial infections.

Follow-up
Follow up weekly as needed for persistent or recurring symptoms.

Complications

Eczema and secondary infections may occur.

Patient teaching

• Tell the patient to wash all clothes, bedding, hats, belts, and scarves in hot water and to dry in hot dryer. If any article can't be washed, put it in a plastic bag, tie the bag off, and set it aside for 10 days.
• Advise the patient to check all household members for symptoms (itching, burrows in the skin).
• Explain that itching is an allergic response to excrement, so itching may persist for several weeks after effective treatment.
• Advise the patient not to self-treat more than twice with scabicides unless advised by a clinician. These medications are harmful when used excessively.

 ALERT Tell the patient to call the primary care provider and report persistent, changing, worsening, anxiety-producing, or specific signs and symptoms, including no improvement within 3 days.

Resources
www.healthtouch.com/level1/leaflets/NIAID/NIAID042.htm

Viral rashes

Many viral infections are accompanied by generalized rashes (exanthems) and mucous membrane eruptions (enanthems). They are all contagious and may be difficult to differentiate. Treatment and complications are, however, similar for most viral rashes.

 ALERT For all viral rashes with fever, tell the patient to call the primary care provider for a rash that turns purple or looks like spots of blood under the skin, rash that lasts longer than 3 days, ear pain or tugging on ears, change in mental status such as increasing sleepiness, and fever that isn't controlled with medication.

Enteroviral rashes

ICD-9-CM coxsackievirus 079.2, echovirus 079.1

• Cause virtually any type of rash, most commonly hand-foot-mouth disease (especially in children) caused by coxsackievirus A16
• Responsible for most viral rashes in late summer and early fall

Transmission and precautions
Transmission: Mostly by the fecal-oral route; also in droplet spray and by direct contact with respiratory secretions
Incubation: 3 to 7 days
Communicable period: Present in feces for several weeks
Isolation: Enteric precautions, prompt handwashing after diaper change and other contact; hot water and soap for soiled items

Signs and symptoms
• Infection may begin with abrupt onset of fever, often along with pharyngitis, cervical lymphadenopathy, myalgia, abdominal pain, and GI symptoms.
• Rash usually begins on the face and, within hours, spreads to the trunk and limbs. Lesions persist for up to 7 days and may be erythema-tous, macular, papular, and urticarial. Some echoviruses produce small blanchable papules with a white halo.
• Hand-foot-and-mouth disease begins with up to 2 days of low-grade fever and malaise before the appearance of small red 1- to 3-cm macules that vesiculate and ulcerate in the mouth, usually sparing the lips; pain may interfere with eating. Dorsal and volar aspects of the hands and feet may be involved. Rash usually resolves in 7 to 10 days.

Treatment and complications
• No antiviral therapy exists.
• For symptomatic relief, give antipyretics and analgesics or nonsteroidal antiinflammatory drugs but *never* aspirin.
• Encourage fluid intake to prevent dehydration, including cool liquids or dairy products that are soothing and nutritious.
• Avoid hot, spicy, salty, or acidic foods to decrease local irritation.
• Advise good oral hygiene, including careful brushing twice daily to decrease the risk of secondary infection. Suggest a mouth rinse of ¼ tsp of salt in a glass of warm water.
• Comfort measures for children include holding, rocking, and distraction.
• Complications aren't common or life-threatening.

Erythema infectiosum

ICD-9-CM 057.0

• Called "slapped cheek" because of its appearance
• Common, benign, self-limited, highly contagious; affects mainly children under age 12
• Caused by human parvovirus B19

Transmission and precautions
Transmission: Primarily by direct contact with respiratory secretions
Incubation: 2 weeks
Communicable period: Highest rate of transmission precedes rash onset; immunocompromised people may remain contagious for months or longer.
Isolation: Most transmission occurs before symptoms occur, and exclusion isn't indicated. However, exclude children from school or day care until fever dissipates.

Signs and symptoms
• A fine, lacy rash appears abruptly on the cheeks, causing a "slapped cheek" or "sunburn" appearance. It intensifies with heat, friction, exercise, or emotional outbursts and disappears in less than 4 days.
• Over a few days, the rash spreads to the rest of the body. Around day six, fading begins with central clearing, leading to a marbled appearance. This may last from 1 to several weeks or may subside and recur intermittently over a 2-month period.
• Other symptoms may include pruritus and arthralgias (more common in adults).

Treatment and complications
• No treatment is necessary except antipyretics for fever and nonsteroidal anti-inflammatories (*never* aspirin) for arthralgias.
• Complications are uncommon except in patients with hemolytic anemias or hydrops fetalis. These patients are at risk for aplastic crisis (symptoms include dyspnea, fatigue, ecchymoses, pallor, and palpitations) and may require transfusion.

Roseola infantum
ICD-9-CM Rose, infantile 057.8, epidemic 056.9

• Common, benign, self-limited; most common viral rash in children under age 3
• Caused by human herpes virus 6

Transmission and precautions
Transmission: Uncertain; believed to be in salivary secretions, primarily by adults
Incubation: 5 to 15 days
Communicable period: Until rash resolves
Isolation: Not recommended

Signs and symptoms
• The prodrome may consist of 3 to 5 days of high fever, mild constitutional symptoms, and pharyngitis, or the patient may be asymptomatic.
• A rash appears abruptly up to 2 days after fever breaks, generally as the patient is feeling better. Lesions are nonpruritic, discrete pink macules and papules, 2 to 5 mm in diameter, mainly on the trunk and neck.
• The rash resolves within hours or up to 2 days; lesions aren't itchy or uncomfortable.
• History and physical examination rule out other sources of fever including otitis media, urinary tract infection, meningitis, and occult bacteremia.

Treatment and complications
• No treatment is necessary except antipyretics (*never* aspirin) for fever.
• Recommend tepid sponge baths for fever that isn't controlled with medication.

Rubella
ICD-9-CM 056

• Also called German measles or 3-day measles
• Typically occurs in childhood or early adulthood

• Dangerous for pregnant women; causes birth defects
• Mild, self-limited, highly contagious
• Caused by rubella virus

Transmission and precautions
Transmission: In droplet spray, by direct contact with respiratory secretions, in urine of infants, and on items soiled with these secretions
Incubation: 14 to 23 days
Communicable period: 1 week before to at least 4 days after rash appears
Isolation: Avoid contact with soiled articles, prevent exposure of nonimmune pregnant women, exclude children from school and adults from work for 7 days after onset of rash

Signs and symptoms
• 80% of cases are asymptomatic.
• Mild upper respiratory and constitutional symptoms may occur, most commonly pain on lateral and upward eye movement.
• Lesions appear as discrete pink-red macules and papules that start on the face, begin clearing within a day, and resolve by day three. They're differentiated from rubeola by pink-red color (rather than purplish-red) and rapid appearance changes, commonly within hours.
• Other symptoms include petechiae on the soft palate and tender lymphadenopathy.

Treatment and complications
• No antiviral treatment exists, but prevention is possible with vaccination.
• Complications include congenital birth defects if a pregnant patient contracts the virus, particularly during the first trimester.
• Report all cases to local health authorities.

Rubeola

ICD-9-CM 055

• Also called measles
• Self-limited, systemic, highly contagious
• Caused by a paramyxovirus

Transmission and precautions
Transmission: In droplet spray, by direct contact with respiratory secretions, and on items freshly soiled with these secretions
Incubation: 7 to 18 days
Communicable period: 2 to 3 days before to 4 days after rash appears
Isolation: Respiratory isolation for 4 days after rash appears; keep children home for at least 4 days after rash appears

Signs and symptoms
• Stage 1: The patient is asymptomatic or shows mild prodromal symptoms.
• Stage 2 (prodrome): Transient Koplik's spots appear, usually preceding rash by 2 days, along with brassy cough, coryza, conjunctivitis, fever, photophobia, and constitutional symptoms.
• Stage 3: Erythematous, macular, but nonpruritic lesions appear at the hairline and spread downward, generally reaching the feet by the day two or three and becoming increasingly papular and confluent.
• Fever and constitutional symptoms peak as rash starts spreading down the body.
• Lesions fade in order of appearance over 3 to 6 days and may leave desquamated areas.

Treatment and complications
• No antiviral therapy exists, however prevention is possible with vaccination.

• Symptomatic relief includes antipyretics and analgesics (but *never* aspirin).
• Encourage fluids to prevent dehydration.
• Complications include otitis media, pneumonia, and encephalitis. Compared to all viral rashes, neurologic complications are most common in rubeola (approximately 2:1,000 cases).
• Report all cases to local health authorities.

CHAPTER

6

Disease management

Initiating a treatment plan

Selected disorders

Angina

ICD-9-CM stable 413, unstable 411.1, Prinzmetal's 413.1

Angina is caused by a net deficit in the oxygen supply and demand of myocardial tissue. Angina is the most common symptom of coronary artery disease (CAD), which is near epidemic in the Western world. Another type of angina follows coronary artery spasm, where the spontaneous, sustained contraction of one or more coronary arteries causes ischemia and dysfunction of the heart muscle. This disorder causes Prinzmetal's angina and can even cause myocardial infarction (MI) in patients with unoccluded coronary arteries.

 SPECIAL POPULATIONS
CAD occurs more often in men than in women, in whites, and in middle-aged and elderly people. In the past, this disorder rarely affected women who were premenopausal; that is no longer the case, perhaps because many women now take oral contraceptives, smoke cigarettes, and are employed in stressful jobs that formerly were held exclusively by men. (See *Preventing heart disease,* pages 162 and 163.)

Causes

Coronary atherosclerosis is angina's usual cause. In this form of arteriosclerosis, fatty, fibrous plaques narrow the coronary artery lumen, reduce the volume of blood flowing through them, and lead to myocardial ischemia. Plaque formation also promotes thrombosis, which can provoke MI.

Uncommon causes of reduced coronary artery blood flow include dissecting aneurysms, infectious vasculitis, syphilis, congenital defects in the coronary vascular system, acute MI, and coronary artery spasms.

The patient history, including the frequency and duration of angina and the presence of associated risk factors, is crucial in evaluating CAD.

Clinical presentation

Angina is usually described as a burning, squeezing, or tight feeling in the substernal or precordial chest that may radiate to the left arm, neck, jaw, or shoulder blade. The patient typically clenches his fist over his chest or rubs his left arm when describing the pain, which may be accompanied by nausea, vomiting, fainting, sweating, and cool extremities. Anginal episodes most often follow physical exertion but may also follow emotional excitement, exposure to cold, or a large meal.

History elicits *O*nset, *L*ocation, *D*uration, *C*haracteristic, *A*ggravating factors, *R*elieving factors, *T*reatments tried, and *S*econdary gains (mnemonic: *OLDCARTS*). Patients with myocardial ischemia usually have exertional discomfort and relief with rest. Angina has three major forms:
• Stable angina causes pain that is predictable in frequency and duration and can be relieved with nitrates and rest.
• Unstable angina causes pain that increases in frequency and duration. It is more easily induced.
• Prinzmetal's angina causes unpredictable coronary artery spasm.

Unstable angina or severe and prolonged anginal pain generally suggests myocardial ischemia, with potentially fatal arrhythmias and mechanical failure.

Examination focuses on differentiating unstable angina.
• *General:* distressed appearance and elevated blood pressure.
• *Skin:* pallor, diaphoresis.

- *Head, eyes, ears, nose, and throat:* retinopathy, jugular vein distention, and thyromegaly.
- *Chest:* 3rd or 4th heart sound, murmur, dyspnea, or crackles.
- *Abdomen:* epigastric discomfort.
- *Extremities:* edema and peripheral pulses.
- *Neurologic:* generalized weakness, change in mental status.

Differential diagnosis

ALERT Myocardial ischemia and MI may present with symptoms, such as a feeling of pressure in the chest, throat or jaw pain, shoulder and back pains, nausea, and shortness of breath. Risk factors for CAD include smoking, diabetes, hypertension, dyslipidemia, and family history.

Exertional pain relieved with rest indicates stable angina or psychogenic pain. Psychogenic pain presents with many noncardiac symptoms as well. Pain aggravated by deep inspiration or cough suggests a pleural, pericardial (pain relieved by leaning forward), or noncardiac muscle cause; focal pain suggests costochondritis. Abrupt onset and dyspnea suggests pneumothorax or pulmonary embolism (particularly if the patient has a high thromboembolitic risk). Abrupt onset of tearing pain suggests dissecting aneurysm, particularly if the person has hypertension.

Other possible causes of chest pain include esophageal spasm, thoracic outlet syndrome, pericarditis, spine disease, pulmonary embolus, pulmonary hypertension, pneumothorax, shoulder arthropathy, peptic ulcer, cholecystitis, costochondritis, and some anxiety and panic disorders. Of course, other causes of decreased blood flow (as discussed above) must be considered also.

Diagnostic tests

- Cardiac enzymes may indicate MI.
- Complete blood count shows anemia, which can exacerbate angina.
- Lipid levels are likely to show high total cholesterol, high low-density lipoproteins, and low high-density lipoproteins.
- Electrocardiography (ECG) during angina may show ischemia and arrhythmias such as premature ventricular contractions, but it is apt to show normal results when the patient is pain-free.
- A treadmill or bicycle exercise test may provoke chest pain and ECG signs of myocardial ischemia (ST segment depression).
- Coronary angiography reveals narrowing or occlusion of the coronary artery, with possible collateral circulation.
- Myocardial perfusion imaging with thallium 201 or Cardiolite during treadmill exercise detects ischemic areas of the myocardium, visualized as "cold spots."
- X-ray may detect fractures, pneumonia, pulmonary embolus, pneumothorax, or tuberculosis.
- Lung ventilation-perfusion scan indicates the probability of a pulmonary embolus.

Management

Acute

Hospitalize patients with unstable angina. Order frequent monitoring of blood pressure and heart rate. Obtain an ECG during anginal episodes and before administering nitroglycerin or other nitrates. Note the duration of pain, amount of medication required to relieve it, and accompanying symptoms.

Obstructive lesions may necessitate coronary artery bypass surgery and the use of vein grafts. Angioplasty may be performed during cardiac

(Text continues on page 164.)

PREVENTING HEART DISEASE

Heart disease in adults can be prevented by primary measures, used for adults without current evidence of heart disease. All adults ages 20 and older should be tested for serum cholesterol levels at least every 5 years. Results of lipoprotein levels and the number of patient risk factors involved help to determine treatment options.

Risk factors include being a male age 45 or older; being a female age 55 or older; having premature menopause without estrogen replacement therapy; a history of myocardial infarction (MI) or sudden death before age 55 in father or other immediate male relative; a history of MI before age 65 in mother or other immediate female relative; current cigarette smoking; the presence of hypertension or diabetes mellitus; or having a low high-density lipoprotein cholesterol (HDL-C) level (below 35 mg/dl).

The diagram below illustrates the steps in primary and secondary prevention in adults. All cholesterol levels are measured in milligrams per deciliter.

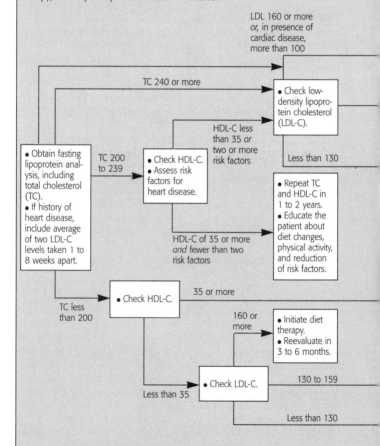

Based on recommendations of the Second Report of the National Cholesterol Education Program Expert Panel on Detection, Evaluation, and Treatment of High Blood Cholesterol in Adults. (*JAMA* 269:3015-23, 1993.)

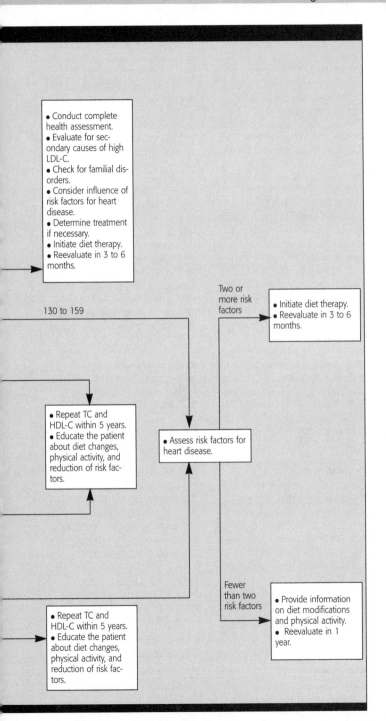

- Conduct complete health assessment.
- Evaluate for secondary causes of high LDL-C.
- Check for familial disorders.
- Consider influence of risk factors for heart disease.
- Determine treatment if necessary.
- Initiate diet therapy.
- Reevaluate in 3 to 6 months.

Two or more risk factors

- Initiate diet therapy.
- Reevaluate in 3 to 6 months.

130 to 159

- Repeat TC and HDL-C within 5 years.
- Educate the patient about diet changes, physical activity, and reduction of risk factors.

- Assess risk factors for heart disease.

Fewer than two risk factors

- Provide information on diet modifications and physical activity.
- Reevaluate in 1 year.

- Repeat TC and HDL-C within 5 years.
- Educate the patient about diet changes, physical activity, and reduction of risk factors.

catheterization to compress fatty deposits and relieve occlusion in patients with no calcification and partial occlusion. A certain risk is associated with this procedure, but its morbidity is lower than that for surgery. Percutaneous transluminal coronary angioplasty may be done in combination with coronary stenting. Stents provide a framework to hold an artery open by securing flaps of tunica media and intima against the artery wall.

After catheterization, review the expected course of treatment with the patient and family. A collagen substance (Vasoseal, Dengroseal) may be used at the femoral arterial puncture site. Tell the patient to expect to feel a hard bump the size of a large pea.

Check for signs of ischemia and arrhythmias. Also, observe for and treat chest pain and possible dye reactions. Order frequent monitoring of the catheter site for bleeding, distal pulse checks, blood pressure, intake and output, breath sounds, chest tube drainage, and ECG. Order plenty of fluids, bed rest for 8 hours, and chest physiotherapy, and guide the patient in coughing and deep-breathing exercises.

General

The goal of treatment in patients with angina is to reduce myocardial oxygen demand or increase oxygen supply. The areas in which to intervene and treat chronic, stable angina, as offered by the American Heart Association and the American College of Cardiology, are summarized by an *ABCDE* mnemonic: *A*spirin and *A*ntianginal therapy, *B*eta-adrenergic blocker and *B*lood pressure, *C*igarettes and *C*holesterol, *D*iet and *D*iabetes, *E*ducation and *E*xercise.

Medication

Therapy consists primarily of nitrates such as nitroglycerin (given sublin-

gually, orally, transdermally, or topically in ointment form), isosorbide dinitrate (given sublingually or orally), beta-adrenergic blockers (atenolol) given orally, or calcium channel blockers (verapamil) given orally. Combination therapy reduces the amount of drug from each class of antihypertensive agent, with the goal of gaining control of blood pressure while minimizing adverse effects.

Other preventive actions include control of hypertension (with centrally acting adrenergic blocking agents such as methyldopa or with diuretics such as hydrochlorothiazide), control of elevated serum cholesterol or triglyceride levels (with antilipemics, such as cerivastatin [Baycol], atorvastatin [Lipitor], pravastatin [Pravachol], or simvastatin [Zocor]), and measures to minimize platelet aggregation and the danger of blood clots (with aspirin).

Referral or consultation

 COLLABORATION Refer the patient immediately to a doctor for suspected MI, dissecting aneurysm, or severe pain and respiratory distress.

Refer to a doctor for major chest trauma, pneumothorax, pulmonary embolus, or severe infection with dehydration or sepsis.

Refer to a cardiologist for evaluation and a treatment plan.

Refer to a physical therapist after the patient is cleared by the cardiologist for an exercise program.

Follow-up

Follow-up is every 3 to 6 months for stable angina, more frequently for changes in the clinical picture.

Complications

Complications of angina include MI, arrhythmia, heart failure, and cardiac arrest.

Patient teaching

- Advise the patient that the primary cause of angina is CAD.
- Stress the need to follow the prescribed drug regimen and to eat a low-fat, low-cholesterol diet.
- Encourage regular, moderate exercise.
- Refer the patient to a self-help program to stop smoking.
- Advise the patient to minimize stress.
- Instruct the patient to keep nitroglycerin available for immediate use.

 ALERT Tell the patient to call the primary care provider to report any chest, arm, and neck pain; dyspnea; diaphoresis; sudden change in mental status; and sudden weakness.

Resources

- American Heart Association: 800-AHA-USA-1 or *www.americanheart.org*
- National Heart, Lung and Blood Institute: 301-251-1222 or *www.nhlbi.nih.gov*

Asthma

ICD-9-CM extrinsic 493.0, intrinsic 493.1

A potentially reversible lung disease, asthma is characterized by obstruction or narrowing of the airways, which are typically inflamed and hyperresponsive to a variety of stimuli. It may resolve spontaneously or with treatment. Its symptoms range from mild wheezing and dyspnea to life-threatening respiratory failure. Symptoms of bronchial airway obstruction may persist between acute episodes.

Causes

Although asthma can strike at any age, half of all cases first occur in children under age 10; in this age-group, asthma affects twice as many boys as girls. Asthma is increasing in prevalence and severity in Black and Hispanic patients.

Extrinsic and intrinsic asthma

Asthma that results from a sensitivity to specific external allergens is known as *extrinsic* or atopic asthma. In cases in which the allergen isn't obvious, asthma is referred to as *intrinsic* or nonatopic. Allergens that cause extrinsic asthma include pollen, animal dander, house dust or mold, kapok or feather pillows, and food additives containing sulfites.

Extrinsic asthma usually begins in childhood and is accompanied by other manifestations of atopy (type 1, immunoglobulin E [IgE]–mediated allergy), such as eczema and allergic rhinitis.

In intrinsic asthma, no extrinsic allergen can be identified. Most cases are preceded by a severe respiratory infection. Irritants, emotional stress, fatigue, exposure to noxious fumes, and endocrine, temperature, and humidity changes may aggravate intrinsic asthma attacks. In many asthmatic patients, intrinsic and extrinsic asthma coexist.

Other asthma triggers

Several drugs and chemicals may provoke an asthma attack without involving the IgE pathway. Apparently, they trigger release of mast-cell mediators through prostaglandin inhibition. Examples of these substances include aspirin, various nonsteroidal anti-inflammatory drugs (such as indomethacin and mefenamic acid), and tartrazine, a yellow food dye.

Exercise may also provoke an asthma attack. In exercise-induced asthma, bronchospasm may follow heat and moisture loss in the upper airways.

Two-phase allergic response

When the patient inhales an allergenic substance, sensitized IgE antibodies trigger mast-cell degranulation in the lung interstitium, thereby releasing histamine, cytokines, prostaglandins, thromboxanes, leukotrienes, and eosinophil chemotactic factors. Histamine then attaches to receptor sites in the larger bronchi, causing irritation, inflammation, and edema. In the late phase, there is an influx of inflammatory cells and eosinophils that provide additional inflammatory mediators and contribute to local injury.

Clinical presentation

An asthma attack may begin dramatically, with simultaneous onset of many severe symptoms, or insidiously, with gradually increasing respiratory distress. It typically includes progressively worsening shortness of breath, cough, wheezing, and chest tightness or some combination of these symptoms.

During an acute attack, the cough sounds tight and dry. As the attack subsides, tenacious mucoid sputum is produced (except in young children, who don't expectorate). Characteristic wheezing may be accompanied by coarse rhonchi, but fine crackles aren't heard unless they're associated with a related complication. Between acute attacks, breath sounds may be normal.

The intensity of breath sounds in symptomatic asthma is typically reduced. A prolonged phase of forced expiration is typical of airflow obstruction. Evidence of lung hyperinflation (use of accessory muscles, for example) is particularly common in children. Acute attacks may be accompanied by tachycardia, tachypnea, and diaphoresis. In severe attacks, the patient may be unable to speak more than a few words without pausing for breath. Cyanosis, confusion, and lethargy indicate the onset of life-threatening status asthmaticus and respiratory failure.

History may reveal a family history of allergies and asthma as well as patterns, such as seasonal or episodic occurrence, occurrence outdoors or with exercise, frequency, impact on daily activities, such trigger factors as pets and exercise, previous treatments and effectiveness of each, and family dynamics. It also may reveal associated conditions, including sinusitis, rhinitis, allergies, atopic dermatitis, nasal polyposis, gastroesophageal reflux disease (GERD) and, usually, a respiratory infection immediately preceding symptom onset.

Examination focuses on severity of respiratory distress first, then differentials.
• *General:* level of distress
• *Skin:* diaphoresis or cyanotic, "allergic shiners" (dark smudges under the eyes)
• *Head, eyes, ears, nose, and throat:* nasal flaring or discharge, frontal and maxillary tenderness, postnasal discharge, pharyngeal cobblestone appearance, unilateral purulent nasal discharge, which suggests presence of a foreign body
• *Chest:* accessory muscle usage, retractions, adventitious breath sounds, prolonged expirations, unilateral wheeze, which suggests an aspirated foreign body

Differential diagnosis

Other conditions to consider include foreign body aspiration (particularly if unilateral wheeze or unilateral nasal mucopurulent drainage is present), cystic fibrosis, tumors of the bronchi or mediastinum, and anxiety and acute viral bronchitis; in adults, other causes include obstructive pulmonary disease, heart failure, pulmonary embolus, tuberculosis, mitral valve prolapse, and epiglottitis.

Diagnostic tests
Laboratory studies in patients with asthma often show abnormalities:
• Arterial blood gas analysis provides the best indications of an attack's severity. In acutely severe asthma, partial pressure of arterial oxygen is less than 60 mm Hg; partial pressure of arterial carbon dioxide ($PaCO_2$) is 40 mm Hg or more, and pH is usually decreased.
• Complete blood count with differential reveals increased eosinophil count.
• Immunoglobulins screen indicates immunodeficiency and allergic bronchopulmonary aspergillosis.
• Purified protein derivative test may detect tuberculosis.
• Peak expiratory flow rate (PEFR) less than 70% of patient's baseline is an indication for treatment.
• Pulmonary function tests (PFTs) reveal signs of airway obstruction (decreased peak expiratory flow rates [PEVR] and forced expiratory volume in 1 second), low-normal or decreased vital capacity, and increased total lung and residual capacity. However, pulmonary function studies may be normal between attacks.
• Pulse oximetry may reveal decreased arterial oxygen saturation.
• Chest X-rays may show hyperinflation with areas of focal atelectasis, or they may be normal.

Management

 ALERT Acute asthma is treated by decreasing bronchoconstriction, reducing bronchial airway edema, and increasing pulmonary ventilation.

(See *Determining asthma attack severity,* page 168.)

 ALERT PEFR less than 60% of patient's baseline indicates the need for emergency care.
Acute attacks that don't respond to self-treatment may require hospital care, beta$_2$-adrenergic agonists by inhalation or subcutaneous injection (in three doses in 60 to 90 minutes), and oxygen for hypoxemia. If the patient responds poorly, call for emergency medical transport to a medical treatment facility.

General
If asthma is known to be caused by a particular antigen, it may be treated by desensitizing the patient through a series of injections of limited amounts of the antigen. The aim is to curb the patient's immune response to the antigen. Develop a prearranged plan with the patient and family for stepwise progression of medications during exacerbations.

Medication
If asthma results from an infection, antibiotics are prescribed. Drug therapy, which is most effective when begun soon after the onset of signs and symptoms, usually includes:
• bronchodilators to decrease bronchoconstriction; for example, the methylxanthines (theophylline and aminophylline) and the beta$_2$-adrenergic agonists (albuterol and terbutaline).
• corticosteroids (hydrocortisone sodium succinate, methylprednisolone, prednisone, and beclomethasone) for their anti-inflammatory and immunosuppressive effects, which decrease inflammation and edema of the airways.
• cromolyn and nedocromil to help prevent the release of the chemical mediators (histamine and leukotrienes) that cause bronchoconstriction.

DETERMINING ASTHMA ATTACK SEVERITY

Mild asthma	Moderate asthma	Severe asthma	Respiratory failure
Signs and symptoms during acute phase			
• Brief wheezing, coughing, dyspnea with activity • Infrequent nocturnal coughing or wheezing • Adequate air exchange • Intermittent, brief (less than 1 hour) wheezing, cough, or dyspnea once or twice a week • Asymptomatic between attacks	• Respiratory distress at rest • Hyperpnea • Marked coughing and wheezing • Air exchange normal or below normal • Exacerbations that may last several days	• Marked respiratory distress • Marked wheezing or absent breath sounds • Pulsus paradoxus greater than 10 mm Hg • Chest wall contractions • Continuous symptoms • Frequent exacerbations	• Severe respiratory distress • Impaired consciousness • Severe wheezing or silent chest • Use of accessory muscles of respiration • Prominent pulsus paradoxus (30 to 50 mm Hg)
Diagnostic test results			
• Forced expiratory volume in 1 second (FEV_1) or peak flow 80% of normal values • pH normal or increased • Partial pressure of arterial oxygen (PaO_2) normal or decreased • Partial pressure of arterial carbon dioxide ($PaCO_2$) normal or decreased • Chest X-ray normal	• FEV_1 or peak flow 60% to 80% of normal values; may vary 20% to 30% with symptoms • pH generally elevated • PaO_2 increased • $PaCO_2$ generally decreased • Chest X-ray shows hyperinflation	• FEV_1 or peak flow < 60% of normal values; may normally vary 20% to 30% with routine medications and up to 50% with exacerbations • pH normal or reduced • PaO_2 decreased • $PaCO_2$ normal or increased • Chest X-ray may show hyperinflation	• FEV_1 or peak flow < 25% of normal values • pH decreased • PaO_2 < 60 mm Hg • $PaCO_2$ > 40 mm Hg
Other assessment findings			
• One attack per week (or none) • Positive response to bronchodilator therapy within 24 hours • No signs of asthma between episodes • No sleep interruption • No hyperventilation • Minimal evidence of airway obstruction • Minimal or no increase in lung volume	• Symptoms occurring more than two times weekly • Coughing and wheezing between episodes • Diminished exercise tolerance • Possible sleep interruption • Increased lung volumes	• Frequent severe attacks • Daily wheezing • Poor exercise tolerance • Frequent sleep interruption • Bronchodilator therapy not completely reversing airway obstruction • Markedly increased lung volumes	• Cyanosis • Tachycardia

- leukotriene-receptor antagonists (zafirlukast, montelukast), which interfere with inflammatory leukotriene response.
- anticholinergic bronchodilators (such as ipratropium), which block acetylcholine, another chemical mediator.

For the most part, medical treatment of asthma attacks must be tailored to each patient. However, the following treatments are generally used.

Chronic mild asthma
- A beta$_2$-adrenergic agonist is given by metered-dose inhaler (alone or with cromolyn) before exercise and exposure to an allergen or other stimuli to prevent symptoms. The drug is used every 3 to 4 hours if symptoms occur.

Chronic moderate asthma
- Initial treatment may include an inhaled beta-adrenergic bronchodilator, an inhaled corticosteroid, and cromolyn. Anticholinergic bronchodilators may also be added. If symptoms persist, inhaled corticosteroid dosage may be increased, and sustained-release theophylline or an oral beta$_2$-adrenergic agonist (or both) may be added. Short courses of oral corticosteroids may also be used.

Chronic severe asthma
- Initially, around-the-clock oral bronchodilator therapy with a long-acting theophylline or a beta$_2$-adrenergic agonist may be required, supplemented with an inhaled beta$_2$-adrenergic agonist and an inhaled corticosteroid with or without cromolyn. An oral corticosteroid such as prednisone may be added in acute exacerbations.

Referral or consultation
 COLLABORATION If the patient has a history of hospitalization for acute exacerbation or a lack of response to treatment, or if he requires additional diagnostic testing, refer him to a pulmonologist.

Follow-up
After initial diagnosis and treatment to achieve a stable clinical picture, see the patient weekly for 2 weeks, every other week for the next two visits, then once every 3 months.

Complications
Atelectasis, pneumonia, pneumothorax, acute exacerbations, and adverse effects of medication are possible complications.

Patient teaching
- If the patient is taking corticosteroids, advise him to minimize adverse effects of long-term use of these drugs by alternate-day dosage or the use of prescribed inhaled corticosteroids.
- If the patient is taking corticosteroids by inhaler, advise him to watch for signs of candidal infection in the mouth and pharynx. Using an extender device and rinsing the mouth afterward may prevent this.
- Teach patients with moderate to severe chronic disease to use an extender device to facilitate delivery of inhaled medications.
- Keep the room temperature comfortable, and use an air conditioner or a fan in hot, humid weather.
- Instruct the patient to control exercise-induced asthma by using a bronchodilator or cromolyn 30 minutes before exercise. Also instruct him to use pursed-lip breathing while exercising.

USING A METERED-DOSE INHALER

When instructing your patient about proper metered-dose inhaler (MDI) use, include these points:

- Shake the MDI well before use.
- Hold the MDI mouthpiece about 1½" to 2" (38 to 51 mm) from the open mouth.
- Exhale normally, then begin slow, steady inspirations through the mouth.
- While inhaling slowly, squeeze firmly on the MDI while continuing to breathe in (one deep steady breath, not several shallow ones).
- Hold the breath for 10 seconds before exhaling.
- Breathe normally for several breaths before administering a second dose.
- After using a corticosteroid MDI, rinse the mouth with water.

Note: When using an extender or spacer device, follow the same routine as above, with the MDI mouthpiece inserted in one end of the spacer and the other end placed in the mouth. Many spacers are equipped with a small whistle that sounds if the dose is being inhaled too fast.

- Teach the patient and his family to avoid known allergens and irritants (pollutants, dust mites, molds, animals).
- Describe prescribed drugs, including their names, dosages, actions, adverse effects, and special instructions.
- Teach the patient diaphragmatic and pursed-lip breathing as well as effective coughing techniques.
- Urge the patient to drink at least 3 qt (3 L) of fluids daily to help loosen secretions and maintain hydration.
- Teach the patient how to use a metered-dose inhaler. (See *Using a metered-dose inhaler.*)
- If the patient has difficulty using an inhaler, he may need an extender device to optimize drug delivery and lower the risk of candidal infection with orally inhaled corticosteroids.
- If the patient has moderate to severe asthma, explain how to use a peak flow meter to measure the degree of airway obstruction. Tell him to keep a record of peak flow readings and to bring it to medical appointments. Explain the importance of calling the doctor immediately if the peak flow drops suddenly. (A drop can signal severe respiratory problems.)
- Instruct the patient on the prearranged plan for exacerbations as defined by PEFR and the patient's baseline.
- Emphasize the need for annual influenza immunization.

 ALERT Tell the patient to call the primary care provider to report any troublesome signs and symptoms, including:
- fever higher than 100° F (37.8° C), chest pain, shortness of breath without coughing or exercising, or uncontrollable coughing (An uncontrollable asthma attack requires immediate attention.)
- PEFR less than 70% of the patient's baseline
- symptoms continuing more than 4 hours despite following the management plan
- fever above 102.5° F (39° C) or cough producing green/brown/dark yellow mucus
- Increasing shortness of breath.

If breathing becomes rapid or increasingly difficult, the patient is extremely drowsy or won't respond, his lips become dusky or blue, or he won't swallow and starts to drool, activate emergency medical services.

Resources

- American Academy of Allergy Asthma and Immunology: 800-822-2762
- American Lung Association: 800-LUNG-USA or *www.lungusa.com*

• Asthma and Allergy Foundation of America: 800-7-ASTHMA
• National Heart, Lung and Blood Institute: 301-251-1222 or *www. nhlbi.nih.gov*

Breast cancer

ICD-9-CM 174.9

Overgrowth of neoplastic cells is classified as invasive (infiltrating) or noninvasive (in situ). Breast cancer is the second most common killer of women ages 35 to 54, but it occurs most commonly after age 50.

Causes

The cause of breast cancer is unknown, but its prevalence in women implicates estrogen. It spreads by way of the lymphatic system and the bloodstream, through the right heart to the lungs, and eventually to the other breast, the chest wall, liver, bone, and brain. Survival time for breast cancer is based on tumor size and spread; the number of involved nodes is the single most important factor in predicting survival time. High risk factors include personal history of breast cancer; atypical hyperplasia on previous biopsy; and a strong maternal family history of breast, ovarian, or prostate cancer. Moderate risk factors include advancing age; menarche before age 12 or menopause after age 55; nulliparity; and first pregnancy after age 30. Other possible risk factors are exogenous estrogen use, high-fat diet, and alcohol or nicotine use.

Clinical presentation

The disease may present with a palpable breast mass or abnormal mammogram without palpable mass, dimpling, nipple changes (retraction, discharge, ulceration), color and skin texture changes (thickened skin with enlarged pores is known as *peau d'orange* [orange peel] sign), breast enlargement, axillary mass, and breast or bone burning or itching.

The patient history includes individual risk factors and use of oral contraceptives. Examination focuses on the suspected mass; illustrate it in the chart and label appropriately to allow future comparisons.

Differential diagnosis

The disease may manifest as a benign, proliferative, or malignant mass. Benign growths include abscesses, hematomas, and fibroadenomas. Proliferative masses include fibrocystic tissue and hyperplasia without malignancy.

The most reliable method of detecting breast cancer is the monthly breast self-examination (BSE), or a significant other may notice or feel a change in breast tissue. Suspicious signs or symptoms should be followed by immediate evaluation.

Diagnostic tests

• Mammography is indicated if physical examination suggests breast cancer. All women should have a baseline mammogram at ages 35 to 39 and then have the test every 1 to 2 years from ages 40 to 49 and annually after age 50. Women who have a family history of breast cancer and those who have had unilateral breast cancer need an annual mammogram.
• Ultrasound of the breast can distinguish a cyst or abscess from a tumor.
• Biopsy can detect and treat intraductal papilloma.
• Fine-needle aspiration can detect fibroadenoma (refer to surgeon).
• BRCA-1 and BRCA-2 genetic testing should be ordered for all women who test positive for cancer; if the test is

positive for the gene, family members should be notified so they can decide whether they wish to be tested.

Management

Acute

Postmastectomy care

Prevent lymphedema of the arm, an early complication of treatments involving lymph node dissection. Teach the patient to prevent lymphedema by exercising the hand and arm and avoiding activities that might cause infection in the affected hand or arm (infection increases the chance of developing lymphedema). Also, avoid using that arm for any I.V. lines, blood sampling, or blood pressure measurements. Such prevention is very important because lymphedema can't be treated effectively. Positioning a small pillow under the arm provides comfort and elevation.

Help the patient contact support groups. The American Cancer Society's Reach to Recovery group can provide instruction, emotional support, and counseling as well as a list of area stores that sell prostheses. Reach for Recovery will visit hospitalized patients.

Reinforce the importance of BSE and annual mammograms.

 COLLABORATION Provide referral to a surgeon, oncologist, or plastic surgeon as needed.

General

Assess the patient's feelings about her illness, and determine what she knows about it and what she expects.

After diagnosis, anticipate the need for a chest X-ray, bone scan and liver imaging, hormonal receptor assay, and axillary lymph node sampling to check for metastasis and determine the best treatment plan.

Much controversy exists over breast cancer treatments. In choosing therapy, the patient and doctor should consider the stage of the disease, the woman's age and menopausal status, and the disfiguring effects of the surgery. Treatment for breast cancer may include one or any combination of the following.

Surgery

• *Mastectomy or lumpectomy:* Radiation therapy is often combined with this surgery.
• *Lumpectomy and dissection of the axillary lymph nodes:* The tumor and axillary lymph nodes are removed, leaving the breast intact.
• *Simple mastectomy:* The breast is removed but not the lymph nodes or pectoral muscles. A *modified radical mastectomy* removes the breast and the axillary lymph nodes. After a mastectomy, reconstructive surgery can create a breast mound if the patient desires it and doesn't have evidence of advanced disease.

Medication

• Cytotoxic chemotherapy (fluorouracil)
• Hormones (tamoxifen)

Radiation

Used before or after tumor removal, primary radiation therapy is effective for small tumors in early stages with no evidence of distant metastasis; it's also used to prevent or treat local recurrence. Presurgical radiation to the breast in inflammatory breast cancer helps make tumors more surgically manageable.

Referral or consultation

Refer the patient to a surgeon with experience in breast surgery for biopsy, needle aspiration for cytologic evaluation, or possible surgery, and refer her to an oncologist for treatment, surgery, and counseling.

Follow-up

Provide follow-up as recommended by the oncologist and with the primary care provider (PCP) as needed.

Patient teaching

• Have the patient demonstrate BSE and correct her technique as needed. Remind the patient to look in a mirror to observe for lesions or skin or breast contour changes.

• Stress the value of BSE. BSE should be done once a month after menses or, if the patient is menopausal, on the same day of each month.

• Teach the patient about diagnosis and treatment options, including combinations of surgery, radiation, chemotherapy, and hormonal therapy. Explain that after mastectomy, an incisional drain or suction device (Hemovac) will be used to remove accumulated serous or sanguineous fluid, lessening the tension on the suture line and promoting healing.

• Advise the patient about reconstructive surgery or advise her to call the local or state medical society for the names of plastic reconstructive surgeons who regularly perform surgery to create breast mounds. In many cases, reconstructive surgery may be planned prior to mastectomy.

• Provide psychological and emotional support. Many patients fear cancer, possible disfigurement, and possible loss of sexual function. Explain that treatments and surgery don't interfere with sexual function.

 ALERT Tell the patient to call the PCP to report any new signs and symtoms, including signs of infection or depression.

Resources

• National Alliance of Breast Cancer Organizations: 212-719-0154

• The Susan G. Komen Breast Cancer Foundation: 800-IM-AWARE

• Y-Me Breast Cancer Organization: 800-221-2141

• American Cancer Society (ask for a Reach for Recovery support group close to patient): 800-ACS-2345

• For patients, caregivers, and professional providers — Association of Cancer Online: *www.acor.org*

Bronchitis

ICD-9-CM 466.0

Bronchitis is an inflammation limited to the tracheobronchial tree, involving the trachea, bronchi, and bronchioles.

Causes

Bronchitis is caused by any number of infections, including viral (adenovirus, influenza, or respiratory syncytial virus), bacterial (*Mycoplasma, Streptococcus pneumoniae, Moraxella catarrhalis,* or *Mycobacterium tuberculosis*) and, rarely, fungal infection. Inflammation of the bronchial tree produces thick secretions that destroy epithelium and inhibit mucociliary function. Other causes of bronchitis include cigarette smoking and exposure to chemicals or smoke.

Clinical presentation

Bronchitis frequently follows a respiratory tract infection, such as a cold and influenza. A nonproductive cough progresses to produce purulent mucus. The patient may also complain of fever, coughing, mucus with traces of blood after coughing spasms, chest pain, dyspnea, and wheezing. History may reveal close contacts who are sick, a smoking habit, or a chronic respiratory disorder.

Examination findings can be non-specific for bronchitis, but they have some typical patterns.

• *General:* fever, lymphadenopathy
• *Head, eyes, ears, nose, and throat:* signs of infection
• *Chest:* chest pain, resonance on percussion, and scattered, coarse crackles (in early inspiration and expiration), wheezes, or rhonchi on auscultation

Differential diagnosis

ALERT History of high fever, rigors, pleuritic chest pain, and hemoptysis suggest pneumonia. Focal dullness on percussion, increased tactile fremitus and transmission of sound, or late inspiratory crackles over the focal dullness suggest pneumonia and requires a chest X-ray or collaboration with a doctor.

Other conditions to consider include bronchopneumonia, acute sinusitis, aspiration, reactive airway disease, or bacterial tracheitis.

Diagnostic tests
• Complete blood count may reveal leukocytosis.
• Sputum culture and sensitivity testing and Gram stain can detect bacterial causes and sensitivities.
• Arterial blood gas analysis detects hypoxemia.
• Viral titers (*Mycoplasma* titer < 1:64) suggests mycoplasma pneumonia; a four-fold rise in titer is diagnostic for the disease.
• Purified protein derivative may detect tuberculosis.
• Chest X-ray may reveal pneumonia.

Management

General
Treatment goals are to treat the infection and relieve symptoms. More aggressive treatment and closer monitoring are recommended for patients who are very young (under age 4 months), elderly, smokers, immunocompromised, have chronic lung disorders, or have severe symptoms (persistent fever higher than 101° F [38° C] in adults or 102.5° F [39° C] in children and purulent discharge).

Medication
• Antiviral medications (amantadine) are most effective if initiated within 48 hours of symptoms.
• If bacterial etiology is suspected or there is a need to prevent secondary infection in high-risk patients (see above), antibiotics (erythromycin, amoxicillin) may help. Culture and sensitivity results will guide drug choice; for example, macrolides (clarithromycin, azithromycin) treat mycoplasma, and tetracyclines (doxycycline) treat chlamydia as well as mycoplasma.
• Cough suppressants and expectorants can help with an ineffective cough by decreasing cough frequency while making mucus less viscous and tenacious. Cough suppressants are contraindicated for patients with chronic obstructive pulmonary disease.
• Antipyretic analgesics, such as nonsteroidal anti-inflammatory drugs and acetaminophen, are recommended for fever and myalgia.
• Bronchodilator and steroid inhalers are indicated for patients with chronic lung problems and for those who develop hyperreactive airways after infection and mucus production have resolved.

Referral or consultation
Refer to a doctor if the patient's condition doesn't improve within 7 days, and refer to a doctor or pulmonologist if bronchitis frequently recurs.

Follow-up

Contact the patient in 2 days to check on fever and response to drugs. See the patient in 1 week to evaluate. If there is no improvement by then, refer or consult. Schedule a weekly visit focusing on lung examination, hyperreactive airways, smoking cessation, and current drugs until the condition resolves.

Complications

Secondary infection, bronchopneumonia, and acute respiratory failure are possible complications.

Patient teaching

• Advise the patient to drink 4 qt (4 L) of fluid per day, eat a balanced diet, avoid stress, and rest as much as possible to help his body fight infection.
• Instruct the patient to use a vaporizer or humidifier or take long, steamy showers to help loosen and thin secretions. (Tell him to breathe in through the nose if it's affected.)
• Suggest antipyretic analgesics to relieve body aches.
• Recommend that the patient gargle with salt water (¼ tsp salt in 8 oz of warm water). For a stuffy nose, the patient may instill saline nose drops (Ocean), leave in for 1 minute, and then blow out, repeating as needed. This may be effective in combination with a hot shower immediately before going to sleep.
• Teach smokers how chemicals in cigarette smoke damage ciliary hairs, decreasing the effectiveness of the ciliary escalator. Viral respiratory infection may last 10 to 14 days versus 7 to 10 days for nonsmokers. Ciliary hairs take about 6 months to grow out. Ineffective ciliary action is part of the reason the patient can expect to have a productive cough that might include "black stuff" (tar) for about 6 months.
• To prevent disease transmission, teach the patient to wash his hands thoroughly and frequently, avoid sharing utensils or beverages, and use disposable tissues.

 ALERT Tell the patient to call the primary care provider (PCP) to report any new signs and symptoms, including the following signs of secondary infection: fever higher than 102.5° F (39° C), mucus color changing to dark yellow, green, or brown; inability to swallow liquids; and new onset of severe ear, throat, or sinus pain. Also tell him to call the PCP if drug intolerance develops or if a new rash appears since starting the drug. Also call the PCP in the event of severe shortness of breath or difficulty breathing.

Cervical cancer

ICD-9-CM 180.0

The third most common cancer of the female reproductive system, cervical cancer is classified as either preinvasive or invasive. Cervical carcinoma ranges from minimal cervical dysplasia, in which the lower third of the epithelium contains abnormal cells (75% to 90% cure rate), to carcinoma in situ, in which the full thickness of epithelium contains abnormal cells.

Causes

Cervical cancer is usually caused by the human papilloma virus (HPV), also called condylomata acuminata or genital warts.

BETHESDA SYSTEM OF CERVICAL CYTOLOGY

The Bethesda System uses diagnostic terminology to indicate the adequacy of Pap test specimens for diagnosis. It can be used to make follow-up recommendations. Determining specimen adequacy is critical to reducing the rate of false-negative results. Pap tests are often inadequate because of obscuring blood or inflammation, sampling done outside the transformation zone.

Adequacy of specimen

Satisfactory for evaluation
Satisfactory for evaluation but limited by . . . (specify reason)
Unsatisfactory for evaluation . . . (specify reason)

General categorization (optional)

Within normal limits
Benign cellular changes; see descriptive diagnosis
Epithelial cell abnormality; see descriptive diagnosis

Descriptive diagnoses

Benign cellular changes
Infection: Treat as needed and repeat Papanicolaou (Pap) test in 6 months.
• *Trichomonas vaginalis;* fungal organisms morphologically consistent with *Candida*; predominance of coccobacilli consistent with shift in vaginal flora; bacteria morphologically consistent with *Actinomyces*; cellular changes associated with herpes simplex virus; other
Reactive changes (hyperkeratosis or parakeratosis): Instruct patient and repeat Pap test in 6 months.
• Reactive cellular changes associated with inflammation (includes typical repair); atrophy with inflammation ("atrophic vaginitis"); radiation; intrauterine contraceptive device (IUD); or diaphragm, pessary, or tampon use within 3 days prior to Pap test

Epithelial cell abnormalities

Atypical squamous cells of undetermined significance (ASCUS)*: Repeat Pap test in 6 months.
• If ASCUS occurrence in a woman with atrophy who isn't on hormone replacement therapy, treated with topical vaginal estrogen; Pap test repeated in 4 to 6 months and, if ASCUS again, referral for colposcopy
• If ASCUS at next Pap test but favoring reactive cells, Pap test repeated again in 6 months
• If ASCUS at next Pap test but favoring dysplasia, referral for colposcopy
Low-grade squamous intraepithelial lesion (LSIL) encompassing HPV** mild dysplasia or cervical intraepithelial neoplasm (CIN 1):
• Globally, LSIL frequently due to the human papilloma virus (HPV); HPV test such as Digene to diagnose and treat as indicated; if cells favor dysplasia, referral for colposcopy also (However, more aggressive follow-up is indicated in some cases.)
• For women who are unlikely to return for follow-up, or who are HIV-positive or otherwise immunocompromised, colposcopy indicated for a single abnormal Pap test
• For women who are likely to have a routine follow-up, have had no abnormal Pap tests in the recent past, and who are immunocompetent, a Pap test every 4 to 6 months for 2 years until there are three consecutive normal findings
High-grade squamous intraepithelial lesion (HSIL) encompassing moderate and severe dysplasia, carcinoma in situ or CIN 2, and CIN 3 or squamous cell carcinoma:
• Colposcopy ALWAYS required; referral to gynecologist-oncologist for treatment and close follow-up
Atypical glandular cell
• Referral to a gynecologist

---

* Atypical squamous or glandular cells of undetermined significance are further qualified by whether a reactive, premalignant, or malignant process is favored.
** Cellular changes of HPV are included in the category of low-grade squamous intraepithelial lesion.

Clinical presentation

Preinvasive cervical cancer produces no symptoms or other clinically apparent changes. Early invasive cervical cancer can cause postcoital spotting, dyspareunia, irregular vaginal bleeding, and malodorous vaginal discharge. In advanced stages, it causes pelvic pain, vaginal leakage of urine and feces from a fistula, hematuria, rectal bleeding, anorexia, weight loss, and anemia.

Risk factors include HPV or human immunodeficiency virus infection, smoking, multiple sexual partners, early age of first coitus, exposure to diethylstilbestrol in utero, and advancing age.

Differential diagnosis

Be aware that a slight daily discharge also occurs with polyps and infection. Bloody flow that has cycles (heavy flow tapering to none for a few days, followed again by heavy flow) also occurs with anovulatory bleeding. Pelvic pain or pressure may suggest corpus luteum cyst, endometrioma, or myoma. Other conditions to consider are cervicitis, cervical polyp, and metastatic carcinoma.

Diagnostic tests
• Urine or serum human chorionic gonadotropin (HCG) test is done on most patients of childbearing age.
• A culture for sexually transmitted illnesses is done as history indicates.
• Papanicolaou (Pap) screening cytologic examination can detect cervical cancer before symptoms appear. Abnormal Pap test specimens must be carefully evaluated. (See *Bethesda System of cervical cytology.*)
• Cervicography provides microscopic visualization to detect abnormalities.
• Colposcopy is indicated for abnormal Pap tests. Consider endocervical sampling in patients over age 40 with possible chronic anovulation and in patients under age 40 with signs or symptoms of hyperplasia or neoplasia. This test can detect the presence and extent of preclinical lesions.
• Cervical cone biopsy is done with colposcopic examination to confirm the diagnosis and determine the extent of invasion. This procedure frequently leads to a cure if the carcinoma is detected early. (See *Cervical cancer staging*, page 178.)
• Laboratory studies include complete blood count (anemia due to blood loss), creatinine (ureteral obstruction), liver function tests (metastases), prolactin, and thyroid panel (may reveal anovulation).
• Computed tomography scans of the abdomen and pelvis can detect lymph node metastases.
• Lymphangiogram is used to detect lymph node metastases.

Management
General
Verify that the patient follows up with a specialist for any abnormality. Use a patient reminder system for follow-up visits for physical examination and pap test.

Surgery
Appropriate treatment depends on accurate clinical staging. Cryosurgery is used in mild dysplasia and cervical intraepithelial neoplasia (CIN 1). All other procedures are used for moderate to severe dysplasia or cancer in situ: laser destruction, conization (and frequent Pap test follow-up) or, rarely, hysterectomy as indicated. Therapy for invasive squamous cell carcinoma may include radical hysterectomy and radiation therapy (internal, external, or both).

Medication
Pharmaceutical treatment includes chemotherapy (fluorouracil, carbo-

CERVICAL CANCER STAGING

Cervical cancer treatment decisions depend on accurate staging. The International Federation of Gynecology and Obstetrics defines cervical cancer stages as follows.

Stage	Description
0	Carcinoma in situ, intraepithelial carcinoma; cases of stage 0 not included in any therapeutic statistics for invasive carcinoma
I	Carcinoma strictly confined to cervix (extension to corpus disregarded)
IA	Invasive cancer identified only microscopically (All gross lesions even with superficial invasion are stage IB cancers. Invasion is limited to measured stromal invasion with maximum depth of 5 mm and no wider than 7 mm. The depth of invasion shouldn't be more than 5 mm taken from the base of the epithelium, either surface or glandular, from which it originates. Vascular space involvement, either venous or lymphatic, shouldn't alter the staging.)
IA1	Measured invasion of stroma no deeper than 3 mm and no wider than 7 mm
IA2	Measured invasion of stroma 3 to 5 mm deep and no wider than 7 mm
IB	Clinical lesions confined to cervix or preclinical lesions greater than stage IA
IB1	Clinical lesions no greater than 4 cm in size
IB2	Clinical lesions greater than 4 cm in size
II	Carcinoma extending beyond cervix but not to pelvic wall; carcinoma involving vagina but not as far as lower third
IIa	No obvious parametrial involvement
IIb	Obvious parametrial involvement
III	Carcinoma extending to pelvic side wall; no cancer-free space between tumor and pelvic wall on rectovaginal examination; tumor involving lower third of vagina (All cases with hydronephrosis or a nonfunctioning kidney should be included unless known to be result of other cause.)
IIIa	No extension to pelvic wall, but involvement of lower third of vagina
IIIb	Extension to pelvic wall, hydronephrosis, or nonfunctioning kidney
IV	Carcinoma extending beyond the true pelvis or clinically involving the mucosa of the bladder or rectum
IVa	Spread of the growth to adjacent organs
IVb	Carcinoma spreading to distant organs

platin) and antiemetics (ondansetron, metoclopramide) to deal with adverse effects of chemotherapy.

Referral or consultation

Refer to a gynecologist or gynecologic oncologist for colposcopy, counseling, or treatment; an urgent appointment is needed for suspected neoplasia. Refer to a psychologist or psychiatrist for counseling or drugs as needed for symptoms of depression or anxiety.

Follow-up

See the patient quarterly for 2 years, semiannually for the next 3 years, and annually after 5 years. Focus on physical examination and Pap test.

For the general population, a Pap test should be done annually for 3 years after the first coitus or age 18; if results are normal and the patient has no risk factors, a Pap test can then be done every 3 years. For all others, annual Pap tests are recommended.

Complications

Ureteral fistula, hydronephrosis, and uremia are possible complications.

Patient teaching

• Teach about diagnosis and treatment options.
• Teach the importance of a regular Pap test. (Schedule depends on age and risk factors.)
• Before a biopsy, explain to the patient that she may feel pressure, minor abdominal cramps, or a pinch from the punch forceps. Reassure her that pain is minimal because the cervix has few nerve endings.
• Before cryosurgery, explain that the procedure takes approximately 15 minutes, during which time refrigerant will be used to freeze the cervix. Warn the patient that she may experience abdominal cramps, headache, and sweating, but reassure her that she'll feel little pain. Cryosurgery will cause a *large* amount of watery discharge for up to 10 days.
• Before laser therapy, explain that the procedure takes approximately 30 minutes and may cause abdominal cramps.
• After any of these procedures, tell the patient to expect a discharge or spotting for about 1 week; also tell her not to douche, use tampons, or engage in sexual intercourse during this time. Tell her to watch for and report signs of infection. Stress the need for a follow-up Pap test and a pelvic examination in 3 months.
• Before radiation therapy, teach the patient to watch for and report discomfort that persists and seems to stay in one area. Radiation may increase susceptibility to infection by lowering the white blood cell count; therefore, the patient should avoid persons with obvious infections during therapy.
• Teach the patient to use a vaginal dilator to prevent vaginal stenosis and to facilitate vaginal examinations and sexual intercourse.
• Reassure the patient that this disease and its treatment shouldn't radically alter her lifestyle or prohibit sexual intimacy.
• Use resources to get educational information (for example, on chemotherapy, support services, and cancer's effect on sexuality).

ALERT Tell the patient to call the primary care provider to report any new signs and symptoms, including postmenopausal bleeding.

Resources
• American Cancer Society: 800-ACS-2345
• Cancer Information Service: 800-4-CANCER
• CHEMOCare: 800-55-CHEMO
• For patients, caregivers, and professional providers — Association of Cancer Online: *www.acor.org*

Chronic obstructive pulmonary disease

ICD-9-CM COPD 496, emphysema 492.8

Chronic obstructive pulmonary disease (COPD) — also called chronic obstructive lung disease — is a chronic airway obstruction that results from emphysema, chronic bronchitis, asthma, or any combination of these disorders. Usually, more than one of these underlying conditions coexist; most often, bronchitis and emphysema occur together. (See *Understanding chronic obstructive pulmonary disease,* pages 182 to 185.)

The most common chronic lung disease, COPD affects an estimated 17 million Americans, and its incidence is rising. It affects men more often than women probably because, until recently, men were more likely to smoke heavily. It doesn't always produce symptoms, and it causes only minimal disability in many patients. However, COPD tends to worsen with time.

Causes

Predisposing factors include cigarette smoking, recurrent or chronic respiratory infections, air pollution, and allergies. Familial and hereditary factors (for example, deficiency of alpha$_1$-antitrypsin) may also predispose a person to COPD.

Smoking is by far the most important of these factors; it impairs ciliary action and macrophage function and causes inflammation in airways, increased mucus production, destruction of alveolar septae, and peribronchiolar fibrosis. Early inflammatory changes may reverse if the patient stops smoking before lung destruction is extensive.

Clinical presentation

The typical patient, a long-term cigarette smoker, has no symptoms until middle age, when his ability to exercise or do strenuous work gradually starts to decline and he begins to develop progressive exertional dyspnea and a productive cough. While subtle at first, these signs become more pronounced as the patient gets older and the disease progresses.

The patient eventually develops dyspnea on minimal exertion, frequent respiratory infections, and intermittent or continuous hypoxemia. Emphysema and bronchitis are both present to varying degrees. In its advanced form, COPD may cause thoracic deformities, overwhelming disability, cor pulmonale, severe respiratory failure, and death.

History may reveal fatigue, weight loss, and decreased libido. Examination may reveal tachypnea, accessory muscle usage, increased anteroposterior diameter, hyperresonance on percussion, decreased heart and lung sounds, and prolonged expirations.

Differential diagnosis

Other conditions that must be considered, particularly if there is a new onset of symptoms, including acute bronchitis, asthma, pulmonary embolism, or pneumothorax. Other differentials include sleep apnea, chronic sinusitis, heart failure, and malignancy.

Diagnostic tests
• Complete blood count may detect polycythemia caused by chronic hypoxemia indicating chronic bronchitis or emphysema.
• Arterial blood gas (ABG) analysis may detect hypercapnia and moderate to severe hypoxia, indicating chronic bronchitis. However, mild hypoxia with a normal partial pressure

of carbon dioxide ($PaCO_2$) indicates emphysema. Eventually, hypoxemia and respiratory acidosis may develop. In more advanced cases, ABG analysis determines oxygen need and helps avoid CO_2 narcosis.

• Pulmonary function testing can diagnose COPD by revealing a forced vital capacity ratio (forced expiratory volume in 1 second divided by forced vital capacity ratio [FEV_1/FVC] less than 70% as well as reduced reversibility achieved with bronchodilators [more than 15%].)

• Chest X-ray is often normal in the course of COPD. However, it's useful in differentiating chronic bronchitis from emphysema. Increased bronchovascular markings and cardiomegaly revealed on X-ray indicate chronic bronchitis, whereas a small heart, hyperinflation, flat diaphragms, and bullous changes suggest emphysema.

Management

Acute

The patient must be hospitalized for respiratory failure, exacerbation, and infection; treatment is dependent on the clinical picture.

General

The main goal of treatment is to relieve symptoms and prevent complications. Effective coughing, postural drainage, and chest physiotherapy can help mobilize secretions.

For patients using metered-dose inhalers, consider using a spacer device to facilitate proper administration. If the patient reports a strong taste in his mouth, he most often is getting the dose in his mouth instead of his lungs, with decreased effectiveness.

Tell the patient to avoid using antihistamines, cough suppressants, sedatives, tranquilizers, beta blockers, and narcotics because of their effects on the respiratory system.

Encourage the patient to participate in local support groups and rehabilitation programs (physical and pulmonary).

Medication

• Bronchodilators can be given by mouth (theophylline), by metered-dose inhalers (beta-adrenergic bronchodilators [albuterol, terbutaline]), or by nebulizer or nasal spray (anticholinergic bronchodilator [ipratropium bromide]), to help alleviate bronchospasm and enhance mucociliary clearance of secretions.

• Theophylline is helpful for nocturnal bronchospasm.

• Corticosteroids (prednisone) are useful as anti-inflammatory agents, with the greatest results noted in early stages when lung tissue reversibility is greatest.

• Pneumococcal vaccination and annual influenza vaccinations are important preventive measures. This is particularly important as more antibiotic-resistant organisms emerge.

• An antiviral (amantadine) is used after exposure to influenza A, for high-risk populations during flu season, and during acute influenza infection.

• Antibiotics are used as needed to treat secondary respiratory infections. For low-risk patients (under age 60, FEV_1 above 50%, and fewer than four acute episodes predicted per year), consider erythromycin or amoxicillin for 10 days. For higher-risk patients, consider clarithromycin or amoxicillin clavulanate for 10 days.

• Low concentrations of oxygen help relieve symptoms. Consider oxygen therapy for patients with a partial pressure of arterial oxygen (PaO_2) less than or equal to 65 mm Hg or an arterial saturation (SaO_2) less than or equal to 88% on room air; for a

(Text continues on page 184.)

UNDERSTANDING CHRONIC OBSTRUCTIVE PULMONARY DISEASE

Disease	Causes and pathophysiology	Clinical features
Emphysema		
• Abnormal irreversible enlargement of air spaces distal to terminal bronchioles due to destruction of alveolar walls, resulting in decreased elastic recoil properties of lungs • Most common cause of death from respiratory disease in the United States	• Cigarette smoking, deficiency of alpha$_1$-antitrypsin • Recurrent inflammation associated with release of proteolytic enzymes from cells in lungs causes bronchiolar and alveolar wall damage and, ultimately, destruction. Loss of lung-supporting structure results in decreased elastic recoil and airway collapse on expiration. Destruction of alveolar walls decreases surface area for gas exchange.	• Insidious onset, with dyspnea the predominant symptom • Other signs and symptoms of long-term disease: chronic cough, anorexia, weight loss, malaise, barrel chest, use of accessory muscles of respiration, prolonged expiratory period with grunting, pursed-lip breathing and tachypnea, and peripheral cyanosis • Complications: recurrent respiratory tract infections, cor pulmonale, and respiratory failure.
Chronic bronchitis		
• Excessive mucus production with productive cough for at least 3 months per year for 2 successive years • Few patients with the clinical syndrome of chronic bronchitis develop significant airway obstruction.	• Severity of disease related to amount and duration of smoking; respiratory infection exacerbates symptoms. • Hypertrophy and hyperplasia of bronchial mucous glands, increased goblet cells, damage to cilia, squamous metaplasia of columnar epithelium, and chronic leukocytic and lymphocytic infiltration of bronchial walls; widespread inflammation, distortion, narrowing of airways, and mucus within the airways produce resistance to small airways and cause ventilation-perfusion imbalance.	• Insidious onset, with productive cough and exertional dyspnea as predominant symptoms • Other signs and symptoms: colds associated with increased sputum production and worsening dyspnea that takes progressively longer to resolve; copious sputum (gray, white, or yellow); weight gain due to edema; cyanosis; tachypnea; wheezing; prolonged expiratory time; use of accessory muscles of respiration

Confirming diagnostic measures	Management
• Physical examination: Hyperresonance on percussion, decreased breath sounds, expiratory prolongation, quiet heart sounds • Chest X-ray: in advanced disease, flattened diaphragm, reduced vascular markings at lung periphery, overaeration of lungs, vertical heart, enlarged anteroposterior chest diameter, large retrosternal air space • Pulmonary function tests (PFTs): increased residual volume, total lung capacity, and compliance; decreased vital capacity, diffusing capacity, and expiratory volumes • Arterial blood gases (ABGs): reduced PO_2 with normal PCO_2 until late in disease • Electrocardiography (ECG): tall, symmetrical P waves in leads II, III, and aV_F; vertical QRS axis; signs of right ventricular hypertrophy late in disease • Red blood cells: increased hemoglobin late in disease when persistent severe hypoxia is present	• Bronchodilators, such as beta-adrenergics and theophylline, to reverse bronchospasm and promote mucociliary clearance • Antibiotics to treat respiratory infection; flu vaccine to prevent influenza; Pneumovax to prevent pneumococcal pneumonia; and mucolytics • Adequate fluid intake and, in selected patients, chest physiotherapy to mobilize secretions • O_2 at low-flow settings to treat hypoxia • Avoidance of smoking and air pollutants • Aerosolized or systemic corticosteroids
• Physical examination: rhonchi and wheezing on auscultation, expiratory prolongation, neck vein distention, pedal edema • Chest X-ray: may show hyperinflation and increased bronchovascular markings • PFTs: increased residual volume, decreased vital capacity and forced expiratory volumes, normal static compliance and diffusing capacity • ABGs: decreased PO_2, normal or increased PCO_2 • Sputum: contains evidence of infection • ECG: may show atrial arrhythmias; peaked P waves in leads II, III, and aV_F; and, occasionally, right ventricular hypertrophy	• Antibiotics for infections • Avoidance of smoking and air pollutants • Bronchodilators to relieve bronchospasm and facilitate mucociliary clearance • Adequate fluid intake and chest physiotherapy to mobilize secretions • Ultrasonic or mechanical nebulizer treatments to loosen secretions and aid in mobilization • Occasionally, corticosteroids • Diuretics for edema • Oxygen for hypoxia

(continued)

UNDERSTANDING CHRONIC OBSTRUCTIVE PULMONARY DISEASE (continued)

Disease	Causes and pathophysiology	Clinical features

Asthma

• Increased bronchial reactivity to a variety of stimuli, which produces episodic bronchospasm and airway obstruction in conjunction with airway inflammation

• Asthma with onset in adulthood: often without distinct allergies; asthma with onset in childhood: often associated with definite allergens. Status asthmaticus is an acute asthma attack with severe bronchospasm that fails to clear with bronchodilator therapy.

• Prognosis: More than half of asthmatic children become asymptomatic as adults; more than half of asthmatics with onset after age 15 have persistent disease with occasional severe attacks.

• Possible mechanisms include allergy (family tendency, seasonal occurrence); allergic reaction results in release of mast cell vasoactive and bronchospastic mediators.

• Upper airway infection, exercise, anxiety and, rarely, coughing or laughing can precipitate an asthma attack; nocturnal flare-ups are common.

• Paroxysmal airway obstruction associated with nasal polyps may be seen in response to aspirin or indomethacin ingestion.

• Airway obstruction from spasm of bronchial smooth muscle narrows airways; inflammatory edema of the bronchial wall and inspissation of tenacious mucoid secretions are also important, particularly in status asthmaticus.

• History of intermittent attacks of dyspnea and wheezing

• Mild wheezing progresses to severe dyspnea, audible wheezing, chest tightness (a feeling of being unable to breathe), and a cough that produces thick mucus.

• Other signs: prolonged expiration, intercostal and supraclavicular retraction on inspiration, use of accessory muscles of respiration, flaring nostrils, tachypnea, tachycardia, perspiration, and flushing; patients often have symptoms of eczema and allergic rhinitis (hay fever).

• Status asthmaticus, unless treated promptly, can progress to respiratory failure.

---

patient with a PaO_2 of 56 to 59 mm Hg or an SaO_2 of 89% with concomitant cor pulmonale or polycythemia; and for those with significant sleep- or exercise-induced hypoxemia that resolves with oxygen therapy.

• In rare cases of alpha$_1$-antitrypsin deficiency, it can be replaced by a weekly I.V. injection of human alpha$_1$ proteinase inhibitor (Prolastin).

Referral or consultation

The patient should be referred to a pulmonologist or doctor if nonresponsive or if his response is unsatisfactory, if the clinical picture is deteriorating rapidly, or if cor pulmonale is present. The patient should get physical therapy to build endurance

and strength after he is cleared medically.

Follow-up

For acute exacerbations, contact the patient in 24 hours to verify improvement. See monthly until the condition is stable, and then every 3 to 6 months as long as the clinical picture remains stable. For patients on theophylline, check the serum level every 2 weeks after each adjustment until the goal is reached and then every 6 months. For patients on home oxygen, reevaluate oxygen need after 3 months — many patients can be weaned. While the patient is on oxygen, check ABG levels annually if sta-

Confirming diagnostic measures	**Management**
• Physical examination: usually normal between attacks; auscultation shows rhonchi and wheezing throughout lung fields on expiration and, at times, inspiration; absent or diminished breath sounds during severe obstruction. Loud bilateral wheezes may be grossly audible; chest is hyperinflated.	• Aerosol containing beta-adrenergic agents, such as metaproterenol or albuterol; also oral beta-adrenergic agents (terbutaline) and oral methylxanthines (theophylline). Many patients require inhaled, oral, or I.V. corticosteroids.
• Chest X-ray: hyperinflated lungs with air trapping during attack; normal during remission	• Emergency treatment: O_2 therapy, corticosteroids, and bronchodilators, such as subcutaneous epinephrine, I.V. theophylline, and inhaled agents (such as metaproterenol, albuterol, or ipratropium bromide).
• Sputum: presence of Curschmann's spirals (casts of airways), Charcot-Leyden crystals, and eosinophils	• Monitor for deteriorating respiratory status and note sputum characteristics; provide adequate fluid intake and oxygen.
• PFTs: during attacks, decreased forced expiratory volumes that improve significantly after inhaled bronchodilator; increased residual volume and, occasionally, total lung capacity; may be normal between attacks	• Prevention: Tell the patient to avoid possible allergens and to use antihistamines, decongestants, cromolyn powder by inhalation, and oral or aerosol bronchodilators as needed. Explain the influence of stress and anxiety on asthma as well as its frequent association with exercise (particularly running), cold air, and nighttime flare-ups.
• ABGs: decreased PO_2; decreased, normal or increased PCO_2 (in severe attack)	
• ECG: sinus tachycardia during an attack; severe attack may produce signs of cor pulmonale (right axis deviation, peaked P wave) that resolve after the attack.	
• Skin tests: may identify allergens	

ble and more often as the clinical picture indicates. Check pulse oximetry every visit.

Complications

Possible complications include hypoxemia, infection, secondary polycythemia, respiratory acidosis, respiratory failure, pulmonary hypertension, malnutrition, cor pulmonale, or left ventricular heart failure.

Patient teaching

• Because most COPD patients receive outpatient treatment, provide comprehensive patient teaching to help them comply with therapy and understand the nature of this chronic, progressive disease.
• Encourage the patient to enroll in available pulmonary rehabilitation programs.
• Encourage exercise, particularly upper extremity and diaphragmatic exercises and pursed-lip breathing.
• Urge the patient to stop smoking.
• Encourage the patient to avoid respiratory irritants and install an air conditioner with an air filter in the home.
• Review the use and adverse effects of drugs.
• Review the signs of infection, and warn the patient to avoid contact with persons who have respiratory infections.

- Review deep breathing, coughing, and chest physiotherapy.
- Encourage fluids and the use of a humidifier to correct dehydration or to thin and loosen thick secretions.
- Emphasize the importance of a balanced diet and small frequent meals to avoid fatigue and to decrease diaphragmatic elevation caused by gastric distention.
- For patients on oxygen, goal levels are PaO_2 equal to or greater than 65 mm Hg or SaO_2 equal to or greater than 90% with activity. If ordering oxygen therapy at home, teach the importance of using equipment correctly. Teach the patient and his family that excessive oxygen therapy may eliminate the hypoxic respiratory drive, causing confusion and drowsiness, which are signs of CO_2 narcosis. Teach the importance of using nasal oxygen while eating.
- Collaborate with the patient and his family on how to adjust their lifestyles to accommodate the limitations imposed by this debilitating chronic disease. Instruct the patient to exercise daily and allow for daily rest periods.
- To help prevent COPD, advise all persons, especially those with a family history of COPD or those in its early stages, not to smoke. Secondhand smoke is especially harmful to this population.

ALERT Tell the patient to call the primary care provider to report any new or persistent signs and symptoms, including fever higher than 101° F (38.3° C) or a cough producing green, brown, or dark yellow mucus; difficulty eating because of shortness of breath; increasing shortness of breath or increasing orthopnea (requiring use of extra pillows to elevate the head in order to sleep); breathing that becomes rapid or increasingly difficult; or unusual drowsiness.

If the patient won't respond, his lips become dusky or blue, or his respirations become very irregular (such as Cheyne-Stokes), activate emergency medical services.

Resources
- American Lung Association: 800-LUNG-USA or *www.lungusa.org*
- National Heart, Lung and Blood Institute: 301-251-1222 (for patient-education pamphlets); *www.nhlbi.nih.gov* (for patients)
- For providers— Drug affordability: *www.needymeds.com* (contains information regarding many drug company programs that provide financial assistance for their drugs)

Colorectal cancer

ICD-9-CM primary 154.0, secondary 197.5, in situ 230.4, benign 211.4, uncertain 235.2

In the United States and Europe, colorectal cancer is the second leading visceral neoplasm. Incidence is equally distributed between men and women, mostly those over age 50, except in familial polyposis. Colorectal malignant tumors are almost always adenocarcinomas. About half of these are sessile lesions (flat-based) of the rectosigmoid area; the rest are pedunculated (stalked) lesions. Sessile lesions are more likely to become malignant.

Colorectal cancer tends to progress slowly and remains localized for a long time. Consequently, it's potentially curable in 75% of patients if an early diagnosis allows resection before nodal involvement. With early diagnosis, the overall 5-year survival rate is nearly 50%. The larger the lesion, the greater the incidence of invasive cancer: (See *Staging colorectal cancer.*)

Causes

While most colorectal cancers arise from adenomas, the exact cause of colorectal cancer is unknown. There are known risk factors. Dietary risk factors include low-fiber and high-fat intake. Other risk factors include a history of inflammatory bowel disease, familial polyposis, a first-degree relative with a history of colon cancer, or adenomatous polyps.

Clinical presentation

Adenomas are precursors for most colorectal cancers. These polyps are treatable lesions but are usually asymptomatic until they're very large. Bleeding from polyps is usually scanty and intermittent. Manifestations of colorectal cancer result from local obstruction and, in later stages, from direct extension to adjacent organs (bladder, prostate, ureters, vagina, sacrum) and distant metastasis (usually to the liver).

In early stages, signs and symptoms are typically vague and depend on the anatomic location and function of the affected bowel segment. Later, they generally include pallor, cachexia, ascites, hepatomegaly, lymphangiectasis (dilation of the lymphatic vessels), fatigue, weakness, iron deficiency anemia, constipation or diarrhea, tenesmus, urgency, and hematochezia.

Cancer on the right side

On the right side of the colon, which absorbs water and electrolytes, early tumor growth causes no signs of obstruction because the tumor tends to grow along the bowel rather than surround the lumen, and the fecal content in this area is normally liquid. It may, however, cause black,

STAGING COLORECTAL CANCER

Named for pathologist Cuthbert Dukes, the Dukes Cancer Classification System assigns tumors to four stages. These stages (with substages) reflect the extent of bowel-mucosa and bowel-wall infiltration, lymph node involvement, and metastasis.

Stage A
Malignant cells are confined to the bowel mucosa, and the lymph nodes contain no cancer cells. If treated promptly, about 80% of these patients remain disease-free 5 years later.

Stage B
Malignant cells extend through the bowel mucosa but remain within the bowel wall. The lymph nodes are normal. In substage B_2, all bowel wall layers and immediately adjacent structures contain malignant cells, but the lymph nodes remain normal. About 50% of patients with substage B_2 cancer survive for 5 or more years.

Stage C
Malignant cells extend into the bowel wall and the lymph nodes. In substage C_2, malignant cells extend through the entire thickness of the bowel wall and into the lymph nodes. The 5-year survival rate for patients with stage C disease is about 25%.

Stage D
Malignant cells have metastasized to distant organs by way of the lymph nodes and mesenteric vessels and typically lodge in the lungs and liver. Only 5% of patients with stage D cancer survive 5 or more years.

tarry stools; anemia; and abdominal aching, pressure, or dull cramps.

As the disease progresses, the patient develops weakness, fatigue, exertional dyspnea, vertigo and, eventually, diarrhea, obstipation (extreme, persistent constipation), anorexia, weight loss, vomiting, and other signs and symptoms of intestinal obstruction. In addition, a tumor on the right side may be palpable.

Cancer on the left side
On the left side, a tumor causes signs and symptoms of an obstruction even in early stages because, in this area, stool is of a formed consistency. A tumor commonly causes rectal bleeding (often ascribed to hemorrhoids), intermittent abdominal fullness or cramping, and rectal pressure.

As the disease progresses, the patient develops obstipation, diarrhea, or "ribbon" (pencil-shaped) stool. Typically, he notices that passage of stool or flatus relieves the pain. At this stage, bleeding from the colon becomes obvious, with dark or bright red blood in the stool and mucus in or on the stool.

Rectal tumor signs
With a rectal tumor, the first symptom is a change in bowel habits, often beginning with an urgent need to defecate on arising ("morning diarrhea") or obstipation alternating with diarrhea. Other indications include blood or mucus in stool and a sense of incomplete evacuation. Late in the disease, pain begins as a feeling of rectal fullness that later progresses into a dull, and sometimes constant, ache confined to the rectum or sacral region.

Differential diagnosis

ALERT Any patient with a GI complaint whose examination reveals an abdominal mass, severe abdominal tenderness, fever, weight loss, or acute onset without obvious cause requires aggressive evaluation. Other red flags include nocturnal wakening due to GI complaints, family history of malignancy, positive fecal occult blood test, and abnormal blood counts.

Other conditions to consider include strictures (hemorrhoids or rectal polyps), rectal fissures, infectious colitis, irritable bowel syndrome, inflammatory bowel disease, other malignancies, and benign adenomas.

Diagnostic tests
Only a tumor biopsy can verify colorectal cancer, but the following tests help detect it:
• Digital rectal examination discovers almost 15% of colorectal cancers by detecting a rectal mass.
• A fecal occult blood test can detect blood in stool but has low specificity for colorectal cancer. Sensitivity is improved with serial testing (three to six specimens).
• Complete blood count detects anemia, which may indicate an occult hemorrhage.
• Carcinoembryonic antigen (CEA), although not specific or sensitive enough for an early diagnosis, is helpful in monitoring patients before and after treatment to detect metastasis or recurrence.
• Urinary 5-hydroxyindoleacetic acid levels may be high in colorectal cancer.
• Proctoscopy or sigmoidoscopy can detect up to 66% of colorectal cancers.
• Colonoscopy permits visual inspection (and photographs) of the colon up to the ileocecal valve and gives access for polypectomies and biopsies of suspected lesions. It's a useful screening tool for high-risk patients.
• Computed tomography scan helps to detect extent of metastasis.
• Barium X-ray, using a dual contrast with air, can locate lesions that are undetectable manually or visually. Barium examination should follow endoscopy or excretory urography

SIGNS AND SYMPTOMS OF PERITONITIS

Use this handy mnemonic device to remember the signs of peritonitis.

P ain
E lectrolytes fall and shock ensues
R igidity (of abdominal wall)
I mmobility
T enderness
O bstruction
N ausea or vomiting
I ncreasing pulse with falling blood pressure
T emperature drops then rises sharply
I ncreasing abdominal girth
S ilent abdomen

because the barium sulfate interferes with these tests.

Management

Acute

The most effective treatment for colorectal cancer is surgery to remove the malignant tumor and adjacent tissues as well as any lymph nodes that may contain cancer cells.

Before surgery

• Order diet modifications, laxatives, enemas, and antibiotics to clean the bowel and to decrease abdominal and perineal cavity contamination during surgery.
• If the patient is having a colostomy, teach him and his family about the procedure.
• Emphasize that the stoma will be red, moist, and swollen and that postoperative swelling will eventually subside.
• Show the patient a diagram of the intestine before and after surgery, stressing how much of the bowel will remain intact. Supplement your teaching with instructional aids if possible. Arrange a postsurgical visit from a recovered ostomate.
• Prepare the patient for postoperative I.V. infusions, a nasogastric tube, and an indwelling urinary catheter.

• Discuss the importance of deep-breathing and coughing exercises, up to 10 exercises per hour.

After surgery

• Explain to the patient's family the importance of their positive reactions to the patient's adjustment.
• Encourage the patient to look at the stoma and participate in its care as soon as possible. Emphasize importance of good hygiene and skin care. Encourage him to shower or bathe as soon as the incision heals.
• Teach the patient to report signs of peritonitis immediately. (See *Signs and symptoms of peritonitis*.)
• If indicated, instruct the patient with a sigmoid colostomy to do his own irrigation as soon as he can after surgery. Advise him to schedule irrigation for the time of day when he normally evacuated before surgery. Many patients find that irrigating every 1 to 3 days is necessary for regularity.
• If flatus, diarrhea, or constipation occurs, eliminate suspected causative foods from the patient's diet. He may reintroduce them later.
• After several months, many ostomates establish control with irrigation and no longer need to wear a pouch. A stoma cap or gauze sponge placed over the stoma protects it and absorbs mucoid secretions.

Physical activity

• Inform the patient that a structured, gradually progressive exercise program to strengthen abdominal muscles may be instituted under medical supervision.
• Before achieving bowel control, the patient can resume physical activities, including sports.
• Avoid injury to the stoma or surrounding abdominal muscles.
• Instruct the patient to avoid heavy lifting because herniation or prolapse may occur through weakened muscles in the abdominal wall.

Medication

Chemotherapy is indicated for patients with metastasis, residual disease, or a recurrent inoperable tumor. Drugs used in such treatment commonly include fluorouracil with levamisole, leucovorin, methotrexate, or streptozocin. Patients whose tumor has extended to regional lymph nodes may receive fluorouracil and levamisole for 1 year postoperatively.

Radiation therapy induces tumor regression and may be used before or after surgery or combined with chemotherapy, especially fluorouracil.

Referral or consultation

Refer the patient to a gastroenterologist or other doctor for colonoscopy, to a gasteroenterologic surgeon and oncologist for evaluation and treatment as indicated, and to a home health agency for follow-up care as needed. The patient should see an enterostomal therapist to set up a colostomy care regimen.

Sexual counseling is important for men because most are impotent after an abdominoperineal resection. Refer the patient to a psychologist or psychiatrist for coping mechanisms to deal with changes in body image.

Follow-up

After resection, monitor CEA levels quarterly. Every 6 months the patient needs serial fecal occult blood tests, examination by a primary care provider (PCP,) chest X-ray, and liver function tests. Colonoscopy is needed yearly for 2 years. If all findings are negative, progress to colonoscopy every 2 to 3 years. If an adenomatous polyp is detected, refer for removal and follow up with colonoscopy in 6 months.

At age 35, patients with two risk factors should have serial fecal occult blood tests and colonoscopy and should start annual digital rectal examination (DRE). All patients need an annual DRE starting at age 40. All patients need serial fecal occult blood tests and either flexible sigmoidoscopy, colonoscopy, or barium enema every 3 years starting at age 50.

Complications

Wound infection, anastomotic problems, pneumonia, urinary tract infection, stomatitis, diarrhea, and temporary alopecia may occur.

Patient teaching

• Teach about the disease process, treatment options, and colostomy care.
• Teach the patient about risk factors (family history of polyposis or colorectal cancer), and reinforce the need for colorectal cancer screening, especially if he's a member of a high-risk group. Recommend a specific screening protocol based on his risk factors.

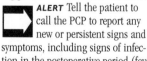 **ALERT** Tell the patient to call the PCP to report any new or persistent signs and symptoms, including signs of infection in the postoperative period (fever higher than 101° F [38.3° C] or increasing pain, swelling, drainage, odor, and wound size); change in

bowel habits or appearance of stool (diarrhea, constipation, blood in stool); palpable mass in abdomen or rectal area; rectal bleeding; and increasing or persistent abdominal pain.

Resources
• American Cancer Society: 800-ACS-2345
• Cancer Information Service: 800-4-CANCER
• Cancer Care: 800-813-HOPE
• CHEMOcare: 800-55-CHEMO
• United Ostomy Association: 800-826-0826
• For patients, caregivers and professional providers — Association of Cancer Online: *www.acor.org*

Depression, major

ICD-9-CM major depressive disorder 296.2, recurrent episode 296.3

Depression is the fourth most common reason patients visit the primary care provider. Depression manifests in many ways, but it occurs when a patient experiences more stress and negative emotions than he can handle. About half of all depressed patients experience a single episode and recover completely. Major depression can profoundly alter a person's ability to function. Suicide is the most serious complication of major depression. Nearly twice as many women as men attempt suicide, but men are far more likely to succeed.

Causes

The exact cause of depression isn't known. Current theory states that each individual is able to handle a certain amount of negative (or positive) stress. The body compensates by altering the rate of uptake of neurotransmitters by synaptic receptors.

When an individual experiences a major stressor (such as the death of a spouse) or a series of smaller stresses (car accident, job insecurity, major expenses, pregnancy), the synapses reset to a lower mood (almost as the adjustment of the thermostat of a house.) After synapses are reset, removing the original stress doesn't necessarily reverse the mood.

Depression commonly occurs secondary to many medical disorders such as cancer. The existence of a reason for the patient to be depressed doesn't stop the diagnosis and shouldn't delay treatment.

Many commonly abused substances (such as alcohol) as well as drugs prescribed for medical and psychiatric conditions can also cause depression. Examples include antihypertensives, psychotropics, narcotic and nonnarcotic analgesics, antiparkinsonian drugs, cardiovascular drugs, oral antidiabetics, antimicrobials, steroids, chemotherapeutic agents, and cimetidine.

Clinical presentation

The primary features of major depression are a predominantly sad mood, a loss of interest or pleasure in daily activities (anhedonia), a significant change in appetite, a sleep disorder (insomnia or hypersomnia), fatigue or loss of energy nearly every day, restlessness, irritability, social withdrawal, perpetual feelings of unworthiness or inappropriate guilt, an inability to concentrate or make decisions, and suicidal ideation. *Dysthymic disorder* is a milder, chronic form of depression.

The patient may report an increase or a decrease in appetite, sleep disturbance, a lack of interest in sexual activity, constipation, or diarrhea. When taking the patient's history, it's important to note affect and inattentiveness. Examination focuses on ruling out suspected causes but frequently reveals other signs, including agitation (such as hand wringing or restlessness) and reduced psychomotor activity (such as slowed speech).

Take special note of high-risk factors for suicide. These include certain age-groups (teenagers and elderly people), recurrent depressive episodes, previous suicide attempt, history of substance abuse (particularly alcohol), thought process disorder (patient hears dead relative calling him), lack of a social support system, lack of a significant other, presence of a chronic or disabling or painful disorder, a specific suicidal plan, giving away of personal belongings, suddenly feeling happy or energetic without cause, or having a family member or friend who has committed suicide. The more risk factors, the more closely the patient should be monitored.

Failure to detect suicidal thoughts early may encourage the patient to attempt suicide. The risk of suicide increases as the depression starts to lift and the patient regains the energy to carry out plans.

If you're uncomfortable in asking about suicidal ideation, practice this approach. After reaching the diagnosis of depression, say, "There is another symptom that you haven't mentioned, but more than 90% of patients with dysthymia have it. Do you ever get the feeling that you and just about everybody else would be better off if you weren't around?" If the patient denies it vehemently or states that their religious convictions are too strong to permit thoughts of suicide, be more concerned than if they state they have the occasional suicidal thoughts. If you are confident the patient isn't actively suicidal, understands the diagnosis and treatment plan, and knows he can contact you any time he feels bad, you can follow up in the office.

Differential diagnosis

 ALERT Insidious onset, inability to answer questions correctly despite extra time allotted, and no improvement with antidepressant medication regimens suggest dementia. You can prompt yourself to consider the causes of these symptoms with the mnemonic DEMENTIA: *D*rugs or alcohol; *E*ye or ear dysfunction; *M*etabolic or endocrine disorders, such as diabetes, hypoxia, chronic obstructive pulmonary disease, liver disease, renal dysfunction, and hypothyroidism; *E*motional problems, such as elder abuse, dysthymia, and chronic pain; *N*eurologic disorders, such as Parkinson's or Alzheimer's disease; *T*umors or trauma; *I*nfection (particularly urinary or respiratory tract in the elderly); and *A*rteriovascular causes, such as anemia or multiple infarcts.

Drugs cause depression in several ways — as an adverse effect or a withdrawal symptom, or from abuse or overdose.

Diagnostic tests
The diagnosis is made on clinical grounds but is supported by psychological tests.
• The Beck Depression Inventory or Children's Depression Inventory may help determine the onset, severity, duration, and progression of depressive symptoms.
• A toxicology screening may suggest drug-induced depression.
• Thyroid-stimulating hormone levels will indicate hypothyroidism.

Management

Acute
If the patient is a danger to himself or others, have someone else activate emergency medical services or get help while you engage the patient in conversation. State that you under-

stand how he feels and express your certainty that this feeling will pass and that there is help and hope.

General

Because of slowed responses, give the patient extra time to answer questions, ask questions, and express feelings. If you act rushed or fail to make eye contact, you may discourage him from confiding in you.

Pharmacologic therapy is usually an adjunct to psychotherapy. Antidepressants may mask deep-rooted problems. Never remove a patient's coping mechanism without giving him an acceptable replacement.

Teach carefully about diagnosis and drugs.

• Patient education increases compliance with management regimen, both pharmacologic and nonpharmacologic measures.

• Dysthymia isn't thoroughly understood, but current theory is that a chemical imbalance develops. Replacing that chemical helps the patient reset the synapses and relieves symptoms.

• Results take 2 to 8 weeks depending on the drug and are gradual.

• The patient may not receive the most effective drug the first time, but with the right drug and the right dose, the patient will feel better.

• The primary care provider will work with the patient until the right drug is found.

You must be willing to work with the patient until he feels better and must be available at all times during an acute episode.

Medication

In depression, drug therapy includes selective serotonin reuptake inhibitors (SSRIs), tricyclic antidepressants (TCAs), monoamine oxidase (MAO) inhibitors, and bupropion.

• SSRIs, including fluoxetine (Prozac), trazodone (Desyrel), paroxetine (Paxil), and sertraline (Zoloft), are increasingly becoming the drugs of choice. They are effective and produce fewer adverse effects than TCAs; however, they're associated with sleep and GI problems and alterations in sexual desire and function.

• TCAs, such as amitriptyline, clomipramine, and desipramine, prevent the reuptake of norepinephrine, serotonin, or both into the presynaptic nerve endings, resulting in increased synaptic concentrations of these neurotransmitters. They also cause a gradual loss in the number of beta-adrenergic receptors.

• MAO inhibitors, such as phenelzine, selegiline, and tranylcypromine, block the enzymatic degradation of norepinephrine and serotonin. These agents often are prescribed for patients with atypical depression (for example, depression marked by an increased appetite and need for sleep, rather than anorexia and insomnia) and for some patients who fail to respond to TCAs.

MAO inhibitors are associated with a high risk of toxicity; patients treated with one of them must be able to comply with the necessary dietary restrictions. Conservative doses of an MAO inhibitor may be combined with a TCA for patients refractory to either drug alone.

The mechanism of action of bupropion is unknown.

After resolution of the acute episode, patients commonly remain on antidepressants for 6 months to 2 years. If depression recurs, the patient may be maintained on low doses of antidepressants.

Referral or consultation

 COLLABORATION If appropriate, refer the patient to a psychiatrist or psychologist whom you know to be reputable and licensed. An appointment is urgent for patients who are in their teens or younger; for those over 64; for those who are pregnant or sexually active without contraceptive measures; for those who are unable to function, have comorbidities, and are nonresponsive to two trials of antidepressant drugs; and for those who are suicidal or having a recurrence of depression.

A counselor can provide the patient with alternatives that others have tried successfully in the past, so the patient won't be limited to coping mechanisms that are already familiar. Support groups specific to the patient's profile (Incest Survivors, Narcotics Anonymous) are useful.

Follow-up

Follow-up should be weekly until improvement is noted (if no improvement occurs in 6 to 8 weeks, consider another drug), then monthly for 3 months, and then quarterly. Focus on the adverse effects, dosage, and effectiveness of the drug regimen.

Complications

Complications include attempted suicide, nonresponsiveness to therapy, and recurrence.

Patient teaching

• Teach the patient that it normally takes 6 to 8 weeks for effects to show. Effects are gradual, not dramatic.
• Help the patient to develop a structured routine, including noncompetitive activities, to build his self-confidence and encourage interaction with others. Urge him to join group activities and to socialize.
• Inform the patient that he can help ease depression by expressing his feelings, participating in pleasurable activities, and improving grooming and hygiene.
• Help him to recognize distorted perceptions that may contribute to

his depression. When he learns to recognize depressive thought patterns, he can consciously begin to substitute self-affirming thoughts.
• Teach the patient about prescribed medications. Stress the need to comply with the drug regimen and to report adverse effects. For drugs with anticholinergic effects, such as amitriptyline and amoxapine, suggest sugarless gum or hard candy to relieve dry mouth.
• Many antidepressants are sedating (for example, amitriptyline and trazodone); warn the patient taking these drugs to avoid activities that require alertness, including driving and operating mechanical equipment, until the central nervous system (CNS) effects of the drug are known.
• Caution the patient taking a TCA to avoid drinking alcoholic beverages or taking other CNS depressants during therapy.
• If the patient is taking an MAO inhibitor, emphasize that he must avoid foods that contain tyramine, caffeine, or tryptophan. The ingestion of tyramine can cause a hypertensive crisis. Examples of foods that contain these substances are cheese, sour cream, pickled herring, liver, canned figs, raisins, bananas, avocados, chocolate, soy sauce, fava beans, yeast extracts, meat tenderizers, coffee, colas, beer, Chianti wine, and sherry.

ALERT Tell the patient to call the primary care provider to report any new or persistent signs and symptoms, including the following: inability to perform daily activities, weight loss, and increasing feelings of frustration, anger, or hopelessness.

Resources
• National Depression Manic Depression Association: 800-82-NDMDA
• National Foundation for Depressive Illness: 800-248-4344

- National Mental Health Services Knowledge Exchange Network: 800-789-CMHS
- For patients—National Mental Health Association: *www.nmha.org*
- For professionals—Health Net's Psych Pharm site: *www.cmhc.com*

Diabetes mellitus

ICD-9-CM 250.0, with nephropathy 250.4, with ophthalmopathy 250.5, with neuropathy 250.6

A chronic disease of absolute or relative insulin deficiency or resistance, diabetes mellitus is characterized by disturbances in carbohydrate, protein, and fat metabolism.

This disorder occurs in two forms: type 1, formerly known as insulin-dependent diabetes mellitus, and the more prevalent type 2, formerly known as non-insulin-dependent diabetes mellitus.

Type 1 usually occurs before age 30 (although it may occur at any age); the patient is usually thin and requires exogenous insulin and dietary management to achieve control. Conversely, type 2 used to be called "adult-onset diabetes" because it occurred mostly in obese adults after age 40. However, changing dietary patterns and increasing rates of obesity are causing type 2 diabetes to develop in younger people, even children. Type 2 diabetes is most often treated with diet, exercise, and antidiabetic drugs, but treatment may include insulin therapy.

Diabetes mellitus affects an estimated 5% of the population of the United States (10 to 12 million people), about half of whom are undiagnosed. Incidence is equal in men and women and rises with age. People are at added risk for developing diabetes if they have a history of gestational diabetes, have given birth to a macrosomic infant (more than 9 lb), or have hypertension, dyslipidemia, or glucose intolerance.

 SPECIAL POPULATIONS
High-risk groups for type 2 diabetes include Blacks, Hispanics, and Native Americans. The incidence of type 2 diabetes has dramatically increased in obese children, particularly among minority populations in North America. Currently, 30% of newly diagnosed diabetics are in their second decade of life.

A leading cause of death by disease in the United States, diabetes contributes to about 50% of myocardial infarctions and about 75% of cerebrovascular accidents as well as to renal failure and peripheral vascular disease. Diabetes is also the leading cause of new blindness in the United States.

Causes

The effects of diabetes mellitus result from insulin deficiency. Insulin transports glucose into the cells for use as energy and storage as glycogen. It also stimulates protein synthesis and free fatty acid storage in the fat deposits. Insulin deficiency compromises the body tissues' access to essential nutrients for fuel and storage.

The cause of both type 1 and type 2 diabetes remains unknown. Genetic factors may play a part in development of all types; autoimmune disease and viral infections may be risk factors in type 1.

Other risk factors include the following:
- Obesity and lower levels of activity contribute to resistance to endogenous insulin.
- Physiologic or emotional stress can cause prolonged elevation of stress hormone levels (cortisol, epinephrine, glucagon, and growth hormone). This raises blood glucose lev-

els, which, in turn, places an increased demand on the pancreas.

• Pregnancy causes weight gain and increases hormonal levels (estrogen, progesterone, prolactin, and human placental lactogen), which cause insulin resistance.

• Some medications can antagonize the effects of insulin, including thiazide diuretics, adrenal corticosteroids, and oral contraceptives.

The patient history should focus on symptoms associated with hyperglycemia and hypoglycemia, reviewing the patient's glucose testing diary, and complications of diabetes. Elicit dietary habits, ideal-weight maintenance attempts, exercise (frequency and duration), and drug treatment and compliance. If the patient is noncompliant due to an inability to pay for medications or supplies, refer to social services or suggest resources. Assess cardiac risk factors: obesity, hypertension, smoking, high triglycerides, high low-density lipoproteins (LDLs), low high-density lipoproteins (HDLs), and stress.

Clinical presentation

In type 1 diabetes, symptomatology may be insidious or dramatic, as with ketoacidosis. The most common symptom is fatigue from energy deficiency and a catabolic state.

Insulin deficiency causes the three P's of diabetes: polyphagia, polydipsia, and polyuria. Hyperglycemia pulls fluid from body tissues, causing osmotic diuresis, polyuria, dehydration, polydipsia, dry mucous membranes, and poor skin turgor. In ketoacidosis and hyperosmolar hyperglycemic nonketotic syndrome (HHNS), dehydration may cause hypovolemia and shock. Wasting of glucose in the urine usually produces weight loss and hunger in type 1 diabetes, even with polyphagia.

ALERT Glucosuria without hyperglycemia is present in benign renal glucosuria and renal tubular disease. Polyuria and polydipsia without hyperglycemia occur in diabetes insipidus. Hyperglycemia and glucosuria are seen in pheochromocytoma, Cushing's syndrome, and acromegaly. Hyperglycemia occurs in acute periods of severe stress from infection, trauma, and burns.

Long-term effects

In diabetes, long-term effects may include cardiovascular problems, retinopathy, nephropathy, atherosclerosis, peripheral and autonomic neuropathy, and an increased susceptibility to infection.

ALERT Macrovascular complications are the major cause of death in diabetics. Additional risk factors exacerbate the problem. These include smoking tobacco, obesity, sedentary lifestyle, hypertension, and dyslipidemia.

A condition known as Syndrome X, or insulin resistance syndrome, occurs if a patient has the all of the following risk factors: obesity, high blood pressure, high triglyceride levels, and low HDL levels (each of which is an independent risk factor for heart disease). Syndrome X is associated with a high risk of developing type 2 diabetes and coronary artery disease. The components (risk factors) of this syndrome are associated with high insulin levels that result from peripheral insulin resistance. Eliminating or reducing any individual component will decrease the overall risk; however, most measures that affect one component will affect the others as well, providing additional risk reduction.

Retinopathy can progress to blindness, nephropathy to kidney failure, and atherosclerosis to cardiovascular events.

Peripheral neuropathy usually affects the hands and feet and may cause numbness or pain. Autonomic neuropathy may manifest itself in several ways, including gastroparesis (leading to delayed gastric emptying and a feeling of nausea and fullness after meals), nocturnal diarrhea, impotence, and orthostatic hypotension.

Because hyperglycemia impairs the patient's resistance to infection, diabetes may result in skin and urinary tract infections (UTIs) and vaginitis. The glucose content of the epidermis and urine encourages bacterial growth.

Differential diagnosis

Other conditions need to be considered before reaching a diagnosis of diabetes. Glucosuria without hyperglycemia can occur in benign renal glucosuria or in renal tubular disease. Diabetes insipidus presents with polyuria and polydipsia but not hyperglycemia. Secondary diabetes may result from endocrine or metabolic disorders that cause hyperglycemia and glucosuria, such as Cushing's syndrome, pheochromocytoma, and acromegaly. Transient hyperglycemia can also occur in severe stress from trauma, burns, or infection.

Diagnostic tests

In nonpregnant adults, one of the following findings confirms diabetes mellitus:

• typical symptoms of uncontrolled diabetes and a random blood glucose level equal to or above 200 mg/dl

• a fasting plasma glucose level equal to or greater than 126 mg/dl on at least two occasions.

• if the fasting glucose test is normal, a blood glucose level above 200 mg/dl during a glucose tolerance test with 75-g glucose load.

An ophthalmologic examination may show diabetic retinopathy. Glycosylated hemoglobin (HgbA1c) reflects glucose control over the previous 3 months; this isn't diagnostic but is useful in long-term management.

Management

General

Types 1 and 2

Effective treatment for both types of diabetes normalizes blood glucose and decreases complications. Therefore, review applicable information about diabetes, self-monitoring, foot care, physical activity, and diet management at each visit.

Treatment of both types of diabetes requires a diet designed to meet nutritional needs, to control blood glucose levels, and to reach and maintain appropriate body weight. For the obese patient with type 2 diabetes, weight reduction is a goal. In type 1, the calorie allotment may be high, depending on growth stage and activity level. For success, the diet must be followed consistently and meals eaten at regular times.

Support groups and classes certified by the American Diabetes Association can help with education, motivation, and compliance.

Researchers are also making progress in gene therapy. Genes have been developed that regulate and produce insulin, but the genes need to be placed in a permanent spot in the deoxyribonucleic acid chain so the effect doesn't die along with the individual cell.

Type 1 diabetes

In insulin-dependent diabetes mellitus, treatment includes insulin replacement. Current forms of insulin replacement include single-dose, mixed-dose, split–mixed dose, and multiple-dose regimens. The multiple-dose regimens may use an insulin pump. Insulin inhalers and insulin patches are being studied.

Insulin may be rapid-acting (Regular), intermediate-acting (NPH), long-acting (Ultralente), or a combination of rapid-acting and intermediate-acting (Mixtard); it may be standard or purified, and it may be derived from beef, pork, or human sources. Purified human insulin is used commonly today.

Pancreas transplantation is experimental and requires chronic immunosuppression.

Type 2 diabetes

Exercise and dietary changes are first-line therapy in many patients with new-onset type 2 diabetes. The success rate of diet and exercise alone is 3% to 5%. Therefore, non-insulin-dependent diabetes mellitus may require oral antidiabetic drugs to stimulate endogenous insulin production, increase insulin sensitivity at the cellular level, delay carbohydrate absorption from the GI tract, and suppress hepatic gluconeogenesis.

Medications for type 2 diabetes include sulfonylureas (tolbutamide, glyburide), which stimulate insulin production; biguanides (metformin), which inhibit hepatic glucose production and increase peripheral insulin sensitivity without increasing insulin levels; alpha-glucosidase inhibitors (acarbose), which decrease the rate of absorption of carbohydrates and so decrease postprandial peaks of blood glucose; and thiazolidinediones (troglitazone), which reduce peripheral insulin resistance. Combination therapy is becoming more common and achieving better control with fewer episodes of hypoglycemia.

Insulin can be added to or temporarily replace oral antidiabetics when maximum dosage or combinations of oral drugs aren't controlling hyperglycemia, during times of major stress or infection, and during pregnancy.

Referral or consultation

The patient should see an endocrinologist for new or poorly controlled diabetes, an ophthalmologist (yearly) for a dilated-eye examination to check for retinopathy, a podiatrist for early intervention with foot disorders, and a dietitian for diet management.

He should be referred to an endocrinologist or another doctor if he has ketosis or uncontrolled blood glucose levels, fails to respond to conventional regimens, switches from oral antidiabetics to insulin, or experiences chest pain, painful neuropathy, mental confusion, or skin ulcers. Genetic counseling may be considered for young adult diabetics who are planning families.

Follow-up

When the drug regimen is changed, see the patient weekly until his glucose level is controlled and then every 2 to 4 months if HgbA1c testing reflects control. Visit frequency is influenced by compliance, metabolic control, and signs of end-organ damage. At each visit review symptoms, blood glucose record, laboratory results, funduscopy, cardiac status (especially blood pressure), and foot status (examine for skin integrity, blood supply, and neuropathy). After 3 years, schedule an annual dilated-eye examination for retinopathy.

Other follow-up includes routine urinalysis for proteinuria and creatinine to detect renal insufficiency, an annual random urine specimen for albumin-to-creatinine ratio, or 24-hour urine collection. (If urinalysis indicates decreased kidney function, repeat twice; if two out of three tests suggest decreased kidney function, the patient should begin taking an angiotensin-converting enzyme inhibitor such as captopril.) Consider scheduling the patient for a periodic lipid panel because diabetics are at high risk for atherosclerosis and cardiac events.

Complications

Treatment of long-term diabetic complications may include transplantation or dialysis for renal failure, photocoagulation for retinopathy, drugs for hypertension and lipid abnormalities, and vascular surgery for large-vessel disease. Tight glucose control is essential in minimizing all of these complications, probably due to decreasing the arterial changes caused by hyperglycemia. Other complications include HHNS, gangrene, glaucoma, cataracts, skin ulceration, and Charcot joints.

The Diabetes Control and Complications Trial has proved that intensive drug therapy that focuses on keeping glucose at near-normal levels for 5 years or more reduces both the onset and progression of retinopathy (by up to 63%), nephropathy (by up to 54%), and neuropathy (by up to 60%).

Patient teaching

• Stress that compliance with the prescribed program is essential. Emphasize the effects of strict blood glucose control on long-term health (delaying or preventing blindness, impotence, stroke, heart attack, and amputation).

 ALERT Teach the patient to always check blood sugar before treating symptoms of hyperglycemia or hypoglycemia because symptoms can be similar.

• Instruct the patient to watch for acute complications of diabetic therapy, especially hypoglycemia (lethargy, dizziness, weakness, pallor, diaphoresis). Check blood glucose levels; if they're low, immediately give carbohydrates in the form of 6 oz fruit juice or one piece of hard candy.

• Be alert for signs of ketoacidosis (acetone breath, dehydration, weak and rapid pulse, Kussmaul's respirations) and HHNS (polyuria, thirst, neurologic abnormalities, and stupor). Check blood glucose levels, and medicate per individualized parameters. If levels exceed the highest range of the personal treatment plan, notify the primary care provider.

• Teach the patient how to manage his diabetes when he has a minor illness, such as a cold, the flu, and an upset stomach.

• Have the patient monitor diabetic control by testing and recording blood glucose levels. Tell him to bring the record and glucometer to the office with each visit; have him demonstrate proper technique and correct as needed.

• Teach the effects of diabetes on the blood vessels, eyes, kidneys, peripheral nervous system, and autonomic nervous system. Reinforce that the best treatment is prevention with close control of blood glucose levels.

• Treat all injuries, cuts, and blisters (particularly on the legs or feet) meticulously.

• Be alert for signs of UTI and renal disease (decreased, concentrated, dark or cloudy urine with or without discomfort).

• Remind the patient of the need for yearly ophthalmologic examinations to detect diabetic retinopathy.

• Teach the patient the signs of diabetic neuropathy (numbness or pain in the hands and feet, footdrop, impotence, neurogenic bladder). Stress the need for personal safety precautions; explain that decreased sensation can mask injuries. Suggest topical anesthetic creams with capsaicin (Zostrix) and gentle massage to relieve discomfort.

• Teach the patient to care for his feet by washing them daily, drying carefully between the toes, and inspecting for corns, calluses, redness, swelling, bruises, and breaks in the skin. Advise him to wear nonconstricting shoes and to avoid walking barefoot.

• To delay the clinical onset of diabetes, teach persons at high risk to avoid risk factors.

ALERT Tell the patient to call the primary care provider to report any new or persistent signs and symptoms, including signs of infection, signs of cardiac distress (chest pain, palpitations, dyspnea, confusion), changes in vision, peripheral numbness or tingling, constipation, anorexia, and blisters or skin openings, particularly on the feet.

Resources

• American Association of Diabetes Educators: 800-338-DMED
• American Diabetes Association: 800-DIABETES or *www.diabetes.org*
• American Diabetes Foundation: 800-232-3472
• Juvenile Diabetes Foundation: 800-223-1138
• Juvenile Diabetes Foundation International: 800-JDF-CURE
• The Neuropathy Association: 800-247-6968 or *www.neuropathy.org*
• Patient information on gestational diabetes: *www.medscape.com*
• For providers — Drug affordability: *www.needymeds.com* (contains information regarding many drug company programs that provide financial assistance for their drugs)

Diverticular disease

ICD-9-CM diverticulosis 562.10, diverticulitis 562.11

In this disorder, bulging pouches (diverticula) in the GI wall push the mucosal lining through the surrounding muscle. The most common site for diverticula is in the sigmoid colon, but they may develop anywhere, from the proximal end of the pharynx to the anus.

Other typical sites are the duodenum, near the pancreatic border (the ampulla of Vater), and the jejunum. Diverticular disease of the stomach is rare and is often a precursor of peptic or neoplastic disease. Diverticular disease of the ileum (Meckel's diverticulum) is the most common congenital anomaly of the GI tract but is rarely symptomatic after age 5.

Diverticular disease has two clinical forms. In *diverticulosis,* diverticula are present but don't cause symptoms. In *diverticulitis,* diverticula are inflamed and may cause potentially fatal obstruction, infection, or hemorrhage.

Causes

Diverticular disease is most prevalent after age 60 and is rare before age 40. Diverticula probably result from high intraluminal pressure on areas of weakness in the GI wall, where blood vessels enter.

Diet may also be a contributing factor because lack of roughage reduces fecal residue, narrows the bowel lumen, and leads to higher intra-abdominal pressure during defecation. The fact that diverticulosis is most prevalent in Western industrialized nations, where processing removes much of the roughage from foods, supports this theory. Diverticulosis is less common in nations where the diet contains more natural bulk and fiber.

In diverticulitis, retained undigested food mixed with bacteria accumulates in the diverticular sac, forming a hard mass (fecalith). This substance cuts off the blood supply to the thin walls of the sac, making them more susceptible to attack by colonic bacteria. Inflammation follows, possibly leading to perforation, abscess, peritonitis, obstruction, or hemorrhage. Occasionally, the inflamed colon segment may form a fistula by adhering to the bladder or other organs.

Clinical presentation

The two forms of diverticular disease produce different clinical effects.

Diverticulosis

Although diverticulosis usually produces no symptoms, the patient may complain of recurrent left lower quadrant pain. Such pain, often accompanied by alternating constipation and diarrhea, is relieved by defecation or the passage of flatus. Symptoms resemble irritable bowel syndrome and suggest that both disorders may coexist.

In older patients, a rare complication of diverticulosis (without diverticulitis) is hemorrhage from colonic diverticula, usually in the right colon. Such hemorrhage is usually mild to moderate and easily controlled, but it may occasionally be massive and life-threatening.

Diverticulitis

Mild diverticulitis produces moderate left lower quadrant pain, gas, and irregular bowel habits. Additionally, the patient may complain of mild nausea, low-grade fever, and leukocytosis.

In severe diverticulitis, the diverticula can rupture and produce abscesses or peritonitis. Rupture occurs in up to 20% of such patients; its symptoms include abdominal rigidity and left lower quadrant pain.

Peritonitis follows the release of fecal material from the rupture site and causes signs of sepsis and shock (high fever, chills, hypotension). Rupture of the diverticulum near a vessel may cause microscopic or massive hemorrhage, depending on the vessel's size.

Chronic diverticulitis may cause fibrosis and adhesions that narrow the bowel's lumen and lead to bowel obstruction. Signs and symptoms of incomplete obstruction include constipation, ribbonlike stools, intermittent diarrhea, and abdominal distention. Signs and symptoms of increasing obstruction include abdominal rigidity and pain, diminishing or absent bowel sounds, nausea, and vomiting.

Differential diagnosis

 ALERT Any patient with a GI complaint whose examination reveals an abdominal mass, severe abdominal tenderness, fever, weight loss, or acute onset without obvious cause requires aggressive evaluation. Other red flags include nocturnal wakening due to GI complaints, family history of malignancy, positive fecal occult blood test, and abnormal blood counts.

Conditions to consider include irritable bowel syndrome, lactose intolerance, colon cancer, ulcerative colitis, Crohn's disease, angiodysplasia (for rectal bleeding), ischemic or infectious colitis, and appendicitis.

Diverticular disease frequently produces no symptoms and is discovered accidentally during an upper GI series.

Diagnostic tests

• White blood cell (WBC) elevation with immature polymorphs indicates diverticulitis.
• A low hemoglobin reading indicates bleeding.
• Erythrocyte sedimentation rate elevation indicates diverticulitis.
• Urinalysis showing WBCs, red blood cells, or pus cells suggests possible fistula formation.

- Urine culture of persistent infection suggests colovesical fistula.
- Blood culture, if positive, indicates diverticulitis with generalized peritonitis.
- An upper GI series confirms or rules out diverticulosis of the esophagus and upper bowel.
- Barium enema confirms or rules out diverticulosis of the lower bowel. Barium-filled diverticula can be single, multiple, or clustered like grapes and may have a wide or narrow mouth. Barium outlines, but doesn't fill, diverticula blocked by impacted feces. In patients with acute diverticulitis, a barium enema may rupture the bowel, so this procedure requires caution.
- Abdominal X-rays may detect peritonitis, perforation and, if irritable bowel syndrome accompanies diverticular disease, colonic spasm.
- Computed tomography (CT) scan with or without contrast is diagnostic for abscess, fistula, and measuring an inflammatory mass.
- Angiography is diagnostic and therapeutic for diverticular bleeding.
- Spiral CT scan with bolus of I.V. contrast may detect bleeding.
- Colonoscopy and flexible sigmoidoscopy may detect cancer and ulcerative or ischemic colitis.
- Cystoscopy is indicated if colovesical fistula is suspected.
- A biopsy rules out cancer; however, a colonoscopic biopsy isn't recommended during acute diverticular disease because of the strenuous bowel preparation it requires.

Management

The two forms of the disease call for different treatment regimens.

Diverticulosis

Asymptomatic diverticulosis generally doesn't require treatment. Intestinal diverticulosis with pain, mild GI distress, constipation, or difficult defecation generally responds to a liquid or bland diet, stool softeners, and occasional doses of mineral oil. These measures relieve symptoms, minimize irritation, and lessen the risk of progression to diverticulitis. After pain subsides, patients also benefit from a high-residue diet and bulk laxatives such as psyllium.

Diverticulitis

Treatment of mild diverticulitis without signs of perforation aims to prevent constipation and combat infection. It may include bed rest, a liquid diet, a broad-spectrum antibiotic (ciprofloxacin), stool softeners, a narcotic pain reliever such as meperidine to control pain and relax smooth muscle, and an antispasmodic, such as hyoscyamine or propantheline, to control muscle spasms.

Diverticulitis that doesn't respond to medical treatment requires a colon resection to remove the involved segment. Perforation, peritonitis, obstruction, or a fistula that accompanies diverticulitis may require a temporary colostomy to drain abscesses and rest the colon, followed by later anastomosis.

Patients who hemorrhage need blood replacement and careful monitoring of fluid and electrolyte balance. Such bleeding usually stops spontaneously. If bleeding continues, angiography may be performed to guide catheter placement for infusing vasopressin into the bleeding vessel.

Referral or consultation

Refer the patient to a gastroenterologist for evaluation and colonoscopy as needed and to a doctor if the condition is nonresponsive in 2 to 3 days. Hospitalization may be needed for toxicity, septicemia, or peritonitis. The patient should see an enterostomal therapist if an ostomy is placed.

Follow-up

See the patient in 2 to 3 days to evaluate response.

Complications

Hemorrhage, perforation, peritonitis, bowel obstruction, abscess, fistula, toxicity, or septicemia may occur.

Patient teaching

If the patient has diverticulosis, include the following points in your teaching:

• Explain what diverticula are and how they form.

• Make sure the patient understands the importance of dietary roughage and the harmful effects of constipation and straining during defecation. Encourage increased intake of foods high in indigestible fiber, including fresh fruits and vegetables, whole-grain bread, and wheat or bran cereals. Warn that a high-fiber diet may temporarily cause flatulence and discomfort.

• Advise the patient to relieve constipation with stool softeners or bulk-forming cathartics. But caution against taking bulk-forming cathartics without plenty of water; if swallowed dry, they may absorb enough moisture in the mouth and throat to swell and obstruct the esophagus or trachea.

 ALERT Tell the patient to call the primary care provider to report any new or persistent signs and symptoms, including abdominal pain that worsens or is nonresponsive to treatment; fever above 101° F (38.3° C); signs of dehydration (light-headedness, voiding small amounts of dark concentrated urine, excessive thirst); vomiting blood or coffee-ground material; bright red, black, tarry, or maroon-colored stools; yellow skin or eyes; or no bowel movement for 5 days.

Resources

• For patient information on irritable bowel syndrome: *www.medscape.com*

Headache

ICD-9-CM headache 784, classic migraine 346.0, unspecified migraine 346.9, tension headache 307.81, cluster headache 346.2

Headache is the most common complaint in primary care. The three most common types are migraine, tension-type, and cluster.

Causes

Most chronic headaches result from tension — muscle contraction — which may be caused by emotional stress, fatigue, menstruation, or environmental stimuli (noise, crowds, bright lights). The cause of migraine headaches isn't known, but they've been linked to constriction and dilation of cranial arteries, indicating a process that causes neurogenic inflammation. One theory stating that disruption of neurotransmitters (serotonin and norepinephrine) occurs during migraines is supported by research findings that antidepressant drugs that regulate neurotransmitters are effective against migraine in some cases.

More than 80% of migraine patients have a family history of migraines, and a chromosomal abnormality has been found in at least one type of migraine. Research suggests that classic migraine, common migraine, and chronic tension-type headache (present more than 15 days a month) are actually variants of the same disorder. This, in turn, is supported by another theory, which states that chronic headaches are caused by a biochemical condition similar to depression.

Other causes of headache include glaucoma; inflammation of the eyes or mucosa of the nasal or paranasal sinuses; diseases of the scalp, teeth, extracranial arteries, and external or middle ear; and muscle spasms of the face, neck, or shoulders.

Headaches may also be secondary to drugs such as vasodilators (nitrates, alcohol, histamine), systemic disease, hypoxia, hypertension, head trauma and tumor, intracranial bleeding, abscess, or aneurysm.

Clinical presentation

The three common categories of headache can be differentiated by presentation.

Migraine

For diagnosis, two of the following characteristics must be present: pulsatile pain, unilateral location, nausea and vomiting, photophobia, or sonophobia. History may reveal that the migraine was preceded by scintillating scotoma (visual aura), hemianopsia, unilateral paresthesia, or speech disorders; aura typically occurs 20 minutes before migraine onset. The patient may experience irritability and anorexia, and may be bedridden. Possible association exists with neck muscle contraction and pain, cervical osteoarthritis, vasodilation, epilepsy, and low plasma serotonin levels. Common migraine is the same as classic migraine but without an aura.

Tension-type headaches

These headaches produce a dull, persistent ache, tender spots on the head and neck, and a feeling of tightness around the head, with a characteristic "hatband" distribution. The pain is often unrelenting and may last a long time, even years (rarely). Examination may reveal associated neck muscle contraction and pain, cervical osteoarthritis, vasodilation, epilepsy, or low plasma serotonin levels.

Cluster headaches

These headaches typically develop within 2 hours of falling asleep. The pain is so excruciating that patients can't sit still. Many patients who use alcohol and tobacco, which trigger these headaches, abstain during attacks. Pain is unilateral during an episode but may switch sides from cycle to cycle. The eye on the affected side is commonly erythematous and edematous. These headaches typically occur in clusters of up to four times a day for 1 to 4 months, disappear completely for 6 months to 2 years, and then the cycle repeats.

An accurate diagnosis requires a history of recurrent headaches and physical examination of the head and neck. Such examination includes percussion, auscultation for bruits, inspection for signs of infection, and palpation for defects (hardened, nonpulsatile temporal arteries), crepitus, or tender spots (especially after trauma). A firm diagnosis also requires a complete neurologic examination and assessment for other systemic diseases (such as hypertension) and depression.

Differential diagnosis

 ALERT Warning signs that suggest a serious underlying cause needing prompt consultation or referral include patient complaints of a cluster, migraine, or chronic tension-type headache for the first time in his life; increasingly frequent and severe headaches; changes in cognition; syncope; seizures; being wakened by a headache; vomiting without nausea; history of recent head injury; tender nonpulsatile temporal arteries; or nuchal rigidity and high fever. More aggressive evaluation is needed if papilledema is observed during funduscopy, if the patient has symptoms suggesting another systemic illness (such as weight loss), or if his headaches fail to respond to treatment.

Specific causes to consider include cervical spondylosis, temporomandibular joint syndrome, caffeine dependence, nonprescription analgesic dependence (due to caffeine content), depression, head injury, severe anemia or polycythemia, uremia, hepatic disorders, toxic effects from drugs or chemical exposure, dental disease, Paget's disease, chronic sinusitis, refractive error, hypertension, hypoxia, temporal arteritis, and lesions of the eye, ear, or oral cavity.

Diagnostic tests

• Elevated sedimentation rate in patients over age 50 may indicate temporal arteritis.
• Complete blood count is done if anemia or polycythemia is suspected.
• Electrolyte and thyroid studies detect metabolic and endocrine disorders.
• X-rays of the cervical spine and sinuses detect arthritis and chronic sinus infection.
• Computed tomography, magnetic resonance imaging, and magnetic resonance angiography are performed for a new onset or change in the headache pattern, or if neurologic abnormalities are found on examination. These tests can detect hemorrhage and tumors.
• Lumbar puncture can reveal infection.

Management

Treatment depends on the length and severity of the headaches. Other measures include identification and elimination of trigger factors and, possibly, psychotherapy if emotional stress is a trigger.

Migraine treatment
Acute
The patient may require hospitalization for severe pain, concurrent medical problems such as dehydration, or medication-withdrawal problems. Urgently institute abortive drug therapy because early intervention assists in management.

General
Explain the diagnosis clearly, and validate the patient's pain. Teach the patient biofeedback techniques so that he can gain conscious control over various autonomic functions with the help of electronic monitors. By observing the fluctuations of a particular bodily function, such as heart rate or blood pressure, on the monitor, he'll eventually learn to adjust his thinking to control that function. For instance, electromyelographic (measuring muscle tension) biofeedback is used for the treatment of muscle contraction headaches.

Massage, gentle exercise, and a balanced diet may help by decreasing overall muscle tension and improving subclinical health problems, such as plaque buildup in arteries and decreasing insulin sensitivity.

Medication
• Abortive drugs include $5HT_1$-receptor agonists (sumatriptan), dihydro-ergotamine, isometheptene-dichloralphenazone-acetaminophen (Midrin), and nonsteroidal anti-inflammatory drugs (NSAIDs). A full daily dose must be given in 1 hour to abort attack. If nausea and vomiting make oral administration impossible, some drugs can be given by alternative routes. Antiemetics (metoclopramide) are a helpful adjunct to other thera-

pies; corticosteroids (prednisone) reduce neurogenic inflammation.
• Preventive drugs include propranolol, atenolol, clonidine, and amitriptyline.

Chronic tension-type headache
• Prophylactic antidepressants (sertraline) are useful.
• For exacerbations, NSAIDs (naproxen) and muscle relaxants (methocarbamol) may be used.

Cluster headache
• Prophylactic drugs include calcium channel blockers (verapamil), corticosteroids (prednisone, tapered over 1 month), and ergotamine vasoconstrictors (methysergide).
• Abortive drugs include oxygen (7 to 10 L by face mask), 5-HT$_1$-receptor agonists (subcutaneous sumatriptan), ergotamine vasoconstrictors (sublingual ergotamine), antimanics (lithium), or local anesthetics (intranasal lidocaine).

Referral or consultation
Refer the patient to a specialist (neurologist, ophthalmologist), as indicated by findings. A psychologist or psychiatrist can assist with biofeedback and pain management. Refer to a primary care provider if you're unsure of diagnosis, for concurrent medical conditions, for drug-seeking behavior, or if the condition is nonresponsive to therapy.

Follow-up
Focus on documenting frequency of attacks, pain behaviors, and medication usage; also stress avoiding triggers through behavior modification.

Complications

Unremitting migraine, cerebral ischemia, adverse effects of medications, and drug dependence are potential complications.

Patient teaching

• Explain to the patient that migraine is a hereditary disorder that affects the blood vessels around the brain. It's treatable but not curable. Drug therapy can decrease the severity and length of migraines, and avoiding trigger factors can reduce their frequency.
• Trigger factors consist of changes in routine: sleep changes, weather changes, a change in caffeine intake (from diet or over-the-counter analgesics), hormonal changes, letdown after stress, and missing meals. If food is a trigger, it will have an effect within 30 minutes to 12 hours after ingestion.
• Encourage the patient to keep a headache diary to help pinpoint individual triggers and most effective therapies. Record the duration and location of the headache; the time of day it usually begins; the nature of the pain; concurrent symptoms such as blurred vision; and precipitating factors, such as tension, menstruation or menopause, loud noises, use of alcohol, use of medications such as oral contraceptives, and prolonged fasting.
• Provide information about the rationale for drug classes, drug actions, and limitations (antidepressants, neurotransmitter regulation, and rebound effects of prolonged use of dihydroergotamine).
• Advise the patient to lie down in a dark, quiet room during an attack and to place ice packs on his forehead or a cold cloth over his eyes.
• Instruct him to take medication at the onset of migraine symptoms.
• Stress that drinking plenty of fluids is important because dehydration is common.

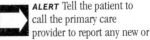 **ALERT** Tell the patient to call the primary care provider to report any new or persistent signs and symptoms,

including headache lasting more than 24 hours despite therapy, difficulty moving extremities, slurred speech, confusion, difficulty walking normally, blurred or double vision, vomiting without nausea, increasing severity or frequency, headaches present on waking (if the patient had a head injury), and fever higher than 101° F (38.3° C) for adults and 102.5° F (39° C) for children ages 4 months to 17 years with a stiff neck. Tell the patient to call during office hours for any other questions or concerns.

Resources

• American Council for Headache Education: 800-255-ACHE
• National Headache Foundation: 800-843-2256
• New England Headache Treatment Program: 800-245-0088
• American Council for Headache Education (a neurologist specializing in headaches serves as an advisor to this site geared toward laypersons): *www.achenet.org*
• Patient information on headaches: *www.medscape.com*

Heart failure

ICD-9-CM congestive heart failure 428.0

A syndrome characterized by myocardial dysfunction, heart failure leads to impaired pump performance (reduced cardiac output) or to frank heart failure and abnormal circulatory congestion. Congestion of systemic venous circulation may result in peripheral edema or hepatomegaly; congestion of pulmonary circulation may cause pulmonary edema, which is an acute, life-threatening emergency.

Pump failure usually occurs in a damaged left ventricle (left-sided

heart failure) but may occur in the right ventricle (right-sided heart failure) either as a primary disorder or secondary to left-sided heart failure. Sometimes left- and right-sided heart failure develop simultaneously.

Although heart failure may be acute (as a direct result of myocardial infarction [MI]), it's generally a chronic disorder associated with retention of sodium and water by the kidneys. Advances in diagnostic and therapeutic techniques have greatly improved the outlook for patients with heart failure, but the prognosis still depends on the underlying cause and its response to treatment.

Causes

Heart failure may result from a primary abnormality of the heart muscle (such as an infarction), inadequate myocardial perfusion due to coronary artery disease, or cardiomyopathy. Other causes include mechanical disturbances in ventricular filling during diastole when there is too little blood for the ventricle to pump, as in mitral stenosis secondary to rheumatic heart disease or constrictive pericarditis, atrial fibrillation, myocarditis, endocarditis, and other arrhythmias. Systolic hemodynamic disturbances, such as excessive cardiac workload due to volume overloading or pressure overload, that limit the heart's pumping ability, also can cause heart failure. Other precipitating causes include infection, anemia, thyrotoxicosis, and pregnancy. These disturbances can result in mitral or aortic insufficiency, which causes volume overloading, and aortic stenosis or systemic hypertension, which results in increased resistance to ventricular emptying.

Reduced cardiac output triggers three compensatory mechanisms — cardiac dilation, ventricular hypertrophy, and increased sympathetic activity. These mechanisms improve cardiac output at the expense of increased ventricular work.

In *cardiac dilation,* an increase in end-diastolic ventricular volume (preload) causes increased stroke work and stroke volume during contraction, stretching cardiac muscle fibers beyond optimal limits and producing pulmonary congestion and pulmonary hypertension, which lead in turn to right-sided heart failure.

In *ventricular hypertrophy,* an increase in muscle mass or the diameter of the left ventricle allows the heart to pump against increased resistance (impedance) to the outflow of blood. However, the increase in ventricular diastolic pressure needed to fill the enlarged ventricle may compromise diastolic coronary blood flow, limiting oxygen supply to the ventricle and causing ischemia and impaired myocardial contractility.

As a response to decreased cardiac output and blood pressure, *increased sympathetic activity* enhances peripheral vascular resistance, contractility, heart rate, and venous return.

Signs of increased sympathetic activity, such as cool extremities and clamminess, may indicate impending heart failure. Increased sympathetic activity also restricts blood flow to the kidneys, which respond by reducing the glomerular filtration rate and increasing tubular reabsorption of sodium and water, in turn expanding the circulating blood volume. This renal mechanism, if unchecked, can aggravate congestion and produce overt edema.

Chronic heart failure may worsen as a result of respiratory tract infections, pulmonary embolism, stress, increased sodium or water intake, and failure to comply with the prescribed treatment regimen.

Clinical presentation

Left-sided heart failure primarily produces pulmonary signs and symptoms; right-sided heart failure primarily produces systemic signs and symptoms. Heart failure often affects both sides of the heart.

Left-sided heart failure

Clinical signs of left-sided heart failure include dyspnea, orthopnea, paroxysmal nocturnal dyspnea, Cheyne-Stokes respirations, crackles, wheezing, hypoxia, respiratory acidosis, cough, cyanosis or pallor, palpitations, arrhythmias, elevated blood pressure, S_3 and S_4 heart sounds, and pulsus alternans.

Right-sided heart failure

Clinical signs of right-sided heart failure include dependent peripheral edema, hepatomegaly, splenomegaly, jugular vein distention (JVD), ascites, slow weight gain, arrhythmias, hepatojugular reflex, abdominal distention, nausea, vomiting, anorexia, jaundice, weakness, fatigue, dizziness, and syncope.

The patient history should elicit previous heart problems, difficulty breathing, cardiac risk factors (smoking, diabetes, hypertension, dyslipidemia), family history of cardiac disorders, drug and alternative therapies tried, and patient response.

Examination focuses on perfusion.
• *General:* level of distress, blood pressure, weight
• *Head, eyes, ears, nose, and throat:* funduscopy, enlarged thyroid, JVD, or hepatojugular reflux
• *Skin:* color, diaphoresis, turgor
• *Chest:* tachycardia, tachypnea, crackles, extra heart sounds, murmurs, point of maximal impulse shifted left and down
• *Abdomen:* hepatomegaly, ascites
• *Extremities:* clubbing, cyanosis, edema

Differential diagnosis

Dyspnea also occurs in asthma and chronic obstructive pulmonary disease. Chest pain is present in pulmonary embolus and endocarditis. Edema is also a sign of renal or liver disease as well as venous insufficiency.

Diagnostic tests

• Echocardiography shows the size and function of ventricles, atria, pericardial effusion, valve deformities, shunts, and wall motions. It may, for instance, reveal left ventricular dysfunction with a reduced ejection fraction.
• Electrocardiography reflects heart strain, enlargement, and ischemia. It may also reveal left ventricular enlargement, tachycardia, and extrasystole.
• Chest X-ray shows increased pulmonary vascular markings, interstitial edema, pleural effusion, and cardiomegaly.
• Pulmonary artery monitoring typically demonstrates elevated pulmonary artery wedge pressures, left ventricular end-diastolic pressure in left-sided heart failure, and elevated right atrial pressure or central venous pressure in right-sided heart failure.
• Urinalysis, blood urea nitrogen (BUN) levels, and serum creatinine levels reveal renal impairment.
• Cardiac enzymes detect MI.
• Liver function tests detect liver impairment.
• Chemistry panel reveals electrolyte imbalance (commonly due to drugs).
• Thyroid-stimulating hormone levels reveal thyroid dysfunction.

Management

General

The aim of therapy is to improve pump function by reversing the compensatory mechanisms that are producing the symptoms. Heart failure can be controlled quickly by treatments that decrease cardiac workload, control salt and water, and increase myocardial contractility.

Check levels of BUN and serum creatinine, potassium, sodium, chloride, and magnesium.

To prevent deep vein thrombosis due to vascular congestion, order range-of-motion exercises, bed rest, and antiembolism stockings. Check regularly for calf pain and tenderness.

Surgical options include cardiac transplantation for end-stage heart failure and ventricular surgery. However, mechanical left ventricular assist devices assist the heart's pumping action and are being studied more intensely because they've been found to allow some damaged cardiac tissue to recover.

Medication

• Diuretics (hydrochlorothiazide) reduce total blood volume and circulatory congestion.
• Cardiac glycosides (digoxin) strengthen myocardial contractility.
• Vasodilators (nitroprusside) and angiotensin-converting enzyme inhibitors (captopril) increase cardiac output by reducing the impedance to ventricular outflow (afterload).

Referral or consultation

After diagnosis, refer the patient to a primary care provider or cardiologist for initial treatment, exacerbations, or noncompliance, and also if he develops ischemic heart disease, arrhythmias, renal insufficiency, liver impairment, or anemia.

 ALERT Refer the patient to a doctor and medical treatment facility at once for suspected cardiogenic shock (severe hypotension, oliguria, change in

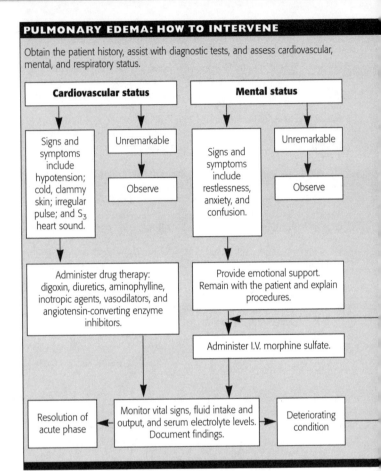

PULMONARY EDEMA: HOW TO INTERVENE

Obtain the patient history, assist with diagnostic tests, and assess cardiovascular, mental, and respiratory status.

Cardiovascular status

- Signs and symptoms include hypotension; cold, clammy skin; irregular pulse; and S_3 heart sound.
- Unremarkable → Observe

Administer drug therapy: digoxin, diuretics, aminophylline, inotropic agents, vasodilators, and angiotensin-converting enzyme inhibitors.

Mental status

- Signs and symptoms include restlessness, anxiety, and confusion.
- Unremarkable → Observe

Provide emotional support. Remain with the patient and explain procedures.

Administer I.V. morphine sulfate.

Monitor vital signs, fluid intake and output, and serum electrolyte levels. Document findings.

Resolution of acute phase

Deteriorating condition

---

mental status) or pulmonary edema with crackles and hypoxia.

Follow-up

If treatment is initiated in the hospital, see the patient in 1 week. If the patient is treated in the office, contact him 1 day after an exacerbation; if his condition hasn't improved, consult a doctor. If his condition has improved, see him every 1 to 2 weeks, depending on the clinical picture, until his symptoms have resolved and his weight goal has been met; afterward, see him monthly for 3 months and then quarterly.

Complications

Complications typically include pulmonary edema, venostasis with a predisposition to thromboembolism (associated primarily with prolonged bed rest), cerebral insufficiency, arrhythmias, protein enteropathy, digitalis toxicity, and renal insufficiency with severe electrolyte imbalance. (See *Pulmonary edema: How to intervene.*)

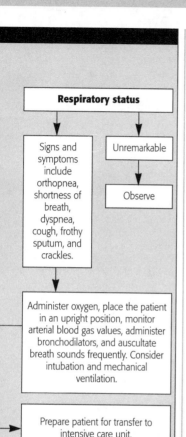

```
┌─────────────────────────────┐
│     Respiratory status      │
└─────────────────────────────┘
         │              │
         ▼              ▼
┌──────────────┐  ┌──────────────┐
│ Signs and    │  │ Unremarkable │
│ symptoms     │  └──────────────┘
│ include      │         │
│ orthopnea,   │         ▼
│ shortness of │  ┌──────────────┐
│ breath,      │  │   Observe    │
│ dyspnea,     │  └──────────────┘
│ cough, frothy│
│ sputum, and  │
│ crackles.    │
└──────────────┘
         │
         ▼
┌───────────────────────────────┐
│ Administer oxygen, place the  │
│ patient in an upright         │
│ position, monitor arterial    │
│ blood gas values, administer  │
│ bronchodilators, and          │
│ auscultate breath sounds      │
│ frequently. Consider          │
│ intubation and mechanical     │
│ ventilation.                  │
└───────────────────────────────┘
         │
         ▼
┌───────────────────────────────┐
│ Prepare patient for transfer  │
│ to intensive care unit.       │
└───────────────────────────────┘
```

Patient teaching

• Explain to the patient how supplemental oxygen and high Fowler's position will help him breathe more easily.
• Explain the rationale for checking daily weights, monitoring intake and output, and checking for peripheral edema.
• Advise the patient to schedule activities to allow adequate rest periods.
• Advise the patient to avoid foods high in sodium, such as canned or commercially prepared foods and dairy products, to curb fluid overload.

• Explain to the patient that the potassium he loses through diuretic therapy must be replaced by taking a prescribed potassium supplement and eating potassium-rich foods, such as bananas, apricots, and orange juice.
• Stress the need for regular follow-up care.
• Emphasize the importance of taking digoxin exactly as prescribed. Tell the patient to watch for and immediately report signs of toxicity, such as anorexia, vomiting, and yellow vision.

 ALERT Tell the patient to call the primary care provider to report pulse irregularities, dizziness, blurred vision, shortness of breath, persistent dry cough, palpitations, increased fatigue, paroxysmal nocturnal dyspnea, swollen ankles, decreased urine output, and rapid weight gain (more than 5 lb [2.25 kg] in a week).

Resources
• American Heart Association: 800-AHA-USA-1 or *www.americanheart.org*
• National Heart, Lung and Blood Institute: for patient-education pamphlets, 301-251-1222 or *www.nhlbi.nih.gov*
• For providers — Drug affordability: *www.needymeds.com* (contains information about many drug company programs that provide financial assistance to patients who need their drugs)

Hepatitis, viral

ICD-9-CM 070.9, type A 070.1, type B acute 070.30, type B chronic 070.32, type B with D 070.31, type C acute 070.51, type C chronic 070.54, type E 070.53, type E prophylaxis V05.3

A fairly common systemic disease, viral hepatitis is marked by hepatic cell destruction, necrosis, and autolysis, leading to anorexia, jaundice, and hepatomegaly. Hepatitis A (HAV) causes no chronic liver disease, and hepatitis E (HEV) is rare. Hepatitis B, C, and D (HBV, HCV, HDV, respectively) cause more severe symptoms plus an increased likelihood of persistent hepatitis and chronic disease, such as cirrhosis and hepatocellular carcinoma. Advanced age and serious underlying disorders such as human immunodeficiency virus make complications more likely. The prognosis is poor if edema and hepatic encephalopathy develop.

Causes

The five major forms of viral hepatitis result from infection with the causative viruses: A, B, C, D, or E. Type G has also been identified. (See *Comparing types of hepatitis*, pages 214 and 215.)

Type A hepatitis

A third of all Americans have antibodies to HAV. This disease is highly contagious and is usually transmitted by the fecal-oral route. Rarely, it's transmitted parenterally. HAV usually results from ingestion of contaminated food, milk, or water. Outbreaks of HAV are often traced to ingestion of seafood from polluted water. An infected person who has poor sanitary habits, performs food preparation, or has close contact with others, when combined with an average incubation period of more than 4 weeks, can cause a widespread outbreak.

Type B hepatitis

Chronic HBV affects about 1 million people in North America. Formerly thought to be transmitted only by direct exchange of contaminated blood or through sexual contact, HBV is now known to be transmitted by body secretions and feces. As a result, nurses, doctors, laboratory technicians, and dentists are frequently exposed to HBV, often as a result of wearing defective gloves. Routine screening of donor blood for the hepatitis B surface antigen (HBsAg) has reduced the incidence of posttransfusion cases, but transmission by needles shared by drug abusers remains a major problem.

Type C hepatitis

Chronic HCV affects about 4 million people in North America—20% of all hepatitis cases. Although the hepatitis C virus has been isolated, few patients have tested positive for it, perhaps reflecting the test's poor specificity. HCV is most often transmitted via transfused blood from asymptomatic donors. In up to 40% of patients, the mode of transmission is unknown.

Type D hepatitis

HDV occurs in 1% of patients with HBV but infects 50% of all who develop fulminant hepatitis, which is associated with a very high mortality rate. HDV is found only in patients with an acute or chronic episode of HBV and requires the presence of HBsAg. HDV depends on the double-shelled type B virus to replicate. For this reason, HDV infection requires prior infection with HBV. Thus, immunization against HBV also protects the patient from HDV.

Type E hepatitis

 SPECIAL POPULATIONS
HEV (formerly grouped with type C under the name non-A, non-B hepatitis) is uncommon in North America, occurring primarily in people who've recently returned from an endemic area, such as India, Africa, Asia, or Central America. It's more common in young adults; 20%

of pregnant women develop fulminant hepatitis. HEV is transmitted enterically, much like HAV. Because this virus is inconsistently shed in feces, detection is difficult.

Type G hepatitis

HGV appears to be transmitted much like HCV and frequently appears as a coinfection with HCV. Not much is known about HGV, but it appears to play a minor role in both acute and chronic hepatitis.

Clinical presentation

Assessment findings are similar for the different types of hepatitis. Typically, signs and symptoms progress in three stages: prodromal (preicteric), clinical (icteric), and recovery (posticteric).

Prodromal stage

In the prodromal stage, the patient typically complains of easy fatigue and anorexia (possibly with mild weight loss), generalized malaise, depression, headache, weakness, arthralgia, myalgia, photophobia, and nausea with vomiting. He also may describe changes in his senses of taste and smell.

Assessment of vital signs may reveal a fever of 100° to 102° F (37.8° to 38.9° C). As the prodromal stage draws to a close, usually 1 to 5 days before the onset of the clinical jaundice stage, inspection of urine and stool specimens may reveal dark-colored urine and clay-colored stools. The patient is most infectious in the 2 weeks prior to the appearance of jaundice.

Clinical stage

If the patient has progressed to the clinical jaundice stage, he may report pruritus, abdominal pain or tenderness, and indigestion. Early in this stage, he may complain of anorexia;

later, his appetite may return. Inspection of the sclerae, mucous membranes, and skin may reveal jaundice, which can last for 1 to 2 weeks. Jaundice indicates that the damaged liver is unable to remove bilirubin from the blood; however, its presence doesn't indicate the severity of the disease. Jaundice typically appears shortly after the most acute phase passes. Occasionally, hepatitis occurs without jaundice.

During the clinical jaundice stage, inspection of the skin may detect rashes, erythematous patches, or urticaria, especially if the patient has HBV or HBC. Palpation may disclose abdominal tenderness in the right upper quadrant, an enlarged and tender liver and, sometimes, splenomegaly and cervical adenopathy.

Recovery stage

During the recovery stage, most of the patient's symptoms decrease or subside. On palpation, a decrease in liver enlargement may be noted. The recovery phase commonly lasts from 2 to 12 weeks, although sometimes this phase lasts longer in patients with HBV, HCV, or HEV.

Differential diagnosis

Conditions to be considered include infectious mononucleosis, primary or secondary hepatic malignancy, ischemic hepatitis, drug-induced hepatitis, alcoholic hepatitis, cytomegalovirus, coxsackievirus, toxoplasmosis, acute cholecystitis, common duct stone, ascending cholangitis, Wilson's disease, rheumatoid disorders, and lupus.

Diagnostic tests

In suspected viral hepatitis, a hepatitis profile is routinely performed. This study identifies antibodies specific to

(Text continues on page 216.)

COMPARING TYPES OF HEPATITIS

	Type A hepatitis (HAV)	Type B hepatitis (HBV)
Incubation	15 to 45 days	30 to 180 days
Onset	Abrupt	Varies
Route of transmission	Fecal-oral, rarely blood or body fluids	Exposure to blood or body fluids
Serum laboratory results	Anti-HAV immunoglobulins IgM* and IgG**	*Acute:* Hepatitis B surface antigen (HBsAg), hepatitis B core antibody (anti-HBc), hepatitis B e antigen (HBeAg) *Chronic:* HBsAg, HBeAg
Chronic state	0%	< 10% of total population, but 90% of infected neonates
Prognosis	Complete resolution, then immune to HAV	Worse with age and additional insults to liver
Risk of hepatocellular cancer	None	Increased if infected during early childhood
Management	None	Interferon 40% effective
Prophylaxis	Anti-HAV vaccine available that provides protection for 20 years (Adults require two injections; children ages 2 to 18 require three injections.)	Hepatitis B series (three shots); postexposure, hepatitis B immune globulin (HBIg), 0.06 ml/kg as soon as possible, followed by hepatitis B series as soon as possible

Type C hepatitis (HCV)	Type D hepatitis (HDV)	Type E hepatitis (HEV)	Type G hepatitis (HGV)
15 to 160 days, more infectious with high viral load or coinfection with human immunodeficiency virus	30 to 180 days	14 to 60 days	Unknown
Insidious	Varies	Abrupt	Varies
Exposure to blood, body fluids, and, especially, liver or renal transplant	Exposure to blood or body fluids	Fecal-oral	Exposure to blood or body fluids
Anti-HCV on enzyme-linked immunosorbent assay, HCV genotyping by recombinant immunoblot assay, anti-HCV by polymerase chain reaction (PCR)	Anti-HDV IgM* and IgG**	Anti-HEV IgM* and IgG** may be detected; levels fall rapidly after resolution	PCR-RNA (ribonucleic acid)
85%	Most	0%	Unknown; often a coinfection with HCV
Progression occurs over decades; rate influenced by subgenotype, viral load, age, and additional insults to liver	Increases severity and progression of hepatitis	Complete resolution common, 1% to 2% fulminant, 20% fulminant if pregnant	Appears to play a minor clinical role in acute or chronic state
Increased	Increased	None	Unknown
Interferon < 15% sustained response	None	None	None
Vaccine available but not feasible because of mutation of genotypes	Hepatitis B series; no vaccine available for patients with HBV	Vaccine under study	No prophylaxis available

*IgM = acute infection   **IgG = previous infection

the causative virus, establishing the type of hepatitis as follows:

• Type A: Detection of an antibody to HAV confirms the diagnosis (anti-HAV immunoglobulin IgM [acute case] or IgG [previous exposure])

• Type B: The presence of HBsAg and HBV antibodies confirms the diagnosis. Anti-hepatitis B surface antigen (anti-HBsAg) and anti-hepatitis B core antigen (anti-HBcAg) IgM reveal the acute stage. IgG and anti-HBcAg reveal a chronic state. Hepatitis B e antigen (HBeAg) reveals the level of viral replication occurring at that moment. Decisions regarding interferon therapy and liver transplant use HBeAg as a parameter.

• Type C: The diagnosis depends on serologic testing for the specific antibody (anti-HCV on enzyme-linked immunosorbent assay) 1 or more months after the onset of acute hepatitis. Until then, the diagnosis is established primarily by obtaining negative test results for HAV, HBV, and HDV. HCV ribonucleic acid (RNA) on polymerase chain reaction (PCR) is the most sensitive test for early stages but is revealed only intermittently in the chronic state. HCV genotypes may be determined by recombinant immunoblot assay (RIBA).

• Type D: The detection of intrahepatic delta antigens or IgM antidelta antigens in acute disease (or IgM and IgG in chronic disease) establishes the diagnosis.

• Type E: IgM anti-HEV and IgG anti-HEV may be detected, but levels rapidly fall after acute infection resolves. These tests aren't routinely done.

• Type G: HGV RNA on PCR may be detected.

The following additional findings from liver function studies support the diagnosis:

• Serum aspartate aminotransferase (AST) and serum alanine aminotransferase (ALT) levels are increased in the prodromal stage of acute viral hepatitis.

• Serum alkaline phosphatase levels are slightly increased.

• Serum bilirubin levels are elevated. Levels may continue to be high late in the disease, especially in severe cases.

• Prothrombin time is prolonged (more than 3 seconds longer than normal indicates severe liver damage).

• White blood cell counts commonly reveal transient neutropenia and lymphopenia followed by lymphocytosis.

• Urinalysis may reveal protein, bilirubin, or both.

• Liver biopsy is performed if chronic hepatitis is suspected (diagnostic for type and reveals extent of liver damage; it's also required before starting interferon).

• Ultrasound may detect ascites or obstruction.

Management

Acute

• Report all newly diagnosed cases to the local health authorities.

• Correct coagulation defects, fluid and electrolyte imbalances, acid-base imbalance, hypoglycemia, and impaired renal function.

• Administer supplemental vitamins and commercial feedings. If symptoms are severe and the patient can't tolerate oral intake, provide I.V. therapy and parenteral nutrition.

• Record the patient's weight daily, and keep intake and output records. Note changes in stool color, consistency, and amount as well as frequency of bowel movements.

• Watch for signs of fluid shift, such as weight gain and orthostasis.

• Watch for signs of hepatic coma, dehydration, pneumonia, vascular problems, and pressure ulcers.

• In fulminant hepatitis, maintain electrolyte balance and a patent airway, prevent infections, and control bleeding. Correct hypoglycemia and any other complications while awaiting liver regeneration and repair.

 ALERT Refer the patient immediately to a doctor for HBV and HCV because there is an increased chance of remission with early treatment. Consultation or referral for HDV is suggested because of the increased probability of fulminant hepatitis.

No specific drug therapy has been developed for hepatitis, with the exception of HBV and HBC, which have been treated somewhat successfully with interferon alfa. Instead, the patient is advised to rest in the early stages of the illness and to combat anorexia by eating small, high-calorie, high-protein meals.

Protein intake should be reduced if signs of precoma — lethargy, confusion, and mental changes — develop. Large meals are usually better tolerated in the morning because many patients experience nausea late in the day.

In acute viral hepatitis, hospitalization usually is required only for patients with severe symptoms or complications. Parenteral nutrition may be required if the patient experiences persistent vomiting and is unable to maintain oral intake.

Antiemetics (trimethobenzamide or benzquinamide) may be given a half-hour before meals to relieve nausea and prevent vomiting; phenothiazines (prochlorperazine [Compazine]) have a cholestatic effect and should be avoided. For severe pruritus, the resin cholestyramine (Questran) may be given. New drugs being tried include amantadine for its antiviral properties in cases of HCV when interferon is ineffective and, also, corticosteroids (Prednisone) in HAV to shorten illness.

Referral or consultation

 COLLABORATION Refer patients with a positive diagnosis as well as all cases of acute hepatitis, to a gastroenterologist or another doctor for evaluation and treatment.

Follow-up

See the patient regularly (exact frequency depends on the clinical picture) and monitor diagnostic tests (serial measurements of serum AST and ALT; serum viral markers as indicated; chemistry panel to detect metabolic complications; complete blood count [platelets if taking interferon]; and liver biopsy). In HCV, HCV-RNA levels monitor the patient's response to treatment; if results are negative after 3 months, an elevated sustained response is likely. In HBV, HbeAg levels indicate increased viral replication and thus an increased viral load. High HBeAg levels are also associated with an increased risk of transmission.

Complications

Acute or subacute necrosis, chronic active or chronic hepatitis, cirrhosis, hepatic failure, and hepatocellular malignancy (HBV, HCV) are possible.

Patient teaching

• Use enteric precautions when caring for patients with HAV or HEV hepatitis. Practice standard precautions for all patients.

• Inform the family and patient about isolation precautions.

• Instruct the patient to allow rest periods throughout the day. He can gradually add activities to his schedule as he begins to recover.

• Encourage the patient to eat small, frequent balanced meals, and encourage plenty of calories and foods high in vitamin K (green, leafy vegetables).

• Force fluids (at least 4,000 ml daily). Encourage the anorectic patient to drink fruit juices. Chipped ice and effervescent soft drinks can hydrate without inducing vomiting.

• Explain the disease process, symptoms, treatment, pros and cons of drugs, and how to prevent transmission. Strongly recommend abstaining from alcohol and medications metabolized by the liver, such as acetaminophen and ibuprofen. Explain to female patients that, because oral contraceptives tend to increase bilirubin levels, they should consider an alternative form of contraception.

ALERT Tell the patient to call the primary care provider to report any new or persistent signs and symptoms, including personality changes (disorientation, forgetfulness, slurred speech), slight tremor, lethargy, and abnormal movements of wrists and fingers (asterixis).

Resources
• American Liver Foundation (Hepatitis): 800-223-0179
• Hepatitis Foundation International: 800-891-0707
• Hepatitis B Foundation: 215-884-8786
• Hepatitis C Foundation: 800-324-7305

Human immunodeficiency virus

ICD-9-CM HIV or AIDS 042, HIV-2 079.53

Currently one of the most widely publicized diseases, acquired immunodeficiency syndrome (AIDS) is marked by progressive failure of the immune system. Although it's characterized by gradual destruction of cell-mediated (T-cell) immunity, it also affects humoral immunity and even autoimmunity because of the central role of the $CD4^+$ T lymphocyte in immune reactions. The resultant immunodeficiency makes the patient susceptible to opportunistic infections, unusual cancers, and other abnormalities that define AIDS.

This syndrome was first described by the Centers for Disease Control and Prevention (CDC) in 1981. Since then, the CDC has declared a case surveillance definition for AIDS and has modified it several times, most recently in 1993.

A retrovirus — the human immunodeficiency virus (HIV) type I — is the primary etiologic agent. Transmission of HIV occurs by contact with infected blood or body fluids and is associated with identifiable high-risk behaviors. It's therefore disproportionately represented in homosexual and bisexual men, I.V. drug users, neonates of HIV-infected women, recipients of contaminated blood or blood products (dramatically decreased since the mid-1980s), and heterosexual partners of persons in the former groups. Because of similar routes of transmission, AIDS shares epidemiologic patterns with hepatitis B and sexually transmitted diseases (STDs).

The natural history of AIDS infection begins with infection by the HIV retrovirus, which is detectable only by laboratory tests, and ends with the severely immunocompromised, terminal stage of this disease. Depending on individual variations and the presence of cofactors that influence progression, the time elapsed from acute HIV infection to the appearance of symptoms (mild to severe) to the diagnosis of AIDS and, eventually, to death varies greatly. Current combination antiretroviral therapy (for example, with zidovudine (AZT), ritonavir, and others) plus treatment and prophylaxis of common opportunistic infections can delay the natural progression of HIV disease and prolong survival.

Causes

AIDS results from infection with HIV, which strikes cells bearing the CD4+ antigen; the latter (normally a receptor for major histocompatibility complex molecules) serves as a receptor for the retrovirus and lets it enter the cell. HIV prefers to infect the CD4+ lymphocyte or macrophage but may also infect other CD4+ antigen-bearing cells of the GI tract, uterine cervical cells, and neuroglial cells. The virus gains access by binding to the CD4+ molecule on the cell surface along with a coreceptor (thought to be the chemokine receptor CCR5).

After invading a cell, HIV replicates, leading to cell death, or becomes latent. HIV infection leads to profound pathology, either directly — through destruction of CD4+ cells, other immune cells, and neuroglial cells — or indirectly — through the secondary effects of CD4+ T-cell dysfunction and resultant immunosuppression.

The infection process takes three forms:
• immunodeficiency (opportunistic infections and unusual cancers)
• autoimmunity (lymphoid interstitial pneumonitis, arthritis, hypergammaglobulinemia, and production of autoimmune antibodies)
• neurologic dysfunction (AIDS dementia complex, HIV encephalopathy, and peripheral neuropathies).

HIV is transmitted by direct inoculation during intimate sexual contact, especially associated with the mucosal trauma of receptive rectal intercourse; transfusion of contaminated blood or blood products (a risk diminished by routine testing of all blood products); sharing of contaminated needles; or transplacental or postpartum transmission from infected mother to fetus (by cervical or blood contact at delivery and in breast milk).

Accumulating evidence suggests that HIV isn't transmitted by casual household or social contact. The average time between exposure to the virus and diagnosis of AIDS is 8 to 10 years, but shorter and longer incubation times have also been recorded.

Clinical presentation

HIV infection manifests itself in many ways. After a high-risk exposure and inoculation, the infected person usually experiences a mononucleosis-like syndrome, which may be attributed to a flu or other virus and then may remain asymptomatic for years. In this latent stage, the only sign of HIV infection is laboratory evidence of seroconversion.

When symptoms appear, they may take many forms:
• persistent generalized adenopathy
• nonspecific symptoms (weight loss, fatigue, night sweats, fevers)
• neurologic symptoms resulting from HIV encephalopathy
• opportunistic infection or cancer.

SPECIAL POPULATIONS The clinical course varies slightly in children with AIDS. Their incubation time is apparently shorter, with a mean of 17 months. Signs and symptoms resemble those of adults, except for findings related to STDs. Children show virtually all of the opportunistic infections observed in adults, with a higher incidence of bacterial infections: otitis media, sepsis, chronic salivary gland enlargement, lymphoid interstitial pneumonia, *Mycobacterium avium* complex function, and pneumonias, including *Pneumocystis carinii*.

The patient history may reveal fevers, night sweats, diarrhea, weight loss, lymphadenopathy, frequent candidal infections, difficulty swallowing, mental status changes, visual changes, and severe headaches. Find out the patient's reason for being tested, current high-risk behaviors, past diagnosis of and treatment for tuberculosis (TB) and hepatitis, and immunization history.

Examination focuses on signs of infection, malignancy, and neurologic involvement.
• *General:* fever, lymphadenopathy
• *Abdomen:* hepatomegaly, splenomegaly
• *Anogenital:* STDs, neoplasia (high risk for cervical carcinoma)
• *Chest:* pneumonia, cardiomyopathy
• *CNS:* mental status changes, other CNS involvement
• *Head, eyes, ears, nose, and throat:* retinopathy, oral lesions
• *Skin:* lesions, including infectious types, such as herpes, autoimmune types, such as psoriasis, and neoplastic types such as Kaposi's sarcoma

Differential diagnosis

The CDC defines AIDS as an illness characterized by one or more "indicator" diseases coexisting with laboratory evidence of HIV infection and other possible causes of immunosuppression. The CDC's current AIDS surveillance case definition requires laboratory confirmation of HIV infection in people who have a CD4+ T-cell count of 200 cells/μl or who have an associated clinical condition or disease. Many conditions can mimic HIV infection. Whenever there is an unexpectedly prolonged or refractive illness, HIV testing is indicated.

Diagnostic tests
• The most commonly performed tests, antibody tests, indicate HIV infection indirectly by revealing HIV antibodies. The recommended protocol requires initial screening of individuals and blood products with an enzyme-linked immunosorbent assay (ELISA) test. A positive ELISA test should be repeated and then confirmed by an alternate method, usually the Western blot or an immunofluorescence assay. However, antibody testing isn't always reliable. Because the body takes a variable amount of time to produce a detectable level of antibodies, a "window" varying from a few weeks to as long as 35 months (in one documented case) allows an HIV-infected person to test negative for HIV antibodies.
• Antibody tests are also unreliable in neonates because transferred maternal antibodies persist for 6 to 10 months. To overcome these problems, direct testing is performed to detect HIV. Direct tests include antigen tests (p24 antigen), HIV cultures, nucleic acid probes of peripheral blood lymphocytes with determination of HIV-1 ribonucleic acid levels, and the polymerase chain reaction (PCR).
• Additional tests to support the diagnosis and help evaluate the severity of immunosuppression include CD4+ and CD8+ T-cell subset counts, erythrocyte sedimentation rate, complete blood cell count, serum beta$_2$-microglobulin, p24 antigen, neopterin levels, and anergy testing. Because many opportunistic infections in AIDS patients are reactivations of previous infections, patients are also tested for syphilis, hepatitis B, tuberculosis, toxoplasmosis and, in some areas, histoplasmosis. When diagnosed with HIV, other needed screening tests include cytomegalovirus (CMV) titer, Papanicolaou (Pap) test, and chest X-ray to detect cancer.

Management

Acute
Treat new interstitial pneumonitis, severe vomiting, or diarrhea with dehydration. Neurologic manifestations

require intensive supportive treatment.

General

Be aware that a diagnosis of AIDS is profoundly distressing because of the disease's social impact and the discouraging prognosis. The patient may lose his job and financial security as well as the support of family and friends. Coping with an altered body image, the emotional burden of serious illness, and the threat of death may overwhelm the patient.

Patients engaging in unprotected sex need family counseling as well as transmission counseling. AZT taken by the mother during pregnancy has decreased vertical transmission but not completely. The probability of a child losing a parent early in life is also an issue.

Medication

No cure has yet been found for AIDS; however, the rate of hospitalization for HIV-related diagnoses declined about 30% between 1995 and 1997, at least partially due to multidrug therapy. Primary therapy for HIV infection includes three types of antiretroviral agents:

• Protease inhibitors (PIs), such as ritonavir, indinavir, nelfinavir, and saquinavir
• Nucleoside reverse transcriptase inhibitors (NRTIs), such as zidovudine, didanosine, zalcitabine, lamivudine, and stavudine
• Nonnucleoside reverse transcriptase inhibitors (NNRTIs), such as nevirapine delavirdine.

HIV treatment is undergoing change so rapidly that new drugs and new information may substantially alter treatment guidelines. However, the founding principles that guide treatment will probably still be applicable. The antiretrovirals, used in various combinations, are designed to inhibit HIV viral replication. Other potential therapies include immunomodulatory agents designed to boost the weakened immune system and anti-infective and antineoplastic agents to combat opportunistic infections and associated cancers. Some of these drugs are used prophylactically to help patients resist opportunistic infections.

Current treatment protocols combine two or more agents in an effort to gain the maximum benefit with the fewest adverse reactions. Such regimens often include one PI plus two NRTIs or one NNRTI plus two NRTIs for persons unable to tolerate a PI or who develop lipodystrophy (abnormal fat distribution). Many variations and drug interactions are under study. Combination therapy helps inhibit the production of resistant, mutant strains. The drug regimen is changed when the patient develops drug toxicity or intolerable adverse effects, or when treatment fails (as indicated by development of opportunistic infections, increasing viral load, or decreasing T-cell count). To prevent cross-resistance, all drugs must be stopped simultaneously when resistance develops to any one drug.

Supportive treatments help maintain nutritional status as well as relieve pain and other distressing physical and psychological symptoms. Many pathogens in AIDS respond to anti-infective drugs but tend to recur after treatment ends. For this reason, most patients need continuous anti-infective treatment, presumably for life or until the drug is no longer tolerated or effective.

Recommended immunizations are pneumonia vaccine, influenza vaccine, tuberculosis booster, and hepatitis B vaccine.

SPECIAL POPULATIONS Administer inactivated polio virus to children.

Treatment with AZT has proved effective in slowing the progression of HIV infection, decreasing opportunistic infections, and prolonging survival. However, it often produces serious adverse reactions and toxicities.

 SPECIAL POPULATIONS AZT is often combined with other agents such as lamivudine, but it has also been used as a single agent for pregnant HIV-positive women.

Referral or consultation

Refer the patient to an infectious disease or HIV/AIDS specialist after diagnosis for evaluation and initial treatment plan as well as for signs of drug failure (opportunistic infection, increasing viral load, decreasing T-cell count). The patient may need to see a neurologist or neurosurgeon for intracranial lesions, a gastroenterologist for intractable diarrhea or painful swallowing not responsive to antifungal drugs, a pulmonologist for interstitial pneumonitis, social services for financial and home care needs, and a psychologist or psychiatrist for counseling and developing coping mechanisms.

Follow-up

See the patient initially every 3 months for viral load and CD4+ count. At each visit, check for shortness of breath, dyspnea on exertion (*Pneumocystis carinii* pneumonia), diarrhea, fever, night sweats (tuberculosis), odynophagia (oral cavity or esophageal candidiasis), neurologic manifestations (infection, cancer, or dementia), and visual changes (retinitis due to CMV). Increase frequency as indicated by clinical picture. Women need a pelvic examination and Pap test every 6 months due to the high risk of cervical carcinoma.

Patients on AZT need a complete blood count and liver function tests every 3 months as well.

Complications

The many possible complications include opportunistic infections and cancers, meningoencephalitis, neuropsychiatric manifestations, thrombocytopenia, wasting syndrome, and premature death.

Patient teaching

• Emphasize that combination antiretroviral therapy aims for maximum suppression of HIV replication, thereby improving survival. Poor drug compliance leads to drug resistance and treatment failure. Patients must understand that medication regimens must be followed closely and may be required for many years, if not throughout life.
• Stress the importance of notifying those who may have been infected.
• Encourage safe sex practices.
• Emphasize that needles must not be shared.
• Stress the importance of good nutrition, vitamin supplements, and regular exercise in maintaining health.
• Advise the patient never to eat raw or possibly contaminated food.
• Inform the patient of national and local support groups and services.
• Explain treatment options, including how drugs work, expected adverse effects, dosage scheduling, and monitoring needed.

 ALERT Tell the patient to call the primary care provider to report any signs and symptoms of infection or cancer (fever higher than 101° F [38.3° C], cloudy or colored discharge, nonhealing wound), chills, weight loss, increasing fatigue, enlarged lymph nodes, mouth sores or painful swallowing, cough, dyspnea, visual changes, headaches, increasing congestion (particularly with purulent drainage), or rash; vomiting or diarrhea with signs of dehydration (fewer than three voidings in 24 hours; dark, concentrated, urine with strong odor; constant thirst; skin tenting); change in mental status or depression; intolerable drug adverse effects; and possible pregnancy.

Resources
• National AIDS Hotline: 800-342-2437; Spanish: 800-342-7432
• National Institutes of Health AIDS Clinical Trials Group: 800-874-2572
• For consumers and providers (site sponsored by the Food and Drug Administration) — Texas AIDS Health Fraud Information Network: *www.tahfin.org*
• For providers — Drug affordability: *www.needymeds.com* (contains information regarding many drug company programs that provide financial assistance for their drugs.)
• The National Nonoccupational HIV Postexposure Prophylaxis (PEP) Registry collects data about type of exposure, decision to use or not use PEP, drugs taken, risk-reduction referrals made, and results of HIV testing. No identifying data are collected. Additional information about the registry is available by calling toll-free: 877-448-1737.

Hypertension, essential

ICD-9-CM essential 401.1

An intermittent or sustained elevation in diastolic or systolic blood pressure of unknown etiology, hypertension affects more than 20% of adults in the United States. If untreated, it carries a high mortality.

Hypertension is a major cause of cerebrovascular accident (CVA), cardiac disease, and renal failure. However, the prognosis is good if this disorder is detected early and if treatment begins before complications develop.

Causes

Increased blood volume, cardiac rate, and stroke volume as well as arteriolar vasoconstriction can raise blood pressure. The link to sustained hypertension, however, is unclear. Hypertension may also result from the failure of the following intrinsic regulatory mechanisms:
• Renal hypoperfusion causes the release of renin, which is converted by angiotensinogen, a liver enzyme, to angiotensin I. Angiotensin I is converted to angiotensin II, a powerful vasoconstrictor. The resulting vasoconstriction increases afterload.
• Angiotensin II stimulates adrenal secretion of aldosterone, which increases sodium reabsorption. Hypertonic-stimulated release of antidiuretic hormone from the pituitary gland follows, increasing water reabsorption, plasma volume, cardiac output, and blood pressure.
• Autoregulation changes the diameter of an artery to maintain perfusion despite fluctuations in systemic blood pressure. The intrinsic mechanisms that are responsible include stress relaxation (vessels gradually dilate when blood pressure rises to reduce peripheral resistance) and capillary fluid shift (plasma moves between vessels and extravascular spaces to maintain intravascular volume).
• When the blood pressure drops, baroreceptors in the aortic arch and carotid sinuses decrease their inhibition of the medulla's vasomotor center, which increases sympathetic stimulation of the heart by norepinephrine. This, in turn, increases

CARDIOVASCULAR RISKS IN HYPERTENSION

Major risk factors
- Smoking
- Dyslipidemia
- Diabetes mellitus
- Age greater than 60 years
- Gender (men and postmenopausal women)
- Family history of cardiovascular disease: women under age 65 or men under age 55

Target organ damage or clinical cardiovascular disease
- Heart diseases
  - Left ventricular hypertrophy
  - Angina/prior myocardial infarction
  - Prior coronary revascularization
  - Heart failure
- Stroke or transient ischemic attack
- Nephropathy
- Peripheral arterial disease
- Retinopathy

Adapted from the National Heart, Lung and Blood Institute. *The Sixth Report of the Joint National Committee on Prevention, Detection, Evaluation and Treatment of High Blood Pressure (JNC VI).* Bethesda, Md.: National Institutes of Health, 1997. Pub #98-4080. Reprinted with permission.

cardiac output by strengthening the contractile force, increasing the heart rate, and augmenting peripheral resistance by vasoconstriction.
- Stress can also stimulate the sympathetic hormones, which increases cardiac output and peripheral vascular resistance.

Risk factors

 SPECIAL POPULATIONS Hypertension is most common in African Americans. Other risk factors include family history, advanced age, stress, obesity, a high intake of saturated fats or sodium, use of tobacco or alcohol, and a sedentary lifestyle. (See *Cardiovascular risks in hypertension.*)

Clinical presentation

Serial blood pressure measurements greater than 140/90 mm Hg confirm hypertension. In those with a high cardiac risk profile, serial readings greater than 135/85 mm Hg confirm hypertension. (See *Classifying blood pressure in adults.*) Auscultation may reveal bruits over the abdominal aorta and the carotid, renal, and femoral arteries; ophthalmoscopy reveals arteriovenous nicking and, in hypertensive encephalopathy, papilledema.

Hypertension is known as the "silent killer" because it usually produces no symptoms until significant damage has occurred. Highly elevated blood pressure damages the intima of small vessels, resulting in fibrin accumulation in the vessels, local edema and, possibly, intravascular clotting.

Symptoms produced by this process depend on the location of the damaged vessels or the target organ.
- *Brain:* cerebrovascular accident, transient ischemic attack
- *Retina:* blindness
- *Heart:* myocardial infarction (MI)
- *Kidneys:* proteinuria, edema and, eventually, renal failure.

Hypertension increases the heart's workload, causing left ventricular hypertrophy. Progressive damage causes left- and right-sided heart failure and pulmonary edema.

Differential diagnosis

 ALERT The following patients need more aggressive evaluation. History revealing new-onset hypertension before age 30 or after age 55; abrupt onset in patients with a history of being normotensive; hypertension resistant

CLASSIFYING BLOOD PRESSURE IN ADULTS*

Category	Systolic		Diastolic (mm Hg)
Optimal †	< 120	and	< 80
Normal	< 130	and	< 85
High-normal	130 to 139	or	85 to 89
Hypertension ‡			
Stage 1	140 to 159	or	90 to 99
Stage 2	160 to 179	or	100 to 109
Stage 3	≥ 180	or	≥ 110

* Not taking antihypertensive drugs and not acutely ill. When systolic and diastolic blood pressures fall into different categories, the higher category should be selected to classify the individual's blood pressure status. For example, 160/92 mm Hg should be classified as stage 2 hypertension, and 174/120 mm Hg should be classified as stage 3 hypertension.

Isolated systolic hypertension is defined as systolic blood pressure of 140 mm Hg or greater and diastolic blood pressure below 90 mm Hg and staged appropriately (for example, 170/82 mm Hg is considered stage 2 isolated systolic hypertension). In addition to classifying stages of hypertension on the basis of average blood pressure levels, clinicians should specify presence or absence of target organ disease and additional risk factors. This specificity is important for risk classification and treatment.
† Optimal blood pressure with respect to cardiovascular risk is below 120/80 mm Hg. However, unusually low readings should be evaluated for clinical significance.
‡ Based on the average of two or more readings taken at each of two or more visits after an initial screening.

Adapted with permission from the National Heart, Lung and Blood Institute. *The Sixth Report of the Joint National Committee on Prevention, Detection, Evaluation and Treatment of High Blood Pressure (JNC VI).* Bethesda, Md.: National Institutes of Health, 1997. Pub #98-4080. Reprinted with permission.

to management despite multiple-drug regimen; or abrupt resistance in patients with previously controlled blood pressure. Examination revealing diastolic pressure greater than 110 mm Hg or ocular hemorrhages, papilledema, punctate hard exudates, tapering, or banking of the blood vessels indicates a need for aggressive evaluation. (See *Blood pressure measurement tips,* page 226.)

Hypertension occurs as two major types: essential (idiopathic) hypertension, the most common, and secondary hypertension, which results from an identifiable cause. Secondary hypertension may result from renal vascular disease (glomerulonephritis, pyelonephritis, polycystic kidneys), endocrine disorders (pheochromocytoma, primary hyperaldosteronism,

Cushing's syndrome, thyroid, pituitary, or parathyroid dysfunction), vascular disease (coarctation of the aorta, renal artery stenosis), and chemical use (oral contraceptives, nonsteroidal anti-inflammatory drugs, decongestants, antidepressants, sympathomimetics, corticosteroids, ergotamine alkaloids, lithium, cocaine, epoetin alfa, cyclosporine, and industrial chemicals). Because of low probability, test for these conditions only if the patient history and physical or laboratory results warrant it.

A patient history revealing paroxysmal headaches, dizziness, perspiration, and palpitations requires more aggressive evaluation to rule out pheochromocytoma.

Examination may also suggest a secondary cause: Weakness and ede-

BLOOD PRESSURE MEASUREMENT TIPS

- The patient should be seated with his back supported and his arm supported at heart level.
- No clothing should come between the stethoscope and the patient's skin.
- Have the patient rest 5 minutes before taking blood pressure.
- Be aware that caffeine, nicotine, and adrenergic stimulants (such as phenylephrine in nasal decongestants) may cause transient elevation.
- The cuff bladder should encompass four-fifths of the arm and be wide enough to cover two-thirds of the distance from the axilla to the antecubital fossa.
- Inflate the cuff to 20 mm Hg above systolic pressure (after disappearance of pulse). Deflate slowly, 2 to 3 mm per second.
- Take blood pressure bilaterally; use higher pressure in decision making.
- Retake blood pressure after the examination is complete and the patient is relaxed. Readings differing more than 5 mm Hg indicate the need for additional measurements.
- Check for orthostatic hypotension in patients over age 65, patients in whom volume loss is suspected, and patients who have diabetes or are taking antihypertensives.
- Document measurements, including cuff size, position, and which arm was used.
- Procure several home blood pressure measurement kits, and lend them to possible hypertensive patients. Have them take and record numerous blood pressures at differing times of day, during different activities, including first thing in the morning. Have them bring back the machine, and their record of measurements at the next visit.
- If the patient is diagnosed with hypertension, advise him to buy a blood pressure monitor. One can be purchased for less than $35.

ma occur in polycystic kidneys. Retinopathy and a lateralizing abdominal bruit are present in renovascular diseases. Decreased femoral pulses, discrepant leg or arm blood pressures, and a precordial murmur suggest coarctation of the aorta. Central obesity, ecchymoses, hirsutism, and purple striae indicate Cushing's syndrome.

Diagnostic tests

- On urinalysis, moderate and higher proteinuria indicates kidney disease.
- Complete blood count baseline is done for comparison.
- Electrolytes may indicate adrenal dysfunction.
- Fasting blood glucose detects diabetes, an additional cardiac risk.
- Elevations in blood urea nitrogen and serum creatinine levels indicate renal disease.
- Lipid panel detects additional cardiac risk factors.
- Electrocardiography detects left ventricular hypertrophy or ischemia.
- Chest X-ray is done if cardiomegaly is suspected.
- Excretory urography is performed if renal atrophy and unilateral renal disease are suspected.

Management

Acute

 ALERT For signs of hypertensive crisis (blood pressure exceeding 180/100 mm Hg), hypertensive encephalopathy, intracranial hemorrhage, unstable angina, acute MI, acute left ventricular failure with pulmonary edema, dissecting aortic aneurysm, eclampsia, or signs associated with optic disk edema or progressive organ damage), treat blood pressure immediately with parenteral or oral drugs. Typically, hypertensive emergencies require parenteral administration of a vasodilator or an adrenergic inhibitor, or oral

administration of a selected drug —
such as nifedipine (do *not* order sublingually), captopril, clonidine, or
labetalol — to rapidly reduce blood
pressure. Have the patient take the
drug in the office, then wait, and
recheck in 1 hour. If there is no
response, refer him to the emergency
department.

General

One episode of high blood pressure
(if lower than 180/110 mm Hg) without risk factors usually isn't treated
but needs referral and follow-up
within 1 week. Round-the-clock
blood pressure monitoring is preferred but not generally available.
Frequent out-of-office measurements
are the next best option. Monitors are
available for less than $35 (consider
keeping a few in the office to lend to
patients). Encourage the patient diagnosed with hypertension to track
and record his daily blood pressure at
home and to bring the written record
to the office on each visit. Home
monitoring lets the patient check early morning blood pressure, which is
usually the highest, and detects
"white-coat hypertension" (readings
that are higher in the health care
provider's office).

The Joint National Committee on
Prevention, Detection, Evaluation
and Treatment of High Blood Pressure recommends the following
stepped-care approach for treating
primary hypertension:
• *Step 1:* Initiate lifestyle changes,
including weight reduction, limited
alcohol, exercise, reduction of sodium intake, and smoking cessation.
• *Step 2:* If insufficient, initiate drug
regimen. *First-line drugs* are long-
acting beta blockers (atenolol) (especially post-MI) and diuretics (hydrochlorothiazide) unless contraindicated (for example, beta blockers mask
symptoms of hypoglycemia, so use
with caution in diabetics). *Alterna-*

tives are angiotensin-converting enzyme inhibitors (captopril) (consider
if renal impairment or diabetes is
present), calcium antagonists
(nifedipine), alpha$_1$- blockers (pra-
zosin) (consider if BPH is present), or
alpha-beta blockers. A new class is
the angiotensin-renin blockers. Although all these drugs reduce blood
pressure, only diuretics and beta
blockers have proved effective in reducing morbidity and mortality.
• *Step 3:* If the patient fails to
achieve the desired blood pressure,
add a drug from a different class,
substitute a drug in the same class,
or increase the drug dosage.
• *Step 4:* If the patient fails to
achieve the desired blood pressure,
add a second or third agent (a diuretic should be part of the regimen).
Second or third agents may include
vasodilators, alpha$_1$-antagonists, and
peripherally acting adrenergic antagonists. (See *Initiating drug treatment for hypertension,* page 228.)

Secondary hypertension treatment
focuses on correcting the underlying
cause and controlling hypertensive
effects. For example, if a younger
woman is on oral contraceptives,
lower the contraceptive dose, and
recheck blood pressure in 3 weeks. If
her blood pressure is still high, discontinue oral contraceptives and discuss other methods of contraception.
Recheck blood pressure in 3 weeks.
Have the patient consider a Depo-
Provera injection (a 150-mg/dose
every 90 days). Recheck her blood
pressure in 3 weeks. If it's still elevated, advise her to use a barrier method
of birth control or an intrauterine device.

Referral or consultation

 COLLABORATION Refer the
patient to a doctor or medical treatment facility if blood
pressure is above 180/110 mm Hg to
prevent end-organ damage. Refer to

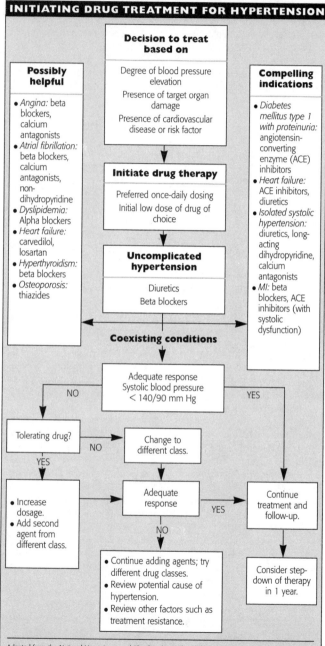

INITIATING DRUG TREATMENT FOR HYPERTENSION

Decision to treat based on

Degree of blood pressure elevation

Presence of target organ damage

Presence of cardiovascular disease or risk factor

Possibly helpful

- *Angina:* beta blockers, calcium antagonists
- *Atrial fibrillation:* beta blockers, calcium antagonists, non-dihydropyridine
- *Dyslipidemia:* Alpha blockers
- *Heart failure:* carvedilol, losartan
- *Hyperthyroidism:* beta blockers
- *Osteoporosis:* thiazides

Initiate drug therapy

Preferred once-daily dosing

Initial low dose of drug of choice

Uncomplicated hypertension

Diuretics

Beta blockers

Coexisting conditions

Compelling indications

- *Diabetes mellitus type 1 with proteinuria:* angiotensin-converting enzyme (ACE) inhibitors
- *Heart failure:* ACE inhibitors, diuretics
- *Isolated systolic hypertension:* diuretics, long-acting dihydropyridine, calcium antagonists
- *MI:* beta blockers, ACE inhibitors (with systolic dysfunction)

Adequate response Systolic blood pressure < 140/90 mm Hg

NO → / YES →

Tolerating drug? —NO→ Change to different class.

YES ↓

- Increase dosage.
- Add second agent from different class.

→ Adequate response —YES→ Continue treatment and follow-up.

NO ↓

- Continue adding agents; try different drug classes.
- Review potential cause of hypertension.
- Review other factors such as treatment resistance.

Consider step-down of therapy in 1 year.

Adapted from the National Heart, Lung, and Blood Institute. *The Sixth Report of the Joint National Committee on Prevention, Detection, Evaluation, and Treatment of High Blood Pressure (JNC VI).* Bethesda, Md.: National Institutes of Health, 1997. Reprinted with permission.

TREATING PATIENTS AT RISK FOR HYPERTENSION*

Blood pressure Stages (mm Hg)	Risk group A (No risk factors, no TOD/CCD)†	Risk group B (At least one risk factor, not including diabetes; no TOD/CCD)	Risk group C (Diabetes with or without TOD/CCD and with or without other risk factors)
High-normal (130–139/85–89)	Lifestyle modification	Lifestyle modification	Drug therapy§
Stage 1 (140–159/90–99)	Lifestyle modification (up to 12 months)	Lifestyle modification‡ (up to 6 months)	Drug therapy
Stages 2 and 3 (≥ 160/≥ 100)	Drug therapy	Drug therapy	Drug therapy

For example, a patient with diabetes and a blood pressure of 142/94 mm Hg plus left ventricular hypertrophy should be classified as having stage 1 hypertension with target organ disease (left ventricular hypertrophy) and with another major risk factor (diabetes). This patient would be categorized as stage 1, risk group C, and recommended for immediate initiation of pharmacologic treatment.

* Lifestyle modification should be adjunctive therapy for all patients recommended for pharmacologic therapy.
† TOD/CCD indicates target organ disease/clinical cardiovascular disease.
‡ For patients with multiple risk factors, clinicians should consider drugs as initial therapy plus lifestyle modifications.
§ For those with heart failure, renal insufficiency, or diabetes.

Adapted from the National Heart, Lung, and Blood Institute. *The Sixth Report of the Joint National Committee on Prevention, Detection, Evaluation and Treatment of High Blood Pressure (JNC VI).* Bethesda, Md.: National Institutes of Health, 1997. Pub #98-4080. Reprinted with permission.

a cardiologist (depending on risk factors) if blood pressure is higher than 160/100 mm Hg and the patient has cardiac risk factors. Follow up within 3 days. Refer to a nephrologist or urologist for indications of primary or secondary renal pathology. Refer to an endocrinologist for endocrine disorders and to another doctor for abnormal electrocardiogram. (See *Treating patients at risk for hypertension.*)

Follow-up

Follow up every 2 weeks until the patient is stable, then quarterly for 1 year. If the goal blood pressure is maintained for 1 year, consider reducing or eliminating drugs. Follow up at least every 3 to 6 months, focusing on behavior and drug compliance, adverse reactions, and quality of life issues (impotence, fatigue). Schedule annual urinalysis and creatinine, potassium, and glucose levels

to monitor kidney function and detect diabetes. (See *Monitoring blood pressure in adults,* page 230.)

Complications

Heart failure, renal failure, MI, CVA, and hypertensive heart disease are complications of high blood pressure.

Patient teaching

• Warn the patient that uncontrolled hypertension may cause stroke and heart attack.
• Help the patient examine and modify his lifestyle, such as by reducing stress and exercising regularly.
• To increase compliance, suggest a daily routine for taking drugs.
• Stress the importance of reporting adverse reactions so drugs can be changed or adjusted to minimize the impact on quality of life.

MONITORING BLOOD PRESSURE IN ADULTS

| Initial blood pressure (mm Hg)* | | Follow-up recommended † |
Systolic	Diastolic	
<130	<85	Recheck in 2 years
130 to 139	85 to 89	Recheck in 1 year‡
140 to 159	90 to 99	Confirm within 2 months‡
160 to 179	100 to 109	Evaluate or refer to source of care within 1 month
≥180	≥110	Evaluate or refer to source of care immediately or within 1 week depending on clinical situation

* If systolic and diastolic categories are different, follow recommendations for shorter time follow-up (for example, 160/86 mm Hg should be evaluated or referred to source of care within 1 month).
† Modify the scheduling of follow-up according to reliable information about past blood pressure measurements, other cardiovascular risk factors, or target organ disease.
‡ Provide advice about lifestyle modifications.

Adapted from the National Heart, Lung, and Blood Institute. *The Sixth Report of the Joint National Committee on Prevention, Detection, Evaluation and Treatment of High Blood Pressure (JNC VI).* Bethesda, Md.: National Institutes of Health, 1997. Pub #98-4080. Reprinted with permission.

• Stress the importance of smoking cessation.
• Emphasize the importance of curbing daily alcohol intake (2 oz hard liquor, 24 oz beer, or 10 oz wine).
• Encourage progressive aerobic exercise, for example, working up to 45 minutes five times weekly.
• Advise the patient to avoid high-sodium antacids and over-the-counter cold and sinus medications, which contain vasoconstrictors.
• Tailor diet to the patient's needs — for example, weight reduction or low saturated fat and cholesterol — as indicated. Urge all patients to avoid high-sodium foods (pickles, potato chips, canned soups, cold cuts) and not to add salt to food. Explain the importance of getting the recommended daily allowance of potassium and magnesium.
• Have the patient keep a record of blood pressure measurements and of drugs used in the past, noting their effectiveness, and bring this record to each visit.

ALERT Tell the patient to call the primary care provider to report any new or persistent signs and symptoms, including signs and symptoms of stroke or MI: severe headache, slurred speech, dizziness, weakness on one side of the body, shortness of breath, excessive sweating and chest pain or pressure that may or may not radiate up to the jaw, neck, or arm. Also tell the patient to call the primary care provider if he can't tolerate the adverse effects of the medications.

Resources
• American Heart Association: 800-AHA-USA-1 or *www.americanheart.org*
• National Kidney Foundation: 800-622-9010
• For providers — Drug affordability: *www.needymeds.com* (contains information regarding many drug company programs that provide financial assistance for their drugs)

Hypothyroidism

ICD-9-CM primary 244.9, postsurgical 244.0

Hypothyroidism, a state of low serum thyroid hormone, results from hypothalamic, pituitary, or thyroid insufficiency. The disorder can progress to life-threatening myxedema coma.

Causes

Hypothyroidism results from inadequate production of thyroid hormone, usually from dysfunction of the thyroid gland due to surgery (thyroidectomy), irradiation therapy, inflammation, chronic autoimmune thyroiditis (Hashimoto's disease) or, rarely, conditions such as amyloidosis and sarcoidosis. It may also result from pituitary failure to produce thyroid-stimulating hormone (TSH), hypothalamic failure to produce thyrotropin-releasing hormone, inborn errors of thyroid hormone synthesis, inability to synthesize thyroid hormone because of iodine deficiency (rare in the United States), or the use of antithyroid drugs such as propylthiouracil. In children, it's a congenital, autoimmune disorder or may be caused by the mother taking antithyroid drugs during pregnancy.

In patients with hypothyroidism, infection, exposure to cold, and sedatives may precipitate myxedema coma.

Clinical presentation

Early clinical features are vague — fatigue, forgetfulness, sensitivity to cold, unexplained weight gain, and constipation. As the disorder progresses, characteristic myxedematous signs appear — decreasing mental stability; dry, flaky, inelastic skin; puffy face, hands, and feet; hoarseness; periorbital edema; ptosis (upper eyelid droop); loss of lateral third of eyebrows; dry, sparse hair; and thick, brittle nails.

Cardiovascular involvement leads to decreased cardiac output, slow pulse rate, signs of poor peripheral circulation and, occasionally, cardiomegaly. Other common effects include anorexia, abdominal distention, menorrhagia, decreased libido, infertility, ataxia, intention tremor, and nystagmus. Reflexes show delayed relaxation time, especially the Achilles tendon.

Progression to myxedema coma is usually gradual, but when stress aggravates severe or prolonged hypothyroidism, coma may develop abruptly. Clinical effects include progressive stupor, hypoventilation, hypoglycemia, hyponatremia, hypotension, and hypothermia.

SPECIAL POPULATIONS
Hypothyroidism is characterized in infants by respiratory difficulties, persistent jaundice, and hoarse crying and in older children by stunted growth, bone and muscle dystrophy, and mental deficiency. If left untreated, children may suffer irreversible mental retardation; skeletal abnormalities are reversible with treatment.

Differential diagnosis

Conditions to consider include depression; euthyroid sick syndrome; thyroid cancer; liver, adrenal, and pituitary disease; nephrotic syndrome; heart failure; primary amyloidosis; and dementia of another cause.

Diagnostic tests

• TSH levels lower than 20 μU/ml are diagnostic of primary hypothyroidism; total serum thyroxine (T_4) is low; triiodothyronine (T_3) resin uptake is high; and the free T_4 index is low.

• High antithyroid titers detect autoimmune thyroiditis. If diagnosis is suspected, test cholesterol, liver enzymes, and electrolytes for baseline (may improve when hypothyroidism is controlled).

Management

Acute
Hypothermia or myxedema coma requires immediate intervention at a medical treatment facility.

Medication
Pharmacologic therapy includes gradual thyroid hormone replacement (levothyroxine, T_4); start low and go slow, particularly in elderly or cardiac patients. Monitor for drug interactions (anticoagulants, hypoglycemics, estrogens, and corticosteroids). Give cathartics and stool softeners as needed.

Referral or consultation
Refer the patient to an endocrinologist if the condition is nonresponsive to treatment and to an endocrinologist or other doctor if the diagnosis is suspected in a child.

Follow-up
Follow up monthly to monitor response and draw TSH. When stable, visits can be every 6 months for examination (focus on cardiac system in elderly patients and patients with a known history of heart disease) and to check TSH level.

Complications

Some complications include treatment-induced heart failure in patients with coronary artery disease, myxedema coma, immunocompromised status, megacolon, organic psychosis, adrenal crisis with rapid increases in thyroid hormone, infertility, bone demineralization (consid-

er hormone replacement therapy, calcium supplements), and hypersensitivity to opiates.

Patient teaching

• Teach the patient about diagnosis and the need for lifelong, uninterrupted therapy, even though symptoms subside.
• Encourage the patient to eat a high-bulk, low-calorie diet and to increase activity to combat constipation and promote weight loss.
• Notify anyone who prescribes drugs of the underlying hypothyroidism.

ALERT Tell the patient to call the primary care provider to report any new or persistent signs and symptoms, including any infection; signs of hyperthyroidism (restlessness, heat intolerance, weight loss despite increased appetite, sweating, diarrhea, tremor, and palpitations) or hypothyroidism (fatigue, cold intolerance, weight gain despite loss of appetite, constipation, and depression); and signs of aggravated cardiovascular disease (chest pain, tachycardia, palpitations, dyspnea).

Resources
• Thyroid Foundation of America, Inc.: 800-832-8321 or *www.thyroid.com*

Iron deficiency anemia

ICD-9-CM 280.9

In iron deficiency anemia, an inadequate supply of iron is available for optimal formation of red blood cells (RBCs). Body stores of iron, including plasma iron, decrease as does transferrin, which binds with and transports iron. Insufficient body stores of iron lead to a depleted RBC mass, which in turn results in a lower hemoglobin concentration (hypochromia) and decreased oxygen-carrying capacity of the blood.

Causes

Iron deficiency anemia may occur because of inadequate dietary intake of iron (less than 2 mg/day), as in prolonged unsupplemented breast- or bottle-feeding, or during periods of stress, such as rapid growth in children and teenagers or poor nutrition in the elderly. Other causes include:

• iron malabsorption, as in chronic diarrhea, partial or total gastrectomy, and malaborption syndromes such as celiac disease

• blood loss secondary to drug-induced GI bleeding (from anticoagulants, aspirin, steroids) or due to heavy menses, hemorrhage from trauma, GI ulcers, cancer, or varices

• pregnancy, which diverts maternal iron to the fetus for erythropoiesis

• intravascular hemolysis-induced hemoglobinuria or paroxysmal nocturnal hemoglobinuria

• mechanical erythrocyte trauma caused by a prosthetic heart valve or vena cava filters.

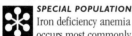 **SPECIAL POPULATIONS** Iron deficiency anemia occurs most commonly in infants (particularly premature or low-birth-weight infants), children, adolescents (especially girls), and premenopausal women.

Clinical presentation

Because of the gradual progression of iron deficiency anemia, many patients are initially asymptomatic, except for symptoms of any underlying condition. They tend not to seek medical treatment until anemia is severe.

At advanced stages, the patient may develop dyspnea on exertion, fatigue, listlessness, pallor, excessive menstrual flow, inability to concentrate, irritability, headache, and a susceptibility to infection. Decreased oxygen perfusion causes compensatory tachycardia and may cause palpitations.

In chronic iron deficiency anemia, the patient may present with koilonychia (nails become spoon-shaped and brittle), cheilosis (the corners of the mouth crack), and a smooth-textured tongue, and the patient complains of dysphagia or may develop pica. Associated neuromuscular effects include vasomotor disturbances, peripheral paresthesias, and neuralgic pain.

Differential diagnosis

It's important to determine the cause of anemia before starting iron because an iron overdose is extremely toxic. Types of anemia include anemias of chronic disease (such as renal disease), aplastic anemia (any condition causing acute or chronic blood loss), hemoglobinopathy (thalassemia, sickle cell), and pernicious anemia (such as vitamin B_{12} deficiency). (See *Differentiating types of anemia,* pages 234 and 235.)

Diagnostic tests

• Complete blood count with differential identifies which type of anemia is present. Indicators of iron deficiency anemia are low RBC count with microcytic, hypochromic cells (in early stages, RBC count may be normal) and decreased mean corpuscular hemoglobin.

• Serum ferritin may detect iron deficiency anemia.

• A high total iron-binding capacity (TIBC) indicates iron deficiency; a low TIBC may indicate chronic disease or malnutrition.

(Text continues on page 236.)

DIFFERENTIATING TYPES OF ANEMIA

To identify the cause of your patient's anemia, use this algorithm to help you order and evaluate appropriate laboratory tests.

Key:

MCV = mean corpusucular volume = cytic/cell size

MCHC = mean corpuscular hemoglobin concentration = chromic/redness

Reticulocytes = immature red blood cellsFerritin = protein that stores iron

TIBC= total iron binding capacity = amount of receptors available for iron

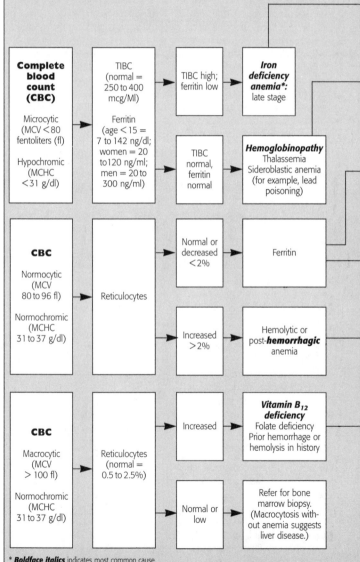

Complete blood count (CBC)

Microcytic (MCV <80 fentoliters (fl)

Hypochromic (MCHC <31 g/dl)

→ TIBC (normal = 250 to 400 mcg/Ml)

Ferritin (age <15 = 7 to 142 ng/dl; women = 20 to120 ng/ml; men = 20 to 300 ng/ml)

→ TIBC high; ferritin low → ***Iron deficiency anemia*:** late stage

→ TIBC normal, ferritin normal → ***Hemoglobinopathy*** Thalassemia Sideroblastic anemia (for example, lead poisoning)

CBC

Normocytic (MCV 80 to 96 fl)

Normochromic (MCHC 31 to 37 g/dl)

→ Reticulocytes

→ Normal or decreased <2% → Ferritin

→ Increased >2% → Hemolytic or post-***hemorrhagic*** anemia

CBC

Macrocytic (MCV > 100 fl)

Normochromic (MCHC 31 to 37 g/dl)

→ Reticulocytes (normal = 0.5 to 2.5%)

→ Increased → ***Vitamin B₁₂ deficiency*** Folate deficiency Prior hemorrhage or hemolysis in history

→ Normal or low → Refer for bone marrow biopsy. (Macrocytosis without anemia suggests liver disease.)

*** *Boldface italics*** indicates most common cause.

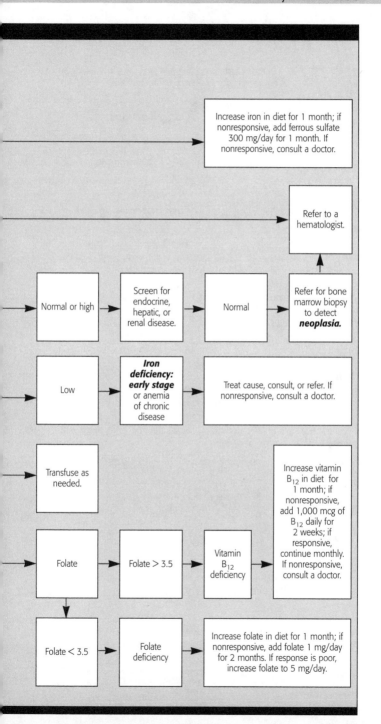

Increase iron in diet for 1 month; if nonresponsive, add ferrous sulfate 300 mg/day for 1 month. If nonresponsive, consult a doctor.

Refer to a hematologist.

Normal or high → Screen for endocrine, hepatic, or renal disease. → Normal → Refer for bone marrow biopsy to detect *neoplasia.*

Low → *Iron deficiency: early stage* or anemia of chronic disease → Treat cause, consult, or refer. If nonresponsive, consult a doctor.

Transfuse as needed.

Increase vitamin B$_{12}$ in diet for 1 month; if nonresponsive, add 1,000 mcg of B$_{12}$ daily for 2 weeks; if responsive, continue monthly. If nonresponsive, consult a doctor.

Folate → Folate > 3.5 → Vitamin B$_{12}$ deficiency

Folate < 3.5 → Folate deficiency → Increase folate in diet for 1 month; if nonresponsive, add folate 1 mg/day for 2 months. If response is poor, increase folate to 5 mg/day.

• Low serum iron indicates iron deficiency, chronic disease, or pernicious anemia.
• Serial fecal occult blood test, endoscopy, or colonoscopy detects occult GI bleeding.
• Bone marrow aspiration detects depleted or absent iron stores and normoblastic hyperplasia.

Management

Acute

 ALERT Hemoglobin levels less than 8 g/dl may require transfusion.

General

Investigate possible sources of bleeding, and correct as indicated. Schedule rest periods to conserve the patient's energy, particularly with low cardiac output, angina, or lightheadedness. Increase dietary iron and ascorbic acid (vitamin C).

Medication

Give ferrous sulfate by mouth in tablets or capsule or use as an elixir. Parenteral administration is available for patients with malabsorption.

 SPECIAL POPULATIONS In pregnant women, give ferrous sulfate twice a day for 2 weeks, then once daily. If hemoglobin levels don't improve, further testing is indicated.

Follow-up

See the patient every 2 weeks for 1 month, monthly for 2 months, then quarterly to semiannually to check for recurrences and reinforce preventive measures. See pregnant women who aren't improved at 2 weeks ; check total iron, TIBC, folate, and vitamin B_{12}. If B_{12} is deficient, she'll need B_{12} injections.

Referral or consultation

Refer the patient to a doctor if you're unable to identify the cause of the anemia or if the condition doesn't respond to treatment.

Complications

Complications include hemorrhage from an unidentified source and not detecting a bleeding malignant tumor.

Patient teaching

• To increase compliance, advise the patient not to stop therapy, even if he feels better, because replacement of iron stores takes time. Tell the patient to report adverse reactions, such as nausea, vomiting, diarrhea, constipation, fever, and severe stomach pain. Inform him that iron may cause stools to turn black.
• Instruct the patient to put iron elixir in a glass of orange juice and to sip it through a straw to prevent staining his teeth.
• Emphasize the need for high-risk individuals, such as premature infants, children under age 2, and pregnant women, to take prophylactic oral iron as ordered. (Children under age 2 should also receive supplemental cereals and formulas high in iron.)
• Tell the patient to avoid dairy products or antacids within 2 hours of taking dietary or supplemental iron because of iron's poor absorption. If GI upset occurs, tell him to take the iron with food (decreases absorption by 50%).
• Heme iron is easily absorbed from meat, poultry, and fish. To increase absorption of nonheme iron from other sources, such as fortified cereal or bread and leafy green vegetables, teach the patient to include vitamin C in the meal, such as from citrus fruits and strawberries.

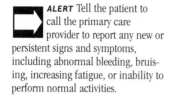 **ALERT** Tell the patient to call the primary care provider to report any new or persistent signs and symptoms, including abnormal bleeding, bruising, increasing fatigue, or inability to perform normal activities.

Resources

• National Heart, Lung and Blood Institute: 301-251-1222 or *www. nhlbi.nih.gov*

Irritable bowel syndrome

ICD-9-CM irritable colon 564.1

Also known as spastic colon or functional bowel pain, irritable bowel syndrome (IBS) is a variable combination of chronic or recurrent GI symptoms with no detectable pathology. The disorder is marked by chronic or periodic diarrhea alternating with constipation and accompanied by gaseousness, straining, and abdominal cramps. The prognosis is good. Supportive treatment or avoidance of a known irritant often relieves symptoms.

Causes

IBS is generally associated with psychological stress. However, this functional disorder may result from physical factors, such as diverticular disease, ingestion of irritants (coffee, raw fruits, or vegetables), or lactose intolerance. Autonomic nervous system abnormalities, genetic and psychosocial factors, and a luminal component (impaired digestion and absorption of certain carbohydrates, such as artificial sweeteners and lactose) may also play a role. Secondary IBS can be caused by abuse of laxatives, food poisoning, or colon cancer.

Clinical presentation

IBS characteristically produces episodes of lower abdominal pain that are usually relieved by bowel movement, or it appears with an alteration in frequency or consistency of stools. Diarrhea is common but typically doesn't disrupt sleep. Stools are often small and contain visible mucus. Dyspepsia, abdominal distention, and feelings of incomplete evacuation may occur.

Patients present with a combination of symptoms, though many state a predominance of either diarrhea, constipation, or abdominal bloating and discomfort. These symptoms alternate with normal bowel function; the presence of symptoms at least 25% of the time without detectable pathology indicates IBS.

Differential diagnosis

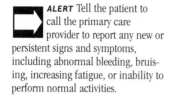 **ALERT** Any patient with a GI complaint whose examination reveals an abdominal mass, severe abdominal tenderness, fever, weight loss, or acute onset without obvious cause requires aggressive evaluation. Other red flags include nocturnal wakening due to GI complaints, family history of cancer, positive fecal occult blood test, and abnormal blood counts.

A careful patient history is required to determine contributing psychological factors such as a recent stressful life change. The diagnosis must also rule out other disorders, such as ulcerative colitis, Crohn's disease, lactose intolerance, infection (such as *Salmonella* and *Clostridium difficile*), drugs (laxative abuse, magnesium-containing antacids), diverticulitis, depression, somatization, endocrine disorders (hypothyroidism, diabetes), colon cancer, or radiation damage to the colon.

Elderly patients need a more intensive evaluation because of their higher risk of certain diagnoses. In addition, some symptoms, such as detection of an abdominal mass, severe abdominal tenderness, recent onset of symptoms, fever, positive fecal occult blood test, weight loss, nocturnal wakening due to bowel movements or pain, and a family history of cancer, also call for a more thorough evaluation.

Diagnostic tests

Appropriate diagnostic procedures to rule out pathology include erythrocyte sedimentation rate (a check for infection, inflammation, and cancer), complete blood count (to check for infection and blood loss), sigmoidoscopy, colonoscopy, barium enema, rectal biopsy, and stool examination for blood, parasites, and bacteria.

Management

The best treatment is education and reassurance. Explain the natural history of IBS. Emphasize that it isn't a mental disorder, but a biological response to stress or irritants and that it affects the quality of life but not longevity.

Therapy aims to relieve symptoms and includes counseling to help the patient understand the relationship between stress and his illness. Studies have found psychological therapy more beneficial than medical therapy in selected patients. Psychological therapy is more beneficial in patients who are aware of the role of stress in their disorder, don't have constant pain, and have fewer pain sites, shorter duration of symptoms, treatable anxiety or depression, and a realistic goal. Rest and heat applied to the abdomen are helpful, as is biofeedback.

Increased fiber (dietary and or supplemental) may be effective for both constipation and diarrhea. Work with the patient to monitor modifications for effectiveness. Patients do better with frequent, supportive contact from the primary care provider.

If the cause of IBS is chronic laxative abuse, bowel training may help correct the condition.

Medication

• Bulk laxative (psyllium) helps prevent constipation and diarrhea.
• Antispasmodics (anticholinergics, including phenobarbital, hyoscyamine, atropine, and hyoscine) relieve spasms.
• Analgesics (Donnatal) may be used for pain but can be addicting.
• Antidiarrheals (loperamide or attapulgite) can be used for diarrhea.
• Osmotic laxatives (magnesium hydroxide) are given for constipation.
• Lactase capsules or tablets counteract milk intolerance.
• Antidepressants (tricyclic antidepressants and serotonin reuptake inhibitors) in low doses may improve GI symptoms.

Referral or consultation

Possible referrals include to a nutritionist for diet counseling, to a psychologist or psychiatrist for counseling and coping mechanisms as needed, and to a gastroenterologist or another doctor for further work-up and management for nonresponsiveness.

Follow-up

See the patient every 2 weeks until condition improves, then every 6 months. If the patient is over age 40, schedule an annual sigmoidoscopy and digital rectal examination because of an increased incidence of diverticulitis and colon cancer.

Complications

Complications include dehydration, laxative abuse, drug dependence, and malnutrition.

Patient teaching

• Emphasize the natural history of the disorder; it affects quality of life but not longevity. This disorder can't be cured, but the patient can control the symptoms to improve quality of life.
• Explain that antidepressants are given for their GI benefits and, in these dosages, generally have no psychotropic effects.
• Recommend a symptom diary to establish a record of association between symptoms and specific foods, stress, and emotional state. This will allow the patient to analyze and modify lifestyle, gaining some control as well as relief of symptoms. It's important not to exclude a food until it's correlated with symptoms at least three times (to avoid the risk of an overly limited diet). Questionable foods include poorly absorbed carbohydrates (such as sorbitol and lactose), high-fat foods, and alcohol.
• Encourage the patient to decrease stress and develop healthy coping mechanisms. Warn him against dependence on sedatives or antispasmodics.
• Encourage regular checkups because IBS is associated with a higher-than-normal incidence of diverticulitis and colon cancer. For patients over age 40, emphasize the need for an annual sigmoidoscopy and rectal examination.

 ALERT Tell the patient to call the primary care provider to report any persistent, changing, worsening, anxiety-producing, or specific signs and symptoms, including fever higher than 101° F (38.3° C), vomiting blood or coffee-ground material, passing tarry black stools or blood, jaundice, and no bowel movements in 5 days.

Resources
• Crohn's and Colitis Foundation of America: 800-343-3637
• For patient information on IBS: *www.medscape.com*

Lumbosacral strain

ICD-9-CM intervertebral disk disorders 722, unspecified backache 724.5

This condition refers to the stretching or tearing of muscles, tendons, ligaments, or the back due to trauma or chronic mechanical stress. Pain can be acute, chronic, or recurring in the lumbosacral spine area. Adults ages 20 to 40 are at greatest risk. Twenty percent of Americans complain of low back pain that is slow to resolve and recurs easily without conscious, daily preventive measures.

Causes

Most acute back pain is caused by muscle strain or spasm of the paraspinal muscles. It can also result from trauma or mechanical causes that tore or physically stressed the structures of the back.

Risk factors include chronic occupational strain, obesity, improper body mechanics when lifting, poor posture, weak back and abdominal muscles, and structural abnormalities, such as an abnormal forward pelvic tilt and unequal leg lengths.

Clinical presentation

Pain is the most significant presenting sign. Onset of pain and stiffness occurs 12 to 36 hours after the injury or activity. Pain is usually moderate to severe, located across the lumbosacral area and down through the buttocks and thighs, and unilateral or bilateral. Aggravating factors include movement, particularly standing and back flexion. Pain and spasm will increase on palpation. Relieving factors are rest and reclining. Muscles spasms may be present and can last several days.

The patient may present with gait and posture that are stiff or slow, and decreased range of motion with increased pain on flexion of the back. Point tenderness and muscle spasm are common. Positive straight-leg raises (elevate each leg passively with flexion at hip and extension of knee) reveal radicular pain when the leg is raised more than 60 degrees. Positive crossed-leg raises (when the patient complains of radicular pain in the leg that isn't raised during a straight-leg raise) strongly suggest a vertebral disk injury. Pain on the Patrick's test (the heel is placed on the opposite knee and lateral force is exerted) suggests hip or sacroiliac disease.

Abnormal reflexes may indicate more serious spinal cord involvement. A lack of sensation of the perineum is a warning sign and indicates further evaluation for cauda equina syndrome. To detect complaints of back pain that have secondary reward (attention-getting behavior) as the root of the problem, do something that should cause no back pain and see if the patient overreacts. For instance, applying slight pressure to the top of the head shouldn't produce pain. Distracting the patient while doing passive tests may elicit a different response.

Differential diagnosis

Initially, differentiate between mechanical and nonmechanical causes of back pain (mechanical is defined as being related to the motion of the body in daily activities and posture). Mechanical causes include strains, disk disease, and spinal stenosis.

It's crucial to consider nonmechanical causes of back pain (which account for 4% of all cases), because sequelae can be life-threatening. These include osteomyelitis, metabolic bone disease, neoplasia, inflammatory disease, spinal cord disease, abdominal aneurysm, pyelonephritis, and spinal instability. Other causes are depression, hysteria, cystitis, prostatitis, endometriosis, osteoarthritis, compression fracture due to osteoporosis, and bursitis.

ALERT More aggressive evaluation is indicated if you suspect a nonmechanical diagnosis; risk factors include age younger than 20 or older than 55, fever, unrelenting pain, extreme hypertension, and abdominal pain.

Diagnostic tests

No tests are routinely indicated for initial presentation with low back pain.

• Complete blood count with elevated white blood cells and an elevated sedimentation rate suggest infection. Low serum calcium may indicate osteoporosis. Alkaline phosphatase can indicate renal disease. Serum immunoelectrophoresis can reveal inflammatory disorders, malignancies, diffuse bone disease, or renal disease. Urinalysis may reveal a urinary tract infection.

• Radiology studies have a high false-positive rate and by themselves are insufficient for diagnosis. They should be done for high-risk groups, such as trauma patients and those suspected of having been abused. X-rays detect fracture in trauma cases (substance abusers may deny or not remember trauma) and pathologic fractures from use of steroids, osteoporosis, or metastasis. They may also detect a malignant tumor (suspect in

patients over age 50 with fever or a recent weight loss).
• Magnetic resonance imaging detects nonmusculoskeletal causes, such as disk disease and neoplasms.
• Bone scan detects malignancy and osteoporosis.

Management

Acute

 ALERT Immediate evaluation is needed for pain extending below the knees, lack of sensation in the perineum, and abnormal findings of motor, sensory and reflex function in the lower extremities.

General
Regardless of the treatment plan, 33% of low back pain cases resolve in 1 week, and 98% resolve within 3 months. Highest patient satisfaction rates result when the patient is provided an explanation and understanding of his back pain.

Initial conservative management of the patient with back pain includes a period of controlled physical activity plus drugs; analgesics should be used only for short periods to avoid risk of drug dependence. Physical therapy must be part of the management plan, including cold and heat treatments to decrease pain and spasm.

Medication
• Nonsteroidal anti-inflammatory drugs (NSAIDs), such as ibuprofen (Motrin) or etodolac (Lodine), can decrease pain and inflammation while the tissues heal. These drugs should be used for a limited time (1 to 2 weeks).
• For back spasms, muscle relaxants, such as cyclobenzaprine (Flexeril) or methocarbamol (Robaxin), are frequently used in conjunction with NSAIDs.

• Narcotics should be prescribed only in severe trauma cases. The patient may resume full activity too soon and cause further injury. There is also a risk of drug dependence because of the chronic nature of the disorder.

Referral or consultation
Refer the patient to an orthopedist if the condition is nonresponsive after 1 week. Refer for physical therapy for back strengthening exercises and proper body mechanics training.

Follow-up
See the patient weekly for evaluation until pain resolves and then at 1 month to reinforce back precautions and exercises.

Complications
Chronic low back pain and narcotics addiction are possible complications.

Patient teaching
• Teach the patient that back pain is slow to ease and can recur with minimal additional stress or injury. It's important to continue back exercises when the pain eases. Most back injuries don't happen suddenly; they're the result of long-term insult (keeping the back in flexion for large amounts of each day for years and poor body mechanics).
• Tell the patient to rest as much as possible on a firm mattress or with a board under the mattress for 24 hours. An alternative is to sleep on the floor, using a comforter or blankets for padding. He should avoid sleeping on a water bed.
• For the first 72 hours, the patient should apply ice packs or cold compresses to the area, no more than 20 minutes at a time, four or more times per day. This will decrease swelling, inflammation, spasms, and pain.

• After 72 hours, the patient can apply a heating pad (set at medium) to the area, no more than 20 minutes at a time (to avoid burns), four or more times per day. This will relax the muscles, enhance blood exchange at the site, and ease stiffness and pain. A hot bath or shower with the water aimed at the site has the same effect.

• Advise the patient to start moving slowly but progressively after the first day, to avoid prolonged sitting or standing (longer than 15 minutes without changing positions), to avoid bending or twisting the back, and to bend at the knees and keep the back straight when lifting. Tell him to begin extension exercises, such as walking or swimming, as soon as pain eases and to progress as tolerated.

• Teach the patient to place a folded towel or lumbar back roll (available at any medical supply house) in the small of the back when sitting for more than 15 minutes at a time or when riding in a car.

• Have the patient learn and practice daily back extension exercises such as the McKenzie exercises. As ambulation increases, decrease medication doses.

• Instruct the patient to avoid strenuous or high-impact activities and actions, such as lifting and pushing, for 6 weeks because healing is a slow process.

• Have the patient decrease his risk of recurrences by reducing weight (if overweight), increasing daily exercise for overall conditioning, and using good body mechanics at all times.

• For patients who need to return to activity early, consider a back support such as a corset. This may provide support but seems to function more by increasing awareness of the back and its relationship with activity. Use of a back support is of questionable use after 3 months and increases the risk of injury after 6 months; patients may attempt more strenuous activities because they feel "protected," and minimizing extension or flexion over long periods tends to weaken the muscles.

ALERT Tell the patient to call the primary care provider to report any new or persistent signs and symptoms, including pain lasting more than 1 week, weakness or numbness in the legs, bowel or bladder dysfunction, or severe pain that is worsened by the management plan.

Resources
• Back Pain Hotline: 800-247-2225
• Arthritis Foundation: 800-283-7800
• McKenzie Institute: 800-635-8380

Osteoporosis

ICD-9-CM 733.0

Osteoporosis is a metabolic bone disorder in which bone absorption outpaces bone formation, causing a net loss of the bony matrix as well as the calcium that adheres to it. Bones become porous, brittle, and abnormally vulnerable to fracture.

Causes

The cause of primary osteoporosis is unknown; however, a mild but prolonged negative calcium balance, resulting from an inadequate dietary intake of calcium, may be an important contributing factor, as may declining ovarian function and a sedentary lifestyle.

Causes of secondary osteoporosis include prolonged therapy with steroids or heparin, metabolic disorders such as hyperthyroidism, and osteogenesis imperfecta.

Risk factors include a positive family history, fair skin color, thin physique, menopause, long-term immobility (such as hemiplegia), malnutrition, lactose intolerance, Scandinavian or Asian descent, and alcohol or tobacco use.

Clinical presentation

Onset of osteoporosis is insidious; it's usually diagnosed when a fracture occurs. Weight-bearing bones are most commonly affected. Compression fracture of the thoracic spine can be asymptomatic or have pain that radiates anteriorly and is aggravated by movement.

Hip fracture generally presents as a minor fall or blow to the area followed by abrupt onset of pain, decreased range of motion of the affected hip, and external rotation of the leg. As vertebral bodies weaken, spontaneous wedge fractures, pathologic fractures of the neck and femur, Colles' fractures after a minor fall, and hip fractures are all common.

Associated signs of osteoporosis are increasing deformity, kyphosis ("dowager's hump"), lordosis, and loss of height.

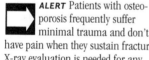 **ALERT** Patients with osteoporosis frequently suffer minimal trauma and don't have pain when they sustain fracture. X-ray evaluation is needed for any suspicion of fracture.

Differential diagnosis

Differential diagnosis includes multiple myeloma, neoplasia, osteomalacia, osteogenesis imperfecta, hyperparathyroidism, and hyperthyroidism.

Diagnostic tests

• Height measurement is taken annually (without shoes) in postmenopausal women.
• Alkaline phosphatase increases transiently after bone fracture.

• Serum or urine protein electrophoresis and urinary free cortisol analysis detect metabolic disorders.
• High levels of serum osteocalcin and urinary calcium, pyridinoline, and N-telopeptide collagen cross-links indicate accelerated demineralization.
• Thyroid-stimulating hormone test may detect hypothyroidism or hyperthyroidism.
• Bone mineral densitometry (BMD or DEXA scan) measures bone density; this screening test is useful in early osteoporosis.
• X-rays show typical degeneration in the lower thoracic and lumbar vertebrae. The vertebral bodies may appear flattened and denser. Loss of bone mineral becomes evident in later stages. X-rays can detect early manifestations (increased width of intervertebral spaces, accentuated cortical plates, vertical striations of vertebral bodies) as well as late manifestations (vertebral compression and multiple fractures of long bones).
• Bone biopsy isn't routinely done, but may detect metabolic bone disorders or quantify bone loss.

Management

 ALERT Acute pain or suspected fracture requires X-rays and immediate evaluation.

Weakened vertebrae should be supported, usually with a back brace. Surgery can correct pathologic fractures of the femur by open reduction and internal fixation. Colles' fracture requires reduction with plaster immobilization for 4 to 10 weeks. Evaluate the patient's skin for redness, warmth, and new sites of pain, which may indicate new fractures.

General

Encourage weight-bearing exercise (build up to walking 2 miles with 1-lb weights five times a week.) The patient should avoid activities that exert stress on vertebrae and long bones. Teach the patient to avoid falls by not using scatter rugs, not rushing to answer the phone, and using handrails in bathroom and on stairs.

Dietary recommendations include the following:

• beginning a reduction diet if overweight
• avoiding a high-protein diet
• avoiding carbonated beverages because excess phosphorus decreases serum calcium.
• ingesting enough calcium (1,000 mg/day after age 24, 1,500 mg/day after menopause, and 2,000 mg/day for patients diagnosed with osteoporosis); all women need at least 600 IU of vitamin D daily (can be obtained by only 10 minutes a week of skin exposure to sun).

Medication

Drug therapy arrests osteoporosis but doesn't cure it.

• Calcium and vitamin D supplements (to reach the recommended daily allowance) to support bone formation are used in conjunction with other therapies (see dietary recommendations above).
• Hormone replacement therapy (estrogen) decreases rate of bone resorption.
• Thyroid hormone (calcitonin inhalant) prevents bone resorption, relieves pain, and may stimulate bone formation.
• Biphosphonates (alendronate) form a bony matrix, which enhances calcium adherence.
• Gonadotropin-releasing hormone analogue (Synarel inhalant) increases ovarian steroid production.

• Selective estrogen receptor modulator (raloxifene) decreases bone demineralization.
• Tamoxifen offers some protection for bone without stimulating breast changes.
• Androgens, steroids, and parathyroid hormone analogues are being researched.

Referral or consultation

Refer the patient to a doctor for back pain due to compression fractures. Refer her to a gynecologist for endometrial evaluation for abnormal vaginal bleeding. Have the patient see a physical therapist for exercises to increase strength, endurance, and proper body mechanics, and an occupational therapist to learn adaptive behaviors and correct technique for the use of braces and other devices.

Follow-up

Follow-up should be monthly during initial treatment, then quarterly. Focus on body mechanics, exercise, compliance with drug regimen, and adverse effects of drugs. The patient will need a Papanicolaou test and pelvic examination, mammography, and BMD examination annually, and vertebral X-rays every 3 years.

Complications

Patients experience severe pain, neurologic deficits due to vertebral fractures, and loss of independence.

Patient teaching

• Stress the importance of physical therapy, emphasizing gentle exercise and activity.
• Promote healthy dietary options, high in nutrients that support skeletal metabolism: calcium, vitamin D, and protein.
• Make sure the person understands the prescribed drug regimen clearly

(for example, take alendronate on an empty stomach with water and then wait at least half an hour before ingesting food or other fluids. Otherwise, absorption drops by more than 60%.)

• Advise the patient to sleep on a firm mattress and avoid excessive bed rest.

• Because an osteoporotic patient's bones fracture very easily, emphasize the importance of moving gently and carefully at all times.

• Teach good body mechanics: stoop before lifting anything and avoid twisting movements and prolonged bending.

• Instruct a woman taking estrogen in breast self-examination. Tell her to perform this examination at least once a month and to report any lumps immediately. Emphasize the need for regular gynecologic examinations. Report abnormal bleeding promptly.

ALERT Tell the patient to call the primary care provider to report any new or persistent signs and symptoms, including new pain, even without trauma; abnormal bleeding; and drug adverse effects (stomach pain, nausea, tarry stools).

Resources

• National Osteoporosis Foundation: 800-223-9994

• Information for those who are newly diagnosed or at high risk: *www.medscape.com*

• For providers — Drug affordability: *www.needymeds.com* (contains information regarding many drug company programs that provide financial assistance for those who need their drugs)

Otitis media

ICD-9-CM acute otitis media 382.0, acute suppurative otitis media 381.0

Inflammation of the middle ear, otitis media may be suppurative or secretory and acute or chronic.

 SPECIAL POPULATIONS Acute otitis media is most common in children; it's also a problem for older adults. Incidence rises during the winter months, paralleling the seasonal rise in nonbacterial respiratory tract infections.

With prompt treatment, the prognosis for acute otitis media is excellent; however, prolonged accumulation of fluid within the middle ear cavity causes chronic otitis media, with possible perforation of the tympanic membrane. Chronic suppurative otitis media may lead to scarring, adhesions, and severe structural or functional ear damage.

Chronic secretory otitis media, with its persistent inflammation and pressure, may cause conductive hearing loss.

Causes

Acute otitis media results from disruption of eustachian tube patency and subsequent inflammation and infection.

Acute otitis media

In the suppurative form of acute otitis media, respiratory tract infection, allergic reaction, nasotracheal intubation, or positional changes allow nasopharyngeal flora to reflux into the eustachian tube and colonize the middle ear. Suppurative otitis media usually results from bacterial infection with pneumococci, *Haemophilus influenzae* (the most common cause in children under age 6), *Moraxella catarrhalis,* beta-hemolytic streptococci, staphylococci (most common cause in children ages 6 and older), or gram-negative bacteria. Predisposing factors include the normally wider, shorter, more horizontal eustachian tubes and increased lymphoid tissue in children as well as anatomic anomalies. Chronic suppurative otitis media results from inadequate treatment of acute otitis media episodes, infection by resistant strains of bacteria or, rarely, tuberculosis.

In the secretory form of acute otitis media, eustachian tube obstruction causes buildup of negative pressure in the middle ear that promotes effusion of sterile serous fluid from blood vessels in the middle ear membrane. This may be secondary to eustachian tube dysfunction from viral infection or allergy. It may also follow barotrauma (pressure injury from inability to equalize pressures between the environment and the middle ear), which can occur during rapid aircraft descent in a person with an upper respiratory tract infection and during rapid underwater ascent in scuba diving (barotitis media). Chronic secretory otitis media follows inadequate treatment of the acute form or persistent eustachian tube dysfunction from mechanical obstruction (adenoidal tissue overgrowth, tumors) or edema (allergic rhinitis, chronic sinus infection).

Clinical presentation

Clinical features vary with the specific type of the disorder.

Acute otitis media
History may reveal tinnitus; severe, deep, throbbing pain (from pressure behind the tympanic membrane); hearing an echo; hearing popping or crackling sounds when moving the jaw; previous occurrences; and preceding illness. Elicit history of aller-

gies, exposure to smoke, and congenital disorders.

Examination of the tympanic membrane usually shows a distorted light reflex, a bulging tympanic membrane with obscured bony landmarks (indicating suppurative acute otitis media) or a retracted tympanic membrane with prominent landmarks (indicating secretory acute otitis media), decreased motility with insufflation (air puffed into the ear), and otorrhea. However, this procedure is painful with an obviously bulging, erythematous tympanic membrane.

Additional signs include signs of upper respiratory tract infection (sneezing, coughing), hearing loss (usually mild and conductive), ear drainage, dizziness, nausea, vomiting, and constitutional symptoms (mild to high fever, irritability).

Chronic otitis media
Cumulative effects of chronic otitis media include thickening and scarring of the tympanic membrane, decreased or absent membrane mobility, cholesteatoma (a cystlike mass in the middle ear) and, in chronic suppurative otitis media, a painless, purulent discharge. The extent of conductive hearing loss varies with the size and type of tympanic membrane perforation and ossicular destruction.

 ALERT If the tympanic membrane has ruptured, the patient may say the pain has suddenly stopped. Complications may include abscesses (brain, subperiosteal, epidural), sigmoid sinus or jugular vein thrombosis, septicemia, meningitis, suppurative labyrinthitis, facial paralysis, and otitis externa.

Differential diagnosis

Conditions to be considered include external otitis media, redness due to crying, cerumen impaction, mastoiditis, trauma, furuncle, temporomandibular joint dysfunction, mumps, dental abscess, tonsillitis, foreign body, and barotrauma.

In patients with chronic otitis media, history discloses recurrent or unresolved otitis media. Otoscopy shows thickening and sometimes scarring and decreased mobility of the tympanic membrane; pneumatoscopy shows decreased or absent tympanic membrane movement. History of recent air travel or scuba diving suggests barotitis media; examination may reveal a blackened tympanic membrane if it has hemorrhaged.

Diagnostic tests

Testing isn't routinely indicated.

ALERT Adults in good health require more aggressive evaluation, because otitis media is an infrequent diagnosis for them. Examination and testing should consider the sinuses, oral cavity with emphasis on teeth, temporomandibular joint, nasopharynx for neoplasia, and cranial nerves for cranial neuralgias.

• Tympanocentesis for culture and sensitivity of middle ear effusion may help in severe cases, persistent or recurrent infections, and immunocompromised patients, and those with .

• Tympanometry may confirm suspicion of fluid behind the tympanic membrane without clinical signs.

• Paranasal sinus X-rays may reveal fracture, Wegener's granulomatosis, neoplasia, cyst, or mucocele and may differentiate acute from chronic sinusitis.

• Audiometry can quantify hearing loss and recovery.

Management

The type of otitis media dictates the treatment guidelines.

Suppurative otitis media

In suppurative acute otitis media, antibiotic therapy includes ampicillin or amoxicillin. In areas with a high incidence of beta-lactamase-producing *Haemophilus influenzae* and in patients who aren't responding to ampicillin or amoxicillin, amoxicillin/clavulanate potassium may be used.

For those who are allergic to penicillin derivatives, therapy may include cefaclor or co-trimoxazole. Broad-spectrum antibiotics can help prevent acute suppurative otitis media in high-risk patients. In patients with recurring otitis, antibiotics must be used with discretion to prevent development of resistant strains of bacteria. Severe, painful bulging of the tympanic membrane usually necessitates myringotomy.

Secretory otitis media

For acute secretory otitis media, inflation of the eustachian tube by performing Valsalva's maneuver several times a day may be the only treatment required. Otherwise, nasopharyngeal decongestant therapy may be helpful. It should continue for at least 2 weeks and sometimes indefinitely, with periodic evaluation.

Surgical treatment

If decongestant therapy fails, myringotomy and aspiration of middle ear fluid are necessary, followed by insertion of a polyethylene tube into the tympanic membrane, for immediate and prolonged equalization of pressure. The tube falls out spontaneously after 9 to 12 months. Concomitant treatment of the underlying cause (such as elimination of allergens or an adenoidectomy for hypertrophied adenoids) may also be helpful in correcting this disorder.

Chronic otitis media

Treatment of chronic otitis media includes broad-spectrum antibiotics, such as amoxicillin/clavulanate potassium or cefuroxime, for exacerbations of acute otitis media; elimination of eustachian tube obstruction; treatment of otitis externa; myringoplasty and tympanoplasty to reconstruct middle ear structures when thickening and scarring are present; and, possibly, mastoidectomy. Cholesteatoma requires excision.

Referral or consultation

Refer the patient to an ear, nose, and throat (ENT) specialist if he has serous otitis media with a hearing loss lasting longer than 6 weeks or a hearing loss that extends bilaterally or exceeds 20 decibels; vertigo or ataxia; or symptoms that worsen after 3 days of treatment. In chronic persistent infections, ENT evaluation is recommended for patients who have significant hearing loss that lasts longer than 3 weeks, infection that fails to resolve after two courses of antibiotics, cholesteatoma formation, or a ruptured tympanic membrane that fails to close.

Follow-up

For acute otitis media, see the patient 3 days after starting treatment if nonresponsive. Otherwise, see a few days after completion of antibiotics to evaluate. For chronic otitis media see every month, focusing on ear examination. For serous otitis media, see the patient 4 to 6 weeks after treatment for evaluation.

Complications

Acute otitis media can be complicated by perforation, otorrhea, acute mastoiditis, facial nerve paralysis, vertigo, ataxia, lateral sinus thrombophlebitis, otitic hydrocephalus, and meningitis. *Chronic* otitis media can be complicated by hearing loss. *Recurrent* otitis media can cause atrophy and scarring of the eardrum, a ruptured tympanic membrane that doesn't close, and otorrhea, cholesteatoma, permanent hearing loss,

chronic mastoiditis, and infection spreading to adjacent intracranial structures.

Patient teaching

• Explain all diagnostic tests and procedures.
• Teach the patient not to place cotton or plugs deep in the ear canal; however, sterile cotton may be placed loosely in the external ear to absorb drainage. To prevent infection, change the cotton whenever it gets damp, and wash hands before and after giving ear care.
• After tympanoplasty, observe for excessive bleeding from the ear canal. Warn the patient against blowing his nose or getting water in the ear.
• Explain the importance of completing a prescribed course of antibiotic treatment. If ordering nasopharyngeal decongestants, teach correct instillation.
• Apply heat to the ear to relieve pain. Advise the patient with acute secretory otitis media to watch for and immediately report pain and fever—signs of secondary infection.
  To prevent otitis media:
• Teach recognition of upper respiratory tract infections and encourage early treatment.
• Instruct parents not to feed their infant in a supine position or put him to bed with a bottle. This prevents reflux of nasopharyngeal flora.
• To promote eustachian tube patency, tell the patient to perform Valsalva's maneuver several times daily.
• Identify and treat allergies.

 ALERT Tell the patient to call the primary care provider to report any new or persistent signs and symptoms, including headache, fever, severe pain, signs of infection (redness, swelling, drainage from ear), and disorientation.

Resources
• American Academy of Pediatrics: 800-433-9016
• Patient information on otitis media: *www.medscape.com*

Parkinson's disease

ICD-9-CM: 332.0

Parkinson's disease is a chronic, progressive, neurodegenerative central nervous system disorder characterized by tremor at rest, rigidity, and bradykinesia. Parkinson's disease strikes 1 in every 100 people over age 60.

Causes

Although the cause of Parkinson's disease is unknown, some theorize accelerated aging, a toxic or infectious cause, or an oxidative mechanism. Regardless, there is a loss of dopamine-producing neurons in the substantia nigra.

Clinical presentation

Disease is of gradual onset; history may reveal recent onset of clumsiness, falling, and a change in handwriting. The cardinal symptoms of Parkinson's disease are muscle rigidity and bradykinesia. The patient typically presents with an insidious tremor that begins in the fingers (unilateral pill-roll tremor), increases during stress or anxiety, and decreases with purposeful movement and sleep.

Muscle rigidity results in resistance to passive muscle stretching, which may be uniform (lead-pipe rigidity) or jerky (cogwheel rigidity). Bradykinesia causes the patient to walk with difficulty (gait lacks normal parallel motion and may be retropulsive or propulsive). The patient has difficulty initiating movement.

Parkinson's disease also produces a monotone voice; drooling; masklike facies; loss of posture control (the patient walks with body bent forward); and dysarthria, dysphagia, or both. Occasionally, bradykinesia may also cause oculogyric crises (eyes are fixed upward, with involuntary tonic movements) or blepharospasm (eyelids are completely closed). In later stages, the patient may exhibit slowed mentation progressing to dementia.

Autonomic dysfunction is evidenced by orthostatic hypotension, constipation, bladder dysfunction, and impotence.

Differential diagnosis

For diagnosis, the patient must have either rest tremor or bradykinesia, plus one of the following: rigidity, flexed posture, loss of postural reflexes, and masklike facies. Slightly hyperactive or hard-to-elicit reflexes, decreased blink reflex, and extraocular movement (EOM) (difficulty with upward gaze) are also common. If EOM elicits disturbance in ocular motility, consider progressive supranuclear palsy.

For differential diagnosis, consider an adverse drug reaction (particularly suspect neuroleptic agents), progressive supranuclear palsy, multisystem atrophy, dementia, depression, Huntington's disease, Creutzfeldt-Jacob disease, Wilson's disease, lacunar infarctions, toxins (such as carbon monoxide, manganese, and cyanide), infections, and benign essential tumor.

Diagnostic tests

No diagnostic tests exist for Parkinson's disease. However, promising research is in progress utilizing a single photon emission computed tomography (SPECT) and altropane or iodine[123] beta-CIT (carbomethoxy-3 [-4-iodophenyl] tropan).

• Conduct a Mini–Mental Status Examination. If the patient scores less than 20, consider a dementia disorder.

• In a younger person, order liver function, serum copper, and ceruloplasmin tests after a doctor's consultation to detect Wilson's disease, which causes excess copper accumulation.

• Consider computed tomography scan or magnetic resonance imaging to detect lacunar infarcts, brain stem atrophy, or cerebellar atrophy if you're unsure of the diagnosis or if the patient is unresponsive to drug therapy.

Management

Treatment is palliative; no curative treatment exists. Acute exacerbation may indicate a secondary cause, depression, or noncompliance. If the condition is drug-induced, symptoms may take months to resolve. Monitor for toxic effects of drugs.

Advise the patient to take small, frequent meals if fatigued by eating. Diet should be high in fluid and fiber intake.

Pallidotomy may be indicated for some patients. Good to excellent mobility has been achieved in 70% of research studies of the surgery. Pallidotomy is generally restricted to one side due to the risk of performing surgery on both sides of the brain.

Medication
• Anticholinergics (trihexyphenidyl hydrochloride, benztropine mesylate)
• Dopamine precursors or agonists (carbidopa-levodopa, generally reserved until other drugs are tried because of decreasing effectiveness after about 5 years of treatment; pramipexole; ropinirole)
• Dopamine receptor agonist (bromocriptine)

• Synthetic cyclic primary amine (amantadine)
• Monoamine oxidase inhibitors (selegiline)
• Catechol-O-methyltransferase inhibitors (tolcapone), used cautiously due to cases of liver injury.

Levodopa, a dopamine replacement that is most effective during early stages, is given in increasing doses until symptoms are relieved or adverse effects appear. Because adverse effects can be serious, levodopa is frequently given in combination with carbidopa to halt peripheral dopamine synthesis. When levodopa proves ineffective or too toxic, alternative drug therapy is initiated.

Referral or consultation
Refer the patient to a neurologist for definitive diagnosis and initial drug regimen, severe disease states that are nonresponsive to drugs, and possible stereotactic neurosurgery such as pallidotomy to relieve symptoms. Physical therapy is complementary to increase strength and endurance and to maintain normal muscle tone and function. This includes active range of motion, passive range of motion, activities of daily living, and massage to help relax muscles. Occupational therapy is important for adjustments in the home (elevated toilet seat, assistive devices for eating and dressing). Speech therapy referral should be made as soon as speech abnormalities are noticed.

Follow-up
Monitor drug treatment so dosage can be adjusted to minimize adverse effects. Evaluate the patient for depression at each visit. See the patient every 2 weeks after any change in drug therapy. During stable periods, see him monthly to quarterly. Lifelong follow-up is needed for drug therapy adjustment and physical therapy.

Complications

Complications of Parkinson's disease include dementia, depression, aspiration pneumonia, falls, freezing (transient paralysis), and dyskinesias. Complications are usually the cause of death.

Patient teaching

• Teach significant others that caring effectively for the patient with Parkinson's disease requires careful monitoring of drug treatment, emphasis on self-reliance, and generous psychological support.

• Teach the patient and the family that this is a progressive disease; the worst prognosis is for older patients with dementia.

• Fatigue may cause the patient to depend more on others; therefore, he should schedule rest periods; eat small, frequent meals; and use assistive devices.

• Teach the family how to prevent pressure ulcers and contractures by proper positioning.

• Establish long- and short-term treatment goals, and be aware of the patient's need for intellectual stimulation and diversion.

• The patient with excessive tremor may achieve partial control of his body by sitting on a chair and using its arms to steady himself.

• Instruct the patient to minimize constipation by drinking at least 2 qt (2 L) of liquids daily and eating high-bulk foods.

 ALERT Tell the patient to call the primary care provider to report any new or persistent signs and symptoms, including lack of improvement with management and signs of stroke, such as mental status change, facial droop, blurred vision, rapidly worsened coordination (especially if unilateral), and seizures.

Resources

• United Parkinson Foundation: 800-344-7872

• American Parkinson's Disease Foundation: 800-223-2732 or *www.apdaparkinson.com*

• National Parkinson Foundation: 800-327-4545 or *www.parkinson.org*

• Parkinson's Disease Foundation: 800-457-6676

• Parkinson's Education Program: 800-344-7872

• Parkinson's Support Groups of America: 301-937-1545

Peptic ulcer

ICD-9-CM duodenal 532.9, gastric 531.9, peptic 536.8

Circumscribed lesions in the mucosal membrane, peptic ulcers can develop in the lower esophagus, stomach, pylorus, duodenum, or jejunum. About 80% of all peptic ulcers are duodenal ulcers, which affect the proximal part of the small intestine and occur most often in men between ages 20 and 50.

Gastric ulcers, which affect the stomach mucosa, are most common in people ages 55 to 70, especially in chronic users of nonsteroidal anti-inflammatory drugs (NSAIDs) or alcohol. *Duodenal ulcers* usually follow a chronic course, with remissions and exacerbations; 5% to 10% of patients develop complications that necessitate surgery.

Causes

Researchers recognize three major causes of peptic ulcer disease: infection with *Helicobacter pylori* (formerly known as *Campylobacter pylori*), use of NSAIDs, and pathologic hypersecretory states such as Zollinger-Ellison syndrome. Regardless of the cause, an imbalance exists between aggressive factors (such as gastric acid) and defensive factors that enhance mucosal integrity (such as mucus, prostaglandins, growth factors, blood flow, bicarbonate, and cell turnover). Gastric acid, which was once considered a primary cause, now appears mainly to contribute to the consequences of infection.

Certain drugs, including salicylates and other NSAIDs, encourage ulcer formation by inhibiting the secretion of prostaglandins (the substances that suppress ulceration). Certain illnesses, such as pancreatitis, hepatic disease, Crohn's disease, preexisting gastritis, and Zollinger-Ellison syndrome, cause hypersecretion of gastric acids.

Predisposing factors

In addition to peptic ulcer's main causes, several predisposing factors are known. They include blood type (gastric ulcers tend to strike people with type A blood; duodenal ulcers tend to afflict people with type O blood) and other genetic factors.

Exposure to irritants, such as alcohol and tobacco, may contribute by accelerating gastric acid emptying and promoting mucosal breakdown. Physical trauma, emotional stress, and normal aging are additional predisposing conditions.

Clinical presentation

Clinical features vary with the area of the GI tract that is affected.

Gastric ulcers

Heartburn and indigestion usually signal the beginning of a gastric ulcer attack. Eating food stretches the gastric wall and may cause — or, in some cases, relieve — pain and a feeling of fullness and distention.

Other typical effects include weight loss and repeated episodes of massive GI bleeding.

Duodenal ulcers

Duodenal ulcers produce heartburn and well-localized midepigastric pain that is relieved by food, antacids, or antisecretory agents; weight gain, because the patient eats to relieve discomfort; and a peculiar sensation of hot water bubbling in the back of the throat. Attacks usually occur about 2 hours after meals, whenever the stomach is empty, or after consumption of orange juice, coffee, aspirin, or alcohol.

Exacerbations tend to recur several times a year and then fade into remission. Vomiting and other digestive disturbances are rare.

Differential diagnosis

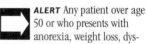
ALERT Any patient over age 50 or who presents with anorexia, weight loss, dysphagia, vomiting, or GI bleeding requires aggressive evaluation. Other red flags include a family history of cancer, positive fecal occult blood test, shortness of breath (may be due to anemia), and abnormal blood counts.

Conditions to consider are gastroesophageal reflux disease, nonulcer dyspepsia, gastric carcinoma, *H. pylori*–associated gastritis, Crohn's disease, pancreatitis, variant angina pectoris, cholecystitis, biliary tract disease, and cardiovascular disease.

Diagnostic tests
• Serologic *H. pylori* or carbon isotope urea breath test detects *H. pylori*. (Breath test yields up to 15% false-negative results.)
• Serial fecal occult blood tests may disclose occult blood in the stools, which requires colonoscopic evaluation. Hemoglobin and hematocrit

values are decreased from GI bleeding (uncommon without hemorrhage).
• An elevated fasting serum gastrin and secretin stimulation test indicates Zollinger-Ellison syndrome.
• Upper GI tract X-rays show mucosal abnormalities; gastric secretory studies show hyperchlorhydria and achlorhydria. Upper GI endoscopy confirms an ulcer, and biopsy rules out *H. pylori* infection and cancer.

Management

Acute

If GI bleeding occurs, emergency treatment begins with passage of a nasogastric tube to allow for iced saline lavage, possibly containing norepinephrine. Gastroscopy allows visualization of the bleeding site and coagulation by laser or cautery to control bleeding. This type of therapy allows postponement of surgery until the patient's condition stabilizes.

Surgery is indicated for perforation, unresponsiveness to conservative treatment, and suspected cancer. Surgical procedures for peptic ulcers include:
• *vagotomy and pyloroplasty:* severing one or more branches of the vagus nerve to reduce hydrochloric acid secretion and refashioning the pylorus to create a larger lumen and facilitate gastric emptying
• *distal subtotal gastrectomy (with or without vagotomy):* excising the antrum of the stomach, thereby removing the hormonal stimulus of the parietal cells, followed by anastomosis of the rest of the stomach to the duodenum or the jejunum.

General

 ALERT Relief of symptoms doesn't rule out cancer.

Medication

Current recommendations include treating every patient at least once to eradicate *H. pylori* because the infection may occur even with other causes such as NSAID use. Although *H. pylori* infection can be eliminated, studies have demonstrated that symptomatic *H. pylori* returns in 80% of patients more than 1 year after treatment.
• Treatment options include acid suppression and a combination of antibiotics (three drugs twice per day for 7 to 10 days). Drug combinations include metronidazole, omeprazole, and clarithromycin; lansoprazole, amoxicillin, and clarithromycin; and ranitidine, bismuth citrate, amoxicillin, and clarithromycin.
• Patients taking NSAIDs may take a prostaglandin analogue (misoprostol) to minimize or prevent ulceration. A histamine-2 (H_2) receptor antagonist (cimetidine or nizatidine) or omeprazole may reduce acid secretion.
• If the condition is uncomplicated, the patient may try antiulcer drugs, including H_2-receptor antagonists (ranitidine, nizatidine), antacids (aluminum hydroxide), or sucralfate for 2 weeks. If the patient isn't responsive, diagnostic studies are indicated. If the patient is responsive, treat him for 8 weeks.

Referral or consultation

Refer the patient to a gastroenterologist for evaluation and GI studies for nonresponsive, recurrent symptoms or for evidence of bleeding.

Follow-up

See the patient in 2 weeks for evaluation. Perform a *Campylobacter*-like organism test biopsy, the urea breath test, or serologic tests if symptoms persist or return. If *H. pylori* returns, treat with a different drug regimen to decrease resistance.

Patients with gastric ulcer need posttreatment endoscopy at 1½ to 3 months to detect cancer or poor healing.

Complications

Both kinds of ulcers may penetrate the pancreas and cause severe back pain. Other complications include hemorrhage, perforation, and gastric outlet obstruction. Dizziness, syncope, hematemesis, or melena suggests hemorrhage.

Patient teaching

• Teach the patient about the adverse effects of H_2-receptor antagonists and omeprazole (dizziness, fatigue, rash, mild diarrhea).
• Advise any patient who uses antacids, has a history of cardiac disease, or follows a sodium-restricted diet, to take only antacids that contain low amounts of sodium.
• Tell the patient to avoid hot, spicy, and high-fat foods.
• Warn the patient to avoid steroids, aspirin, and NSAIDs because they decrease protective factors. For the same reason, warn the patient to avoid stressful situations, smoking, excessive intake of coffee, and ingestion of alcoholic beverages during exacerbations of peptic ulcer disease.
• Inform the patient of the potential adverse effects of antibiotic therapy (superinfection, diarrhea).
• Emphasize need for follow-up testing to confirm eradication of *H. pylori* infection.
• Tell the patient taking bismuth subsalicylate that this drug may cause constipation and very dark stools.

ALERT Tell the patient to call the primary care provider to report any new or persistent signs and symptoms, including abdominal pain that worsens or fails to respond to treatment; fever above 101° F (38.3° C); bloody or coffee-ground vomitus; and bright-red, black, tarry, or maroon-colored stools.

Pneumonia

ICD-9-CM 486, aspiration 507.0, atypical 486, with influenza 487.0, bacterial 482.9, pneumo-coccal/streptococcal 481, interstitial 516.8, mycoplasma 483, Pneumocystis carinii 136.3, viral 480.9

An acute infection of the lung parenchyma, pneumonia often impairs gas exchange. The prognosis is generally good for people who have normal lungs and adequate host defenses before the onset of pneumonia; however, pneumonia is the sixth leading cause of death in the United States.

 SPECIAL POPULATIONS Adults over age 65 with bacterial pneumonia are at higher risk for death because clinical presentation is often atypical or obscured, and may even be asymptomatic.

Causes

The causes of pneumonia are reflected in the way the disease is classified:
• by microbiological etiology — Pneumonia can be viral, bacterial, fungal, protozoal, mycobacterial, mycoplasmal, or rickettsial in origin.
• by type — Primary pneumonia results from inhalation or aspiration of a pathogen and includes pneumococcal and viral pneumonia. Secondary pneumonia may follow initial lung damage from a noxious chemical or other insult (superinfection), or it may result from hematogenous spread of bacteria from a distant focus (See *Types of pneumonia*, pages 256 to 259.)

• by location — Bronchopneumonia involves distal airways and alveoli; lobular pneumonia, part of a lobe; and lobar pneumonia, an entire lobe.

Predisposing factors

Predisposing factors to bacterial and viral pneumonia include age extremes, chronic illness and debilitation, cancer (particularly lung cancer), abdominal and thoracic surgery, atelectasis, common colds or other viral respiratory infections, chronic respiratory disease (chronic obstructive pulmonary disease [COPD], asthma, bronchiectasis, cystic fibrosis), influenza, smoking, malnutrition, alcoholism, sickle cell disease, tracheostomy, exposure to noxious gases, aspiration, and immunosuppressant therapy.

Predisposing factors to aspiration pneumonia include old age, debilitation, nasogastric tube feedings, impaired gag reflex, poor oral hygiene, and decreased level of consciousness.

Clinical presentation

The patient history may elicit the five cardinal symptoms of early bacterial pneumonia: coughing, sputum production, pleuritic chest pain, rigors, and high fever.

Examination that yields focal dullness on percussion, increased tactile fremitus and transmission of sound, or late inspiratory crackles over the focal dullness suggests pneumonia and requires a chest X-ray or a consultation with a doctor.

Differential diagnosis

Other conditions to consider include pneumothorax, COPD, heart failure, atelectasis, infectious pneumonitis, pulmonary embolus, pulmonary contusion, tuberculosis, and cancer.

Diagnostic tests

• Complete blood count may reveal leukocytosis.
• Chest X-ray showing infiltrates and sputum smear demonstrating acute inflammatory cells support the diagnosis. Chest X-ray may also reveal lobar or segmental consolidation, bronchopneumonia, pleural effusion, or air bronchogram.
• Positive blood cultures in patients with pulmonary infiltrates strongly suggest pneumonia produced by the organisms isolated from the blood cultures.
• Pleural effusions, if present, should be tapped and the fluid analyzed for evidence of infection in the pleural space. Occasionally, a transtracheal aspirate of tracheobronchial secretions or bronchoscopy with brushings or washings may be done to obtain material for smear and culture.
• The patient's response to antimicrobial therapy also provides important evidence of the presence of pneumonia.

Management

Acute

Hospitalization is indicated for children younger than 4 months, for elderly patients, and for those with significant comorbidity or a severe infection.

General

Outpatient treatment involves supportive measures and follow-up to ensure effectiveness of management plan.

Medication

Antimicrobial therapy varies with the causative agent. Besides the clinical picture, it's important to know what types of respiratory infections (influenza or bacterial strains) are currently affecting your local area (com-

(Text continues on page 258.)

TYPES OF PNEUMONIA

Type	Signs and symptoms
Viral	
Influenza (prognosis poor even with treatment; 50% mortality)	• Cough (initially nonproductive; later, purulent sputum), marked cyanosis, dyspnea, high fever, chills, substernal pain and discomfort, moist crackles, frontal headache, myalgia • Death from cardiopulmonary collapse
Adenovirus (insidious onset; generally affects young adults)	• Sore throat, fever, cough, chills, malaise, small amounts of mucoid sputum, retrosternal chest pain, anorexia, rhinitis, adenopathy, scattered crackles, and rhonchi
Respiratory syncytial virus (RSV; most prevalent in infants and children)	• Listlessness, irritability, tachypnea with retraction of intercostal muscles, slight sputum production, fine moist crackles, fever, severe malaise and, possibly, cough or croup
Measles (rubeola)	• Fever, dyspnea, cough, small amounts of sputum, coryza, skin rash, and cervical adenopathy
Chickenpox (varicella; uncommon in children but present in 30% of adults with varicella)	• Cough, dyspnea, cyanosis, tachypnea, pleuritic chest pain, hemoptysis, and rhonchi 1 to 6 days after onset of rash
Cytomegalovirus (CMV)	• Difficult to distinguish from other nonbacterial pneumonias • Fever, cough, shaking chills, dyspnea, cyanosis, weakness, and diffuse crackles • Occurs in neonates as devastating multisystemic infection; in normal adults, resembles mononucleosis; in immunocompromised hosts, varies from clinically inapparent to devastating infection
Bacterial	
Streptococcus (Diplococcus pneumoniae)	• Sudden onset of a single, shaking chill and sustained temperature of 102° to 104° F (38.9° to 40° C), often preceded by upper respiratory tract infection
Klebsiella	• Fever and recurrent chills; cough producing rusty, bloody, viscous sputum (currant jelly); cyanosis of lips and nail beds due to hypoxemia; shallow, grunting respirations • Likely in patients with chronic alcoholism, pulmonary disease, and diabetes

Diagnosis	Treatment
• *Chest X-ray:* diffuse bilateral bronchopneumonia from hilus • *White blood cell (WBC) count:* normal to slightly elevated • *Sputum smears:* no specific organisms	• *Supportive:* for respiratory failure, endotracheal intubation and ventilator assistance; for fever, hypothermia blanket or antipyretics; for influenza A, amantadine or rimantadine
• *Chest X-ray:* patchy distribution of pneumonia, more severe than indicated by physical examination • *WBC count:* normal to slightly elevated	• Symptomatic treatment only. • Mortality low; usually clears with no residual effects
• *Chest X-ray:* patchy bilateral consolidation • *WBC count:* normal to slightly elevated	• *Supportive:* humidified air, oxygen, antimicrobials often given until viral etiology confirmed, aerosolized ribavirin • Complete recovery in 1 to 3 weeks
• *Chest X-ray:* reticular infiltrates, sometimes with hilar lymph node enlargement • *Lung tissue specimen:* characteristic giant cells	• *Supportive:* bed rest, adequate hydration, antimicrobials; assisted ventilation, if necessary
• *Chest X-ray:* shows more extensive pneumonia than indicated by physical examination, and shows bilateral, patchy, diffuse, nodular infiltrates • *Sputum analysis:* predominant mononuclear cells and characteristic intranuclear inclusion bodies with skin rash (confirm diagnosis)	• *Supportive:* adequate hydration, oxygen therapy in critically ill patients • Therapy with I.V. acyclovir
• *Chest X-ray:* in early stages, variable patchy infiltrates; later, bilateral, nodular, and more predominant in lower lobes • *Percutaneous aspiration of lung tissue, transbronchial biopsy, or open lung biopsy:* microscopic examination shows intranuclear and cytoplasmic inclusions; can culture virus from lung tissue	• *Supportive:* adequate hydration and nutrition, oxygen therapy, bed rest • Generally, benign and self-limiting in mononucleosis-like form • In immunosuppressed patients, disease more severe and possibly fatal; ganciclovir or foscarnet treatment warranted
• *Chest X-ray:* areas of consolidation, often lobar • WBC count: elevated • *Sputum culture:* may show gram-positive *Streptococcus pneumoniae*; this organism not always recovered	• *Antimicrobial therapy:* macrolide for 7 to 10 days (Therapy begins after obtaining culture specimen but without waiting for results.)
• *Chest X-ray:* typically, but not always, consolidation in the upper lobe that causes bulging of fissures • *WBC count:* elevated • *Sputum culture and Gram stain:* may show gram-negative cocci *(Klebsiella)*	• *Antimicrobial therapy:* an aminoglycoside and a cephalosporin

(continued)

TYPES OF PNEUMONIA *(continued)*

Type	Signs and symptoms
Bacterial *(continued)*	
Staphylococcus	• Temperature of 102° to 104° F (38.9° to 40° C), recurrent shaking chills, bloody sputum, dyspnea, tachypnea, and hypoxemia • Should be suspected with viral illness, such as influenza and measles, and in patients with cystic fibrosis
Aspiration	
Results from vomiting and aspiration of gastric or oropharyngeal contents into trachea and lungs	• Noncardiogenic pulmonary edema possibly following damage to respiratory epithelium from contact with stomach acid. • Crackles, dyspnea, cyanosis, hypotension, and tachycardia • May be subacute pneumonia with cavity formation; lung abscess possible if foreign body is present

munity biography profile). Therapy should be reevaluated early in the course of treatment for effectiveness.
• Antivirals (amantadine) are most effective if started within 48 hours of symptom onset. For cytomegalovirus or herpes simplex virus, ganciclovir is beneficial; for *Hantavirus* and influenza B virus, ribavirin.
• Antibiotics are ordered empirically then adjusted as culture and sensitivity results indicate. For instance, co-trimoxazole treats *Pneumocystis carinii* pneumonia or *Haemophilus influenzae,* erythromycin treats mycoplasma, and penicillin G treats streptococcal and most aspiration pneumonias.
• Cough suppressants should be used sparingly, at bedtime, as needed for sleep.
• Bronchodilator puffs (albuterol) relieve wheezing.

Referral or consultation
Refer the patient to a doctor for distressed appearance, hemoptysis, history of lung disease or immunocompromise, unresponsiveness, or hospitalization. Refer to an infectious disease specialist as indicated.

Follow-up
Contact the patient by phone within 48 hours; if his condition has improved, see him in 1 week. See him again in 4 to 6 weeks and order a chest X-ray if he smokes, is over age 40, or still has symptoms.

Complications
Reactive airway disease, respiratory distress syndrome, hemolytic anemia, erythema multiforme, pericarditis, myocarditis, arthralgia, hypoxemia, pleural effusion, empyema, and bacteremia are possible complications.

Patient teaching
• Teach the patient that self-care measures can increase comfort, prevent complications, and speed recovery.
• Advise the patient of the importance of increasing fluid intake to at least 2 qt (2 L) per day and of getting adequate rest.
• Teach the patient how to cough and perform deep-breathing exercises to clear secretions, and advise him to do so often.

Diagnosis	Treatment
• *Chest X-ray:* multiple abscesses and infiltrates; high incidence of empyema • *WBC count:* elevated • *Sputum culture and Gram stain:* may show gram-positive staphylococci	• *Antimicrobial therapy:* nafcillin or oxacillin for 14 days if staphylococci are penicillinase producing • Chest tube drainage of empyema
• *Chest X-ray:* locates areas of infiltrates, which suggest diagnosis	• *Antimicrobial therapy:* penicillin G or clindamycin • *Supportive:* oxygen therapy, suctioning, coughing, deep breathing, adequate hydration

• Instruct the patient about precautionary measures — washing hands frequently, not sharing tissues or utensils, and disposing of soiled tissues properly.
• Teach the patient about the drugs ordered and associated adverse effects.
• Instruct the patient how to use a vaporizer or humidifier to thin secretions. If these devices aren't available, encourage a long steamy shower with deep breathing before bedtime.

To prevent pneumonia:
• Advise the patient to avoid using antibiotics indiscriminately during minor viral infections; this may result in upper airway colonization with antibiotic-resistant bacteria. If the patient then develops pneumonia, the organisms producing the pneumonia may require treatment with more toxic antibiotics.
• Encourage annual influenza vaccination, plus *Haemophilus pneumoniae* immunization for patients over age 65 and those with COPD, chronic heart disease, or sickle cell disease. Repeat *H. pneumoniae* immunization as indicated.

ALERT Tell the patient to call the primary care provider to report any new or persistent signs and symptoms, including fever higher than 101° F (38.3° C) and cough producing a change in sputum color (to green, brown, or dark yellow); difficulty eating due to shortness of breath; severe throat pain and difficulty swallowing; earache or sinus pain; increasing shortness of breath and increasing orthopnea (number of pillows elevating head in order to sleep); breathing that becomes rapid or increasingly difficult, or unusual drowsiness.

If the patient fails to respond, his lips become dusky or blue, or his respirations become very irregular (as occurs in Cheyne-Stokes respirations), activate emergency medical services.

Resources
• American Lung Association: 800-LUNG-USA or *www.lungusa.org*
• Patient information on viral pneumonia: *www.medscape.com*

Prostate cancer

ICD-9-CM primary 185, secondary 198.82, in situ 233.4 benign 222.2, uncertain 236.5

Prostate cancer is the second most common neoplasm found in men over age 50. Adenocarcinoma is its most common form; sarcoma occurs only rarely. Most prostatic carcinomas originate in the posterior prostate gland; the rest originate near the urethra. Malignant prostatic tumors seldom result from the benign hyperplastic enlargement that commonly develops around the prostatic urethra in elderly men. Prostate cancer seldom produces symptoms until it's advanced.

Causes

Although androgens regulate prostate growth and function and may also speed tumor growth, no definite link between increased androgen levels and prostate cancer has been found. When primary prostatic lesions metastasize, they typically invade the prostatic capsule and spread along the ejaculatory ducts in the space between the seminal vesicles or perivesicular fascia.

 SPECIAL POPULATIONS Prostate cancer accounts for about 18% of all cancers. Incidence is highest in Blacks and lowest in Asians. Incidence also increases with age far more than any other cancer.

Clinical presentation

Manifestations of prostate cancer appear only in the advanced stages and include difficulty initiating a urinary stream, dribbling, urine retention, unexplained cystitis and, rarely, hematuria. Lymph node metastases can lead to lower extremity lymph-

edema. Skeletal metastases can present as back pain or pathologic fractures. Neurologic involvement may result in epidural compression and cord compression.

Differential diagnosis

Conditions to consider include benign prostatic hypertrophy, prostatitis, bladder cancer, and prostatic calculi.

Diagnostic tests

• A digital rectal examination that reveals a small, hard nodule may help diagnose prostate cancer.
• Biopsy confirms the diagnosis.
• Prostate-specific antigen (PSA) levels will be elevated in most men with prostate cancer, and serum acid phosphatase levels will be elevated in two-thirds of men with metastatic prostate cancer. Therapy aims to return the serum acid phosphatase level to normal; a subsequent rise points to recurrence.
• Magnetic resonance imaging (MRI), computed tomography scan, and excretory urography may also aid the diagnosis. Complete blood count that detects anemia as well as elevated acid phosphatase and alkaline phosphatase and may indicate metastasis. At that point, MRI, bone scan, and transrectal ultrasound are used to detect metastasis.

Management

➡ **ALERT** The urge to void and inability to void for more than 8 hours despite fluid intake is a medical emergency. If left untreated, renal damage can occur.

General

Management of prostate cancer depends on clinical assessment, tolerance of therapy, expected life span, and the stage of the disease. (See *Staging prostate cancer.*) Treatment

STAGING PROSTATE CANCER

The American Joint Committee on Cancer recognizes the TNM (tumor, node, metastasis) cancer staging system for assessing prostatic cancer.

Primary tumor

TX — primary tumor not able to be assessed

T0 — no evidence of primary tumor

T1 — tumor an incidental histologic finding

T1a — three or fewer microscopic foci of cancer

T1b — more than three microscopic foci of cancer

T2 — tumor limited to the prostate gland

T2a — tumor less than 1.5 cm in greatest dimension, with normal tissue on at least three sides

T2b — tumor larger than 1.5 cm in greatest dimension or present in more than one lobe

T3 — unfixed tumor extending into the prostatic apex or into or beyond the prostatic capsule, bladder neck, or seminal vesicle

T4 — tumor fixed or invading adjacent structures not listed in T3

Regional lymph nodes

NX — regional lymph nodes able to be assessed

N0 — no evidence of regional lymph node metastasis

N1 — metastasis in a single lymph node, 2 cm or less in greatest dimension

N2 — metastasis in a single lymph node, between 2 and 5 cm in greatest dimension, or metastasis to several lymph nodes, none more than 5 cm in greatest dimension

N3 — metastasis in a lymph node, more than 5 cm in greatest dimension

Distant metastasis

MX — distant metastasis not able to be assessed

M0 — no known distant metastasis

MI — distant metastasis

Staging categories

Prostate cancer progresses from mild to severe as follows:

Stage 0 or Stage I — T1a, N0, M0; T2a, N0, M0

Stage II — T1b, N0, M0; T21b, N0, M0

Stage III— T3, N0, M0

Stage IV — T4, N0, M0; any T, N1, M0; any T, N2, M0; any T, N3, M0; any T, any N, M1

---

must be chosen carefully because prostate cancer usually affects older men, who commonly have coexisting disorders, such as hypertension, diabetes, and cardiac disease. It's important to discuss with the patient the disease process, prognosis, and advantages and disadvantages of treatment options. It's even more important to support the patient's decisions about the extent of treatment he'll receive.

Therapy varies with each stage of the disease and generally includes radiation, prostatectomy, orchiectomy to reduce androgen production, and hormone therapy with synthetic estrogen (diethylstilbestrol) and antiandrogens, such as cyproterone, megestrol, and flutamide. Radical prostatectomy is usually effective for localized lesions.

Radiation therapy is used to cure some locally invasive lesions and to relieve pain from metastatic bone involvement. A single injection of the radionuclide strontium 89 is also used to treat pain caused by bone metastasis.

If hormone therapy, surgery, and radiation therapy aren't feasible or successful, chemotherapy (using combinations of cyclophosphamide, doxorubicin, fluorouracil, cisplatin, etoposide, and vindesine) may be tried. However, current drug therapy offers little benefit. Combining several treatment methods may be most effective.

Referral or consultation

If PSA levels are elevated or a prostatic mass is found, refer the patient to a urologist and anticipate a transurethral ultrasonogram. After being diagnosed, the patient will be referred to an oncologist for evaluation and treatment.

Follow-up

See the patient quarterly to annually, depending on the clinical picture. Incorporate specialists' recommendations into routine visits. Focus on the patient's response to treatment and changes in urination. Ask about any type of pain in the pubic area or lower abdomen or any unusual bone pain.

 SPECIAL POPULATIONS The American Cancer Society advises a yearly digital examination for men over age 40. For black men starting at age 40 and for all others starting at age 50, a yearly blood test is recommended to detect PSA.

Complications

Complications of prostate cancer include urinary outflow obstruction, metastasis (particularly to bone), and cardiac failure.

Patient teaching

• Explain the expected effects of surgery, such as impotence and incontinence, and of radiation treatments, such as diarrhea, bladder spasms, and urinary frequency.

• Teach the patient to do perineal exercises 1 to 10 times an hour, starting 24 hours after surgery. Have him squeeze his buttocks together, hold this position for a few seconds, and then relax.

After transurethral prostatic resection:
• Check for signs of urethral stricture: dysuria, decreased force and caliber of urinary stream, straining to urinate, and abdominal distention.

After radiation therapy:
• Check for common adverse effects: proctitis, diarrhea, bladder spasms, and urinary frequency. Internal radiation usually results in cystitis in the first 2 to 3 weeks.

• Advise the patient to drink at least 2 qt (2 L) of fluids per day but to avoid alcohol, caffeinated beverages, and decongestants because they can cause spasms and discomfort.

• Order analgesics (such as acetaminophen plus codeine) as needed to relieve pain.

ALERT Tell the patient to call the primary care provider to report any new or persistent signs and symptoms, including signs and symptoms of urinary tract infection (pain or burning on urination, urinary frequency, urinary urgency, blood in urine, cloudy or odorous urine, fever higher than 101° F [38.3° C], drainage from penis), the urge to void and the inability to void for more than 8 hours despite good fluid intake, increased pain in the pubic or lower abdominal area, and difficulty starting a stream of urine, decreased force of the urine stream, or a feeling of incomplete emptying.

Resources
• US TOO International (Prostate Cancer/BPH): 800-808-7866
• American Cancer Society: 800-ACS-2345

• Cancer Information Service: 800-4-CANCER
• Cancer Care: 800-813-HOPE
• Patient information on prostate cancer: *www.medscape.com*
• For patients, caregivers, and professional providers — Association of Cancer Online: *www.acor.org*

Sexually transmitted diseases

*ICD-9-CM (*See *Identifying sexually transmitted diseases,* pages 264 to 269.)

Sexually transmitted disease (STDs) are a group of infections with similar manifestations that aren't linked to a single organism. They cause urethritis in males, vaginitis and cervicitis in females. These primarily sexually transmitted infections have become more prevalent since the mid-1960s.

Gonorrhea and chlamydia are the most common STDs in the United States at this time. Treatment, duration of contagion, and prognosis depend on which organism is involved. The biggest risk is that any patient with one STD is at higher risk for developing another STD, the most serious being the human immunodeficiency virus (HIV).

Causes

STDs are spread primarily through sexual intercourse. The causative organisms are bacterial, viral, and fungal.

Clinical presentation

Signs and symptoms vary depending on the causative organism but typically include mucopurulent urethral discharge, variable dysuria, pruritus, lesions, and occasional hematuria. Subclinical STDs may be found on physical examination, especially if the patient's sexual partner has a positive diagnosis.

Both males and females may be asymptomatic or show signs of urethral, vaginal, or cervical infection on physical examination.

Differential diagnosis

(See *Identifying sexually transmitted diseases*, pages 264 to 269.)

Management

Recommend screening tests for anyone suspected of having an STD. All patients whose symptoms suggest infection require education about STDs and HIV, regardless of test results. Patients are usually more receptive at this time because of the perceived risk.

Patient teaching

• Tell women to clean the pubic area before applying vaginal medications and to avoid using tampons during treatment.
• Make sure the patient understands the dosage schedule for all prescribed medications clearly and follows it strictly.
• Teach him about the incubation, duration, transmission, recurrence, and complications of his specific STD.
• Teach the patient how to prevent genitourinary infections.
To prevent genitourinary infections:
• Tell patients to abstain from sexual contact with infected partners, to use condoms during every sexual encounter and follow appropriate hygienic measures afterward, and to void before and after intercourse. As appropriate, instruct on use of condoms and vaginal dams.

(Text continues on page 268.)

IDENTIFYING SEXUALLY TRANSMITTED DISEASES

Although these diseases are usually transmitted sexually, other forms of transmission are possible. For example, the etiology of bacterial vaginosis isn't completely understood, but sexual transmission is now considered unlikely. The chart below provides a quick overview of diagnosis and treatment of common genital infections.

Disease and ICD-9-CM code	Clinical presentation and time from contact to symptom	Diagnosis
Bacterial vaginosis (616.10)	• White, malodorous, "fishy" discharge; itching; burning on urination; genital redness • time frame not applicable	Examination, culture, wet mount preparation: Clue cells, "fishy" odor produced by a drop of potassium hydroxide
Chlamydia (vaginitis 099.53; urethritis 099.41); also known as nongonococcal urethritis	• Thin, clear, malodorous discharge; postcoital bleeding; dyspareunia; or patient possibly asymptomatic. • Varies (1 to 3 weeks)	Examination; deoxyribonucleic acid (DNA) assay probe to check for gonorrhea and chlamydia
Gonorrhea (098.0; in eye 098.40)	• Yellowish-green genital discharge; burning on urination; occasionally asymptomatic in men; frequently asymptomatic in women; partner possibly diagnosed first • 2 to 10 (up to 30) days	Examination; DNA probe assay to check for gonorrhea and chlamydia; possibly endocervical, conjunctival, rectal, or oral culture
Herpes simplex (054.10)	• Swollen, tender, painful blisters on genitals or lips • Up to 2 weeks	Papanicolaou (Pap) test, examination, herpes culture
Human immunodeficiency virus (HIV) infection or acquired immunodeficiency syndrome (042)	• Purplish discolorations on skin, unexplained weight loss, persistent cough, anorexia, fever, fatigue • 2 years or more	Tests for cancer and superinfection, as indicated by examination

Cause and treatment	Complications	Follow-up and referral
• Bacteria or chemical irritation; curable • *Orally:* metronidazole 500 mg b.i.d. for 7 days or 750 mg for 7 days *Intravaginally:* metronidazole gel, 1 applicator h.s. for 5 days or clindamycin 2%, 1 applicator h.s. for 5 days (may use during pregnancy)	Not known	• If condition recurs, consider need to treat sexual partners.
• Mycoplasma; curable • *Orally:* azithromycin 1 g in a single dose (best treatment for pregnant women); doxycycline 100 mg b.i.d. for 7days	Pelvic inflammatory disease (PID), sterility, tubal pregnancy, scar tissue, possible eye infections or pneumonia in newborns	• Follow up in 2 to 4 weeks for test of cure to determine antibody resistance or reinfection. • Ensure that partners are treated.
• Bacterium; curable • Same treatment as for Chlamydia • *Alternative:* P.O. spectinomycin 2 g in a single dose • *Disseminated infection:* ceftriaxone 1g I.M. or I.V. q 24 hr until 2nd day after improvement begins, then P.O. cefixime or ciprofloxacin for total of 7 days of therapy	PID, ectopic pregnancy, sterility, arthritis, blindness, eye infection in newborns	• Follow up in 2 to 4 weeks for test of cure to check for reinfection. • Ensure that partners are treated. • Report to local health authority; if a child, report to child abuse authorities.
• Virus; no cure • *Supportive:* intermittent, cool, moist dressings with Burow's solution	Strong association with cervical cancer; severe central nervous system damage or death in infants infected during birth	• Follow up for recurrences and annual Pap test.
• Virus; no cure • Supportive and antiviral	Severe medical and psychiatric problems; death	• Refer to a psychotherapist for counseling and to an HIV specialist.

(continued)

IDENTIFYING SEXUALLY TRANSMITTED DISEASES
(continued)

Disease and ICD-9-CM code	Clinical presentation and time from contact to symptoms	Diagnosis
Pediculosis pubis (132.2; infestation 132.9)	• Intense itching, pinhead blood spots on underwear; small eggs or nits (white, light gray, or honey-colored ovals on hair shaft) • 3 to 14 days	Examination
Scabies (133.0)	• Severe nocturnal itching; raised lines in skin where mite burrows; may infest elbows, hands, web spaces, breasts, buttocks, and genitalia • 4 to 6 weeks	Examination, fountain-pen ink applied to infested skin concentrates in grooves under the skin, easing identification of burrows
Syphilis (090.0-097.9)	• First stage: painless lesions of long duration on genitalia, fingers, lips, and breasts that resolve without treatment; second stage: rash, fever, flu-like symptoms; latent stage: asymptomatic • 10 to 90 days; average 21 days	Examination, rapid plasma reagin (RPR) positive, fluorescent treponemal antibody (FTA) positive
Trichomoniasis (131.9)	• Green, frothy, malodorous discharge; intense itching, burning, and redness of genitalia and thighs; dyspareunia; men usually asymptomatic • Varies (1 to 4 weeks)	Pap test, examination, urinalysis, wet mount preparation: trichomonads present (motile with flagella)
Venereal warts (*Condylomata acuminata*) (078.19)	• Local irritation, itching, pink or red cauliflower-like lesions; can look like ordinary warts • Varies (1 to 8 months, average 2 months)	Pap test, examination, application of acetic acid (5% vinegar) to area, which will turn bluish-white. (Scrapings of area turn white with acetic acid application.)

Cause and treatment	Complications	Follow-up and referral
• Louse; curable • *Topical:* permethrin, pyrethrins, lindane (follow directions on bottle); wash and dry all cloth on hot settings; if unable to wash items, dry-clean or seal in plastic bag for 2 weeks; 1:1 vinegar to water solution in hair every 15 minutes to ease nit removal	Secondary infection from scratching	• Follow up if unresponsive or symptoms recur. • Ensure that partners are treated.
• Itch mite; curable • *Topical:* lindane, permethrin (follow directions on bottle); itching may continue up to 14 days after successful treatment due to allergic reaction to mite and excrement; same clothing and bedding measures as for lice except no need to dry-clean and only 1 week sealed in bag	Secondary infection from scratching	• Follow up in 2 weeks to verify resolution. • Ensure that partners are treated.
• Spirochete; curable until stage 3 (latent) • Benzathine penicillin G 2.4 million U I.M. for primary, secondary, or latent < 1 year; if latent > 1 year or if unknown, benzathine penicillin G 2.4 million U I.M. weekly for 3 weeks; see Centers for Disease Control and Prevention guidelines for options	Brain damage, insanity, paralysis, heart disease, death; damage to skin, bones, eyes, liver, and teeth of fetus and newborns	• Venereal Disease Research Laboratory test at 3, 6, 12, and 24 months to detect relapse; if latent, test every 6 months for 2 years. • Report to local health authority.
• Protozoa; curable • Same treatment as for bacterial vaginosis • *Alternative:* P.O. metronidazole 2 g in a single dose (for compliance)	Gland infections in females; prostatitis	• Follow up in 2 weeks. • Ensure that partners are treated.
• Virus; no cure • 85% trichloracetic acid applied to lesions by primary care provider, repeated weekly until resolved • Podofilox 0.5% cream (Condylox) applied to warts b.i.d. for 3 days, rest 4 days, then repeated for 4 cycles (may be used in pregnancy) • If warts > 1", referral for laser treatment, cryosurgery, or electrocautery	Highly contagious; if large enough, possible blockage of vaginal opening (90% of women with cervical cancer have evidence of venereal warts.)	• Follow up every 2 weeks until no visible warts; annual Pap test.

(continued)

IDENTIFYING SEXUALLY TRANSMITTED DISEASES (continued)		
Disease and ICD-9-CM code	**Clinical presentation/ Time from contact to symptoms**	**Diagnosis**
Vulvovaginal candidiasis (112.1)	• Severe vaginal itching, vulvar inflammation, cheesy discharge, yeastlike odor (like raw bread dough) • Varies	Examination, culture, wet mount preparation

• Encourage patients to maintain adequate fluid intake.

• Advise women to avoid routinely using douches and feminine hygiene sprays, wearing tight-fitting pants and panty hose, and inserting foreign objects into the vagina.

• Suggest that women wear cotton underpants and remove them before going to bed.

Resources

• National STD Hotline: 800-227-8922.

• Planned Parenthood: *www. plannedparenthood.org* (includes section for teen issues); for Spanish-speaking patients: *www. plannedparenthood.org/ESPANOL/ INDEX.html*

• Patient information on sexual assault: *www.cs.utk.edu/~bartley/ saInfoPage.html*

Sinusitis

ICD-9-CM 473.9, with influenza 487.1, acute 461.9, allergic 477.9

Inflammation of the paranasal sinuses may be acute, chronic, allergic, or hyperplastic. Acute sinusitis usually results from the common cold and lingers in only about 10% of patients.

Chronic sinusitis follows persistent bacterial infection; allergic sinusitis accompanies allergic rhinitis; hyperplastic sinusitis is a combination of purulent acute sinusitis and allergic sinusitis or rhinitis. The prognosis is good for all types.

Causes

Sinusitis usually results from viral or bacterial infection. The bacteria responsible for acute sinusitis are usually pneumococci, other streptococci, *Haemophilus influenzae,* and *Moraxella catarrhalis.* Staphylococci and gram-negative bacteria are more likely to occur in chronic cases or in patients in intensive care.

On rare occasions, fungi can also be an etiologic factor. *Aspergillus fumigatus* is the fungus most frequently associated with sinus disease.

Predisposing factors include any condition that interferes with drainage and ventilation of the sinuses, such as chronic nasal edema, deviated septum, viscous mucus, nasal polyps, allergic rhinitis, nasal intubation, nasogastric tubes, and debilitation related to chemotherapy, malnutrition, diabetes, blood dyscrasias, chronic use of steroids, or immunodeficiency.

Cause and treatment	Complications	Follow-up and referral
• Fungus; curable • *Intravaginally:* 2% miconazole cream 5 g h.s. for 7 days, terconazole 4% cream for 7 days, 8% cream 5 g for 3 days • *Orally:* fluconazole 150 mg in a single dose, then repeated in 3 days	None known	• For recurrent infections, consider HIV and diabetes mellitus testing.

Bacterial invasion commonly occurs from the conditions listed above or after a viral infection. It may also result from swimming in contaminated water.

Clinical presentation

Signs and symptoms vary with sinusitis type. In acute sinusitis, the primary symptom is nasal congestion, followed by a gradual buildup of pressure in the affected sinus. For 24 to 48 hours after onset, nasal discharge may be present and later may become purulent. Associated symptoms include malaise, sore throat, headache, low-grade fever (temperature of 99° to 99.5° F [37.2° to 37.5° C]), malodorous breath, painless morning periorbital swelling, and a sense of facial fullness.

Characteristic pain depends on the affected sinus: maxillary sinusitis causes pain over the cheeks and upper teeth; ethmoid sinusitis, pain over the eyes; frontal sinusitis, pain over the eyebrows; and sphenoid sinusitis (rare), pain behind the eyes.

Purulent nasal drainage that continues for longer than 3 weeks after an acute infection subsides suggests lingering acute sinusitis. Other clinical features include a stuffy nose, vague facial discomfort, fatigue, and a nonproductive cough.

Other forms of sinusitis tend to be chronic, with symptoms similar to those of acute sinusitis, but with a continuous mucopurulent discharge. The effects of *allergic* sinusitis are predominantly those of allergic rhinitis — sneezing, frontal headache, watery nasal discharge, and a stuffy, burning, itchy nose. However, in *hyperplastic* sinusitis, bacterial growth on the diseased tissue causes pronounced tissue edema. This thickening of the mucosal lining and the development of mucosal polyps, combine to produce chronic stuffiness of the nose as well as headaches.

Differential diagnosis

Other conditions to consider are rhinitis, tumors, cysts, foreign bodies (particularly in children), and Wegener's granulomatosis. The following measures are useful:
• Nasal examination reveals inflammation and pus, which indicate sinusitis.
• Sinus X-rays reveal cloudiness in the affected sinus, air and fluid, and any thickening of the mucosal lining.
• Antral puncture promotes drainage of purulent material but is rarely

done. It may also be used to provide a specimen for culture and sensitivity testing of the infecting organism.

• Ultrasonography and computed tomography (CT) scan aid in diagnosing suspected complications. CT scans are more sensitive than routine X-rays in detecting sinusitis.

Management

For acute sinusitis, local decongestants usually are tried before systemic decongestants; steam inhalation may also be helpful. Local application of heat may help to relieve pain and congestion.

Treatment of allergic sinusitis may include identification of allergens by skin testing and desensitization by immunotherapy. If irrigation fails to relieve symptoms, one or more sinuses may require surgery.

Medication

Antibiotics are necessary to combat purulent or persistent infection resulting from acute sinusitis. Amoxicillin, ampicillin, and amoxicillin-clavulanate potassium are the drugs of choice. Because sinusitis is a deep infection, antibiotics should be given for 2 to 3 weeks. Analgesics (ibuprofen, acetaminophen) and antihistamines (diphenhydramine) are given as needed.

In chronic and hyperplastic sinusitis, antihistamines (loratidine), antibiotics (guided by culture and sensitivity tests), and a steroid nasal spray (triamcinolone) may relieve pain and congestion. Severe allergic symptoms may require treatment with corticosteroids (cortisone) and bronchodilators (epinephrine).

Referral or consultation

Refer the patient to an otolaryngologist or another doctor for a condition that is chronic, complex, or unresponsive after 3 weeks; refer him to a surgeon if necessary.

Follow-up

See the patient in 2 to 3 days to evaluate the effectiveness of treatment, and again in 2 weeks.

Complications

Osteomyelitis, orbital or facial cellulitis, or central nervous system complications may occur.

Patient teaching

• Encourage the patient to rest and to drink plenty of fluids to promote drainage. The patient should place an extra pillow under the head and shoulders or place bricks or books under the head of the bed to promote drainage.

• Teach the patient to relieve pain and promote drainage by applying warm compresses.

• Urge the patient to finish the prescribed antibiotics, even if his symptoms disappear.

• Warn that vasoconstrictive nose drops and spray are associated with rebound edema if used for more than 5 to 7 days.

 ALERT Tell the patient to call the primary care provider to report any new or persistent signs and symptoms, including vomiting, chills, fever, edema of the forehead or eyelids, blurred or double vision, and personality changes.

Tuberculosis

ICD-9-CM 011.9

An acute or chronic infection caused by *Mycobacterium tuberculosis,* tuberculosis (TB) is characterized by pulmonary infiltrates, formation of granulomas with caseation, fibrosis, and cavitation. People who live in crowded, poorly ventilated conditions are most likely to become infected with TB.

In patients with strains that are sensitive to the usual antitubercular agents, the prognosis is excellent with correct treatment. However, in patients infected with drug-resistant strains, mortality is 50%.

 SPECIAL POPULATIONS In the United States, more than 66% of reported TB cases are among nonwhite persons.

Causes

After exposure to *M. tuberculosis,* roughly 5% of infected people develop active TB within 1 year; in the remainder, bacilli cause a latent infection. The host's immune system usually controls the tubercle bacillus by killing it or walling it up in a tiny nodule (tubercle). However, the bacillus may lie dormant within the tubercle for years and later reactivate and spread.

TB is transmitted by droplet nuclei produced when infected persons cough or sneeze. After inhalation, if a tubercle bacillus settles in an alveolus, infection occurs. Cell-mediated immunity to the mycobacteria, which develops about 3 to 6 weeks later, usually contains the infection and arrests the disease.

Although mycobacteria primarily infect the lungs, they commonly exist in other parts of the body. A number of factors increase the risk of infection reactivation: gastrectomy, uncontrolled diabetes mellitus, Hodgkin's disease, leukemia, silicosis, acquired immunodeficiency syndrome, and treatment with corticosteroids or immunosuppressants.

If the infection becomes reactivated, the body's response characteristically leads to caseation—the conversion of necrotic tissue to a cheese-like material. The caseum may localize, undergo fibrosis, or excavate and form cavities, the walls of which are studded with multiplying tubercle bacilli. If this happens, infected caseous debris may spread throughout the lungs by the tracheobronchial tree.

Sites of extrapulmonary TB include the pleura, meninges, joints, lymph nodes, peritoneum, genitourinary tract, and bowel.

Clinical presentation

In primary infection, after an incubation period of 4 to 8 weeks, TB is usually asymptomatic but may produce nonspecific symptoms, such as fatigue, weakness, anorexia, weight loss, night sweats, and low-grade fever. The patient history should also elicit TB exposure, previous TB, other chronic diseases, and immunocompromised status. In TB reactivation, symptoms may include a cough that produces mucopurulent sputum, occasional hemoptysis, and pleuritic chest pains.

On examination, auscultation detects crepitant crackles, bronchial breath sounds, wheezes, and whispered pectoriloquy (sound transmission through the chest wall). Chest percussion detects a dullness over the affected area, indicating consolidation or pleural fluid.

Differential diagnosis

Conditions to consider include malignant tumors and pulmonary infections, such as pneumoconiosis, pneumonia, lung abscess, and fungal infection. In some situations, with an initial negative reaction, the tuberculin skin test may be repeated. In this two-step test, the first injection shows no response but sensitizes persons with decreased immune systems;

the second injection elicits a visible response.

Diagnostic tests
• Chest X-ray shows nodular lesions, patchy infiltrates (mainly in upper lobes), cavity formation, scar tissue, and calcium deposits; however, it may not be able to distinguish active TB from inactive TB.
• Tuberculin skin test detects TB infection. Intermediate-strength purified protein derivative or 5 tuberculin units (0.1 ml) are injected intracutaneously on the forearm. The test results are read in 48 to 72 hours; a positive reaction (induration of 5 to 15 mm or more, depending on risk factors) develops 2 to 10 weeks after infection in both active and inactive TB. However, severely immunosuppressed patients may never develop a positive reaction.
• Stains and cultures (of sputum, cerebrospinal fluid, urine, drainage from abscess, or pleural fluid) show heat-sensitive, nonmotile, aerobic, acid-fast bacilli.

Management

General
All cases of newly diagnosed TB must be reported to the local health authority. Before initiating drug treatment, obtain baseline laboratory values: liver function studies, bilirubin, serum creatinine, complete blood count, platelet count, serum uric acid (if the patient is to receive pyrazinamide), and visual acuity plus red-green color perception (if the patient is to receive ethambutol).

Medication
• Daily oral doses of isoniazid, rifampin, and pyrazinamide (and sometimes ethambutol or streptomycin) for at least 6 months usually cures TB. After 2 to 4 weeks, the disease generally is no longer infectious.

The patient can resume his normal lifestyle while taking the drugs.
• Because isoniazid sometimes leads to hepatitis or peripheral neuritis, monitor closely. To prevent or treat peripheral neuritis, give pyridoxine (vitamin B_6).
• Patients with atypical mycobacterial disease or drug-resistant TB may require treatment with second-line drugs, such as capreomycin, streptomycin, para-aminosalicylic acid, cycloserine, amikacin, and quinolones.

Referral or consultation
Refer the patient to a doctor specializing in TB if treatment has failed after 3 months.

Follow-up
For patients who need direct observation therapy, follow-up is two to three times weekly by office staff or home visit, every 2 weeks for the next two visits, then monthly for two visits, and finally monthly for the remainder of treatment. Focus on compliance, toxicity and adverse effects of drugs, plus a monthly chest X-ray.

For patients taking ethambutol, watch for optic neuritis; if it develops, discontinue the drug. If the patient takes rifampin, watch for hepatitis and purpura. Because isoniazid sometimes leads to hepatitis or peripheral neuritis, monitor aspartate aminotransferase and alanine aminotransferase levels monthly; if levels exceed three times normal, consider changing the drug.

After 3 months of treatment and at the conclusion of therapy, repeat the chest X-ray, acid-fast smear, and culture.

Complications

Complications of TB include secondary bacterial infection of cavitary lesions, metastasis, and drug resistance.

Patient teaching

• Teach the patient to cough and sneeze into tissues and to dispose of all secretions properly.
• Remind the patient to get plenty of rest and to eat balanced meals. If the patient is anorectic, urge him to eat small meals throughout the day. Record weight weekly.
• Advise him of drug adverse effects.
• Emphasize the importance of regular follow-up examinations, and instruct the patient and his family concerning the signs and symptoms of recurring TB.
• Advise persons who have been exposed to infected patients to receive tuberculin tests and, if necessary, chest X-rays and prophylactic isoniazid.

 ALERT Tell the patient to call the primary care provider to report any persistent, changing, worsening, anxiety-producing, or specific signs and symptoms, including signs of secondary infection or drug intolerance (fever, malaise, anorexia, nausea, yellowed skin) or starting to cough up blood.

Resources

• American Lung Association: 800-LUNG-USA
• For providers — Drug affordability: *www.needymeds.com* (contains information regarding many drug company programs that provide financial assistance to those who need their drugs)

Urinary tract infection

ICD-9-CM urinary infection 599.0 (may request organism specific code), cystitis 595

Cystitis and urethritis, the two forms of lower urinary tract infection (UTI), are nearly 10 times more common in women than in men and affect approximately 10% to 20% of all women at least once. Lower UTI is also a prevalent bacterial disease in children, with girls also more commonly affected.

In men and children, lower UTIs are frequently related to anatomic or physiologic abnormalities and therefore require extremely close evaluation. UTIs often respond readily to treatment, but recurrence and resistant bacterial flare-up during therapy are possible. (See *Treating and preventing urinary tract infections*, page 274.)

Causes

Most UTIs result from ascending infection by a single gram-negative enteric bacteria, such as *Escherichia coli, Klebsiella, Proteus, Enterobacter, Pseudomonas,* or *Serratia*. In a patient with neurogenic bladder, an indwelling urinary catheter, or a fistula between the intestine and bladder, UTI may result from simultaneous infection with multiple pathogens. An anatomic or functional abnormality may predispose the patient to infection.

Recent studies suggest that infection results from a breakdown in local defense mechanisms in the bladder that allow bacteria to invade the bladder mucosa and multiply. These bacteria can't be readily eliminated by normal micturition.

Bacterial flare-up

During treatment, bacterial flare-up is generally caused by the pathogenic organism's resistance to the prescribed antimicrobial therapy. The presence of even a small number (less than 10,000/ml) of bacteria in a midstream urine sample obtained during treatment casts doubt on the effectiveness of treatment.

TREATING AND PREVENTING URINARY TRACT INFECTIONS

Teach the female patient how to clean the perineum properly and keep the labia separated during voiding to collect a clean, midstream urine specimen. Explain that a noncontaminated midstream specimen is essential for accurate diagnosis.

Treatment
• Explain the nature and purpose of antimicrobial therapy. Emphasize the importance of completing the prescribed course of therapy or, with long-term prophylaxis, of adhering strictly to ordered dosage.
• Recommend taking nitrofurantoin macrocrystals with milk or a meal to prevent GI distress. If therapy includes phenazopyridine, warn the patient that this drug may turn urine red-orange.
• Urge the patient to drink at least eight glasses of water a day. Stress the need to maintain a consistent daily fluid intake of about 2 qt (2 L). More or less than this amount may alter the effect of the prescribed antimicrobial.
• Tell the patient that fruit juices, especially cranberry juice, and oral doses of vitamin C may help acidify the urine and enhance the action of the medication.
• Suggest warm sitz baths for relief of perineal discomfort.

Prevention
To prevent recurrent infections in men, urge prompt treatment of predisposing conditions such as chronic prostatitis.

To prevent recurrent infections in women, teach the patient to:
• wipe the perineum carefully from front to back and to clean it thoroughly with soap and water after defecation
• void immediately after sexual intercourse, drink plenty of fluids routinely, and avoid postponing urination. Recommend frequent comfort stops during long car trips, and stress the need to empty the bladder completely.

Recurrent UTI
In 99% of patients, recurrent UTI results from reinfection by the same organism or from some new pathogen; in the remaining 1%, recurrence reflects persistent infection, usually from renal calculi, chronic bacterial prostatitis, or a structural anomaly that may become a source of infection.

 SPECIAL POPULATIONS The high incidence of UTI among women may result from the shortness of the female urethra (1.5″ to 2″ [3 to 5 cm]), which predisposes women to infection caused by bacteria from the vagina, perineum, rectum, or a sexual partner.

Men are less vulnerable to UTIs because their urethras are longer (7¾″ [19.7 cm]) and their prostatic fluid serves as an antibacterial shield.

Clinical presentation

UTIs usually produce urgency, frequency, dysuria, spasms of the bladder, itching, burning on urination, hematuria, sensation of incomplete bladder emptying, and fever. The urine may be dark, cloudy, and malodorous. Other symptoms include low back pain, malaise, nausea, vomiting, abdominal pain or tenderness over the bladder area, costovertebral angle tenderness, rigors, and flank pain.

The history may elicit chronic predisposing diseases (such as diabetes mellitus, multiple sclerosis, frequent UTIs, and immunocompromise), structural anomalies, methods of birth control and last menstrual period, constitutional symptoms (fever, rigor), and (in mature men) symptoms of prostatic hypertrophy.

Differential diagnosis

Conditions to consider include vaginitis, hematuria from noninfectious causes, and urethritis or pyuria secondary to sexually-transmitted disease.

 ALERT A history of gradual onset, intermittent symptoms, dysuria as urine passes over the labia (suggests candida or herpes simplex), penile discharge, vaginal discharge with bleeding, or lower abdominal pain requires aggressive evaluation to rule out an STD. A finding of pyuria without significant bacteriuria also suggests an STD.

Diagnostic tests

• A clean midstream urine specimen revealing a bacterial count of more than 100,000/ml (pyuria) confirms the diagnosis. Lower counts don't necessarily rule out infection, especially if the patient is voiding frequently, because bacteria require 30 to 45 minutes to reproduce in urine.
• Culture and sensitivity testing determines the appropriate therapeutic antimicrobial agent. Suspect specimen contamination when multiple types of bacteria are detected. Consider urethral catheterization.
• Voiding cystoureterography or excretory urography may detect congenital anomalies that predispose the patient to recurrent UTIs.
• If the patient history and physical examination warrant, a blood test and stained smear of the discharge rules out a sexually transmitted disease (such as gonorrhea, chlamydia, syphilis, and human immunodeficiency virus).

Management

General

Encourage the patient to drink plenty of fluids (2 qt [2 L] per day).

Medication

• Antimicrobials (co-trimoxazole, fluoroquinolone) are the treatment of choice for most initial UTIs. For uncomplicated, infrequent UTIs, a 3-day antibiotic regimen is prescribed. All others receive a 10- to 14-day regimen and follow-up urine cultures for test of cure.
• If the urine isn't sterile, bacterial resistance has probably occurred, requiring change to a different antimicrobial. Recurrent infections due to infected renal calculi, chronic prostatitis, or structural abnormality may necessitate surgery; prostatitis also requires long-term antibiotic therapy. In patients without these predisposing conditions, long-term, low-dosage antibiotic therapy is the treatment of choice.

Referral or consultation

Make a referral to a physician or urologist for conditions that are nonresponsive within 3 days of treatment with a bacteria-sensitive antibiotic, for frequent recurrences, for suspected anatomic abnormality, for diabetes, for a history of nephrolithiasis, or if follow-up culture detects the same pathogen.

Follow-up

See the patient in 1 to 2 weeks. Perform a urine culture at this time to verify that the infection has been eradicated.

Complications

Pyelonephritis, cystitis, or renal abscess may occur.

Patient teaching

• Tell the patient to watch for GI disturbances from antimicrobial therapy, and to take drugs on an empty stomach with 8 oz (236 ml) water if possible.

• Explain that forcing fluids flushes bacteria out and cranberry juice changes pH of urine so bacteria can't survive.

• Instruct the patient to avoid alcohol, caffeine, and cold medications with decongestants because they can cause bladder spasms.

• Teach women to decrease the risk of infection by wiping from front to back after urination and by choosing a form of contraception other than a diaphragm.

• Tell the patient not to go long periods without voiding.

• Explain that voiding immediately postcoitally flushes bacteria out. If STD is suspected, instruct the female patient to avoid intercourse.

• Teach comfort measures, such as taking a sitz bath, pouring warm water over the meatus during urination, washing with mild soap and water, not rubbing or scrubbing the area, and patting it dry.

ALERT Tell the patient to call the primary care provider to report any new or persistent signs and symptoms, including symptoms that aren't mostly resolved within 48 hours, or high fever, chills, flank pain, inability to urinate for more than 8 hours despite the urge to void, increased pain in the pubic area or lower abdomen, and abnormal vaginal discharge.

Resources

• Patient information on urinary tract infections: *www.medscape. com*

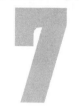

Emergency care

Responding swiftly and accurately

Common types of trauma

The best way to deal with emergencies is to prevent them. To accomplish this, you must have full knowledge of your patient's health history, be mindful of physical and behavioral changes that foretell an emergency, and know the appropriate steps to take at any turn. This chapter details history questions to identify patient risk, precautions to avoid an emergency, signs and symptoms to guide diagnosis, and appropriate responses for situations requiring quick action. Finally, it provides patient teaching regarding when to contact a primary care provider or activate the emergency medical services. If an emergency does occur, this serves as a guide to ensure a response that is quick, competent, and ensures appropriate follow-up care.

Anaphylaxis

ICD-9-CM due to: food 995.60, immunization 999.4, overdose or wrong substance given/taken 977.9

Anaphylaxis is an acute, life-threatening allergic reaction to a sensitizing substance. When severe, it may trigger vascular collapse, leading to systemic shock and possibly death.

Severe anaphylaxis causes physical distress, such as hives and respiratory distress, within seconds or minutes after exposure to the sensitizing substance. The sooner the reaction starts, the more severe it will be; death from vascular collapse and shock may occur within minutes or hours. A delayed or persistent reaction can occur for up to 24 hours after exposure to an allergen. (See *How anaphylaxis occurs.*)

Sometimes anaphylaxis takes a milder form, causing only hives or a rash, or an intermediate form marked by a fever and swollen glands.

Causes

Anaphylaxis results from ingestion or other systemic exposure to a substance that activates a hypersensitive immunoglobulin E or M response. Drugs that can trigger anaphylaxis include:
- anesthetics (cocaine, lidocaine, procaine, thiopental)
- antibiotics (most notably penicillin)
- sulfonamides
- local anesthetics
- serums (usually horse serum)
- blood and blood products
- vaccines
- hormones
- narcotic analgesics (morphine, codeine, meprobamate)
- nonsteroidal anti-inflammatory drugs (salicylates, indomethacin).

Other sensitizing substances may include diagnostic chemicals, such as sulfobromophthalein and radiographic contrast media; foods, such as nuts, legumes, berries, seafood, and egg albumin; sulfite-containing food additives, as in wines; pollens; and venoms from insects (bees, wasps, hornets, and yellow jackets), spiders, snakes, and jellyfish.

Clinical presentation

The history may reveal feelings of weakness, fright, or impending doom; frequent sneezing; and an itchy, runny, or stuffy nose. The patient may also complain of dizziness or light-headedness, severe stomach cramps, nausea, diarrhea, urgent urination, or loss of bladder control.

Examination findings include hives, wheezing, diaphoresis, pruritic skin rash, and swelling (especially of

HOW ANAPHYLAXIS OCCURS

An anaphylactic reaction occurs only in a person who has been previously exposed, or sensitized, to a drug or other substance, called an antigen. The initial exposure leads to the production of specific immunoglobulin E (IgE) antibodies by plasma cells. IgE antibodies then bind to membrane receptors on mast cells.

The next time the person is exposed to the antigen, an antigen-antibody immune reaction may occur. The antigen binds to adjacent IgE antibodies or cross-linked IgE receptors, activating a series of cellular reactions that trigger degranulation (release of powerful chemical mediators from mast cell stores). Two other types of chemical mediators, bradykinin and leukotrienes, impair the circulatory system and drastically lower the blood pressure. Death may follow quickly.

---

the face, neck, lips, throat, hands, and feet). Some patients develop arrhythmias, hypotension, and shock.

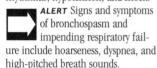 **ALERT** Signs and symptoms of bronchospasm and impending respiratory failure include hoarseness, dyspnea, and high-pitched breath sounds.

Management

The first priority is to remove the underlying cause, if possible; subsequent priorities are to ensure adequate oxygenation, correct metabolic abnormalities, and support hemodynamic functions.

Immediate actions

Get emergency assistance immediately if a patient experiences signs or symptoms of anaphylaxis moments after taking a drug, eating, or being bitten or stung by an insect. Then check his airway, breathing, and circulation. If pulse and breathing are absent, start cardiopulmonary resuscitation (CPR).

If the patient doesn't require CPR, administer epinephrine (Adrenalin) as needed.

Keep the patient quiet. If possible, help him to an upright position to ease breathing. If he becomes dizzy, faints, or experiences nausea, have him lie down with his feet slightly elevated. Watch for signs and symptoms of throat swelling and respiratory distress. If these occur, an artificial airway and supplemental oxygen should be considered.

Pharmacologic treatment options include epinephrine subcutaneously, I.V., or I.V. drip; diphenhydramine I.V.; albuterol aerosol in saline solution; methylprednisolone I.V.; and cimetidine I.V.

Later actions

If the patient is conscious and has normal blood pressure, give epinnephrine I.M. or S.C. immediately to reduce airway edema; repeat every 5 to 20 minutes, as needed. Additional therapy depends on how the patient responds to initial treatment. When the acute phase of the emergency passes, consider using longer-acting steroids (prednisolone P.O.) and antihistamines (diphenhydramine) to ease breathing, or aminophylline (Aminophyllin) to treat bronchospasm.

If anaphylaxis is related to medication, consider stopping the drug, reducing the drug dosage, or stopping the drug and substituting another drug.

Follow up within 2 days. Consider providing an emergency anaphylaxis kit, such as EpiPen or Ana-Kit, as well as medical identification jewelry.

Referral or consultation

 COLLABORATION A patient in shock requires emergency medical transport to an emergency department.

Patient teaching

 ALERT Tell the patient to call the primary care provider to report appearance of a rash after beginning a new medication (before taking another dose).

 ALERT Tell the patient to call emergency medical services for severe difficulty breathing (including rapid onset of progressive wheezing or stridor), facial swelling, severe mental status change, or a loss of consciousness.

Burns

ICD-9-CM (for first, second, and third degree, add .1, .2, .3 suffix to site code): arm 943, back 942.04, cornea 940.4, digits 944.03, face 941, leg 945, external genitalia 942.05, tongue 947

A burn is an injury to tissues caused by a chemical, gas, electricity, abrasion, or heat. Most burns occur in the home and the workplace. Usually these are minor and can be treated on an outpatient basis.

Causes

Chemical burns occur when a caustic or corrosive substance comes in contact with the skin. Typically, these burns result from touching, eating, inhaling, or injecting an acid such as battery acid, an alkali such as lye, or a vesicant (blistering agent). Alkali burns are more serious than acid burns because alkalis (producing liquefaction necrosis) penetrate deeper into the skin and burn longer than acids (which produce coagulation necrosis).

Inhalation burns come from inhaling smoke (gases) or certain chemicals—especially in an enclosed space.

Electrical burns arise from contact with electric current, such as from touching faulty electrical wiring or a high-voltage power line or being struck by lightning. Even a relatively low current can be fatal. (See *What happens in electrical burns,* page 282.)

Thermal burns, the most common type of burn, commonly result from fires, motor vehicle accidents, playing with matches, improperly stored gasoline, space heater mishaps, handling explosives or firecrackers, and scalding accidents.

Clinical presentation

Signs and symptoms vary with the type of burn. History reveals when the burn happened, the location of contact (arms, lungs by inhalation), characteristics of the agent (name, concentration, quantity, mechanism of action [acid, alkali]), what therapeutic action was taken, and if the burn was an intentional act.

External chemical burns

External chemical burns may turn the skin red or discolored, raw, white, soft, or mushy. The patient may report severe pain and general weakness, although he'll feel no pain at all if the burn has completely destroyed nerve endings. Dyspnea or loss of consciousness may also occur.

Inhalation burns

For inhalation burns, the history may reveal light-headedness, nausea, chest pain, dyspnea, loss of consciousness, and a burning sensation of the eyes or mouth. Examination may detect facial burns and laryngeal edema.

Electrical burns

For electrical burns, the history may reveal severe pain or no pain at either the entrance or exit burn.

Examination may reveal rapid, shallow breathing or absence of breathing; rapid, irregular, or absent pulse; extensive skin injuries; damage to bones, joints, and tendons; spinal injuries; paralysis; seizures; sluggishness; stupor; loss of consciousness; and loss of hearing (50% will have ruptured tympanic membrane).

An electrical burn can damage the nervous system, the cardiovascular system, and the kidneys. It may lead to seizures, coma, respiratory arrest, or even paralysis if the spinal cord is damaged; arrhythmias and possible cardiac arrest; renal failure; and massive bleeding.

In addition to causing the signs and symptoms listed above, a *lightning burn* may cause swollen, charred, or reddened skin around the entrance wound and a burn pattern resembling a tree branch. Permanent neurologic changes, including neuralgia and paresis, may also result.

Thermal burns

Thermal burns are classified by depth.

First-degree burns, also called superficial burns, injure only the epidermis, the top layer of the skin. Examples include minor sunburn and burns from brief contact with a hot iron. The burned area usually is tender, reddened, painful, and has little or no swelling and no blistering. Erythema resolves in 1 to 2 days without scarring.

Second-degree burns, also called partial-thickness burns, damage both the epidermis and dermis, the skin layer below the epidermis. Examples include deep sunburns, short expo-

sure to flame, and burns caused by hot liquids. Usually, the burn causes pronounced pain, and the burned area blisters or the epidermis may be broken. The skin will be edematous, and the burn may weep. The skin may appear red, streaked, or splotchy; although it may heal in 10 days to 4 weeks, it remains discolored.

Third-degree burns, also called full-thickness burns, destroy all skin layers and may damage subcutaneous muscle tissue, fat, and bone. The skin appears leathery and charred, edematous, with a dry surface. This type of burn commonly comes from a fire, electricity, or prolonged contact with a hot object. A warning sign is the absence of pain due to nerve damage. Other signs include loss of consciousness, respiratory distress (from lung injury due to smoke inhalation), tissue necrosis, and white, reddened, grayish, or darkened skin with ulceration. Because this tissue cannot regenerate, autografting is indicated.

Fourth-degree burns are full-thickness burns marked by the presence of charred skin; they extend deep into muscle or bone and may require amputation.

Sometimes fatal and often permanently disfiguring, chemical and thermal burns can cause tremendous physical and emotional suffering. Inhalation burns may lead to airway edema, resulting in respiratory distress, airway obstruction, and death. Chemical irritants can also disrupt normal lung function and allow fluids and protein to build up in the lungs, causing adult respiratory distress syndrome, which can lead to death within days of the accident.

Chemical and thermal burns harm the skin, the body's first line of defense. For this reason, a patient with extensive burns is severely immunocompromised.

WHAT HAPPENS IN ELECTRICAL BURNS

Electric current — whether machine-generated or natural (lightning) — can cause a wide range of injuries. When the current contacts the skin, three types of injury can occur:
• heat burns on the skin surface from flames that accompany the current
• arc or flash burns from current that doesn't pass through the body
• so-called true electrical injury from current that does pass through the body.

True electrical injury is more like a crush injury than a thermal burn, often destroying muscle tissue and affecting internal organs.

The most dangerous burns

Some electrical burns are more dangerous than others. Here are the factors that come into play.

Intensity of voltage and amperage
Lightning is measured in millions of volts and from 12,000 to 200,000 amperes. In contrast, common household electricity generates 110 or 220 volts. The higher the voltage, the greater the potential for damage.

Types of current
Alternating current (AC) such as household current is much more dangerous than direct current (DC), such as from lightning or a car battery.

Tissue resistance
Wet skin is much less resistant to electric current than dry skin. That is why a typical bathtub accident — when someone drops a low-voltage appliance into the water — often causes death.

Length of contact with the body
The longer the person touches the source of the electrical burn, the greater the damage.

Current's route through the body
The most serious injuries occur from electric current passing through vital organs. For example, a current that moves from one hand to the other passes through the heart. This can cause a fatal arrhythmia or cardiac arrest.

Management

Immediate actions

Actions depend on the type and severity of the burn. (See *When not to flush a chemical burn.*)

Don't use soap if the burn came from an alkali or if you're not sure which chemical caused the burn. Soap will increase pain and irritation from an alkali.

Don't let burned body surfaces touch because this increases irritation, pain, and the risk of infection. (Instead, for instance, place a clean towel between the inside of the patient's arm and the side of the body.)

Thermal burns

First-degree burns. Apply a cold pack immediately until pain is relieved. *Don't* put ice or ice water on the burn because this will cause rapid chilling and further tissue injury. *Don't* put ointments, creams, butter, or sprays on the burn because they trap heat inside and increase tissue damage.

Don't apply a dressing or prescription antibiotic ointment; neither are necessary.

For sunburn, a topical corticosteroid can be ordered; a short course of methylprednisolone may be considered for extensive sunburn.

The patient may take aspirin or ibuprofen for symptomatic relief; these medications will also help with inflammation.

The patient should be instructed to return if the skin blisters.

WHEN NOT TO FLUSH A CHEMICAL BURN

Most often, a chemical burn is immediately rinsed with copious amounts of water for at least 15 minutes. If it's a dry chemical, the substance should be brushed off first. Sometimes, rinsing does more harm than good because certain chemicals react when mixed with water. Read the chart below to learn when not to rinse—and what to do instead.

Chemical	Reaction with water	Intervention
Dry lime	Becomes more corrosive	Wearing gloves, remove the patient's clothes and brush off the lime; then flush the burn with water for 30 minutes.
Sodium	May explode	Cover the burn with oil.
Hydrofluoric acid	Causes continuing tissue destruction	Make sure the patient gets a calcium gluconate injection.

Second-degree burns. Wash the area gently with soap and water. After washing, irrigate the wound with sterile saline. Silver sulfadiazine (Silvadene) cream can be applied to allow the wound a better chance of healing without infection. Silver sulfadiazine cream is contraindicated in patients who are pregnant, breast-feeding, or allergic to sulfonamides.

Apply a thick sterile dressing to protect the area.

Treatment of blisters is often left to the discretion of the caregiver; if the blister is small and has a thick wall, it's usually left intact; if it's thin-walled and appears liable to rupture, it should be lanced and covered with a nonadherent dressing.

Pharmacologic treatment options include:
• oral narcotic analgesics (acetaminophen with codeine or propoxyphene): as needed for pain relief. If the patient doesn't have a painful burn, nonsteroidal anti-inflammatory drugs or aspirin are preferred.
• tetanus prophylaxis: 0.5 ml of tetanus toxoid I.M. in patients who have been immunized in the past but haven't had a booster within the past 5 years; 0.5 ml of tetanus toxoid and tetanus immune globulin in patients who haven't had an initial immunization series.

There is no need to prescribe systemic antibiotics for second-degree burns unless secondary cellulitis develops.

 COLLABORATION An electrical burn, an external chemical burn, a chemical burn to the eye, and a third- or fourth-degree thermal burn need emergency medical transport to an emergency department from the trauma scene. For electrical burn, locate entrance and exit wounds. If oral or nasal mucosa is edematous or burned, aggressive management to maintain respiratory status is needed, including oxygen or intubation; if the patient is unresponsive to oxygen and his color is very red, consider cyanide poisoning from burning carpet or plastic. Inform emergency medical services personnel of pertinent information, including the patient's condition when you first saw him, his medical history, allergies, and the name of the primary care provider (PCP).

Follow-up for first-degree burns is needed only if the skin blisters. All other burns require follow-up within 2 days, with a focus on preventing infection. For patients struck by lightning, eye, ear, nose, and throat evaluation is needed because of the high risk of tympanic membrane rupture.

The Rule of Nines helps determine percentage of body surface affected by burns (head 9%, trunk and back 18%, chest and abdomen 18%, arms 9%, legs 18%). Burn involvement can also be estimated based on the patient's palm size equaling 1% of his body surface. If, for example, a burn on the back covers the same area as five of the patient's palms, the burn covers 5% of the total body surface area.

Referral or consultation

Surgical consultation is indicated if burns are greater than 10% of body surface or full-thickness burns are greater than 3% of body surface.

Hospital admission and surgical consultation are needed for patients with circumferential burns and burns involving the perineum, hand, or organs of sensation. Hospital admission is required if smoke inhalation injury is suspected.

Patient teaching

• Instruct the patient to check for signs and symptoms of infection and impaired circulation.
• Instruct the patient to change the dressing on second-degree burns daily for 5 to 7 days; before replacing the dressing, the wound should be gently cleaned with soap and water and silver sulfadiazine cream should be reapplied in a layer thick enough to cover the burn. When the wound has healed, he should apply moisturizing cream to prevent skin cracking.
• Instruct the patient regarding burn prevention—appliances properly installed with grounding, rubber gloves and dry shoes used when working

with electric circuits, unused wall sockets capped, and extension cords unplugged when not in use. Teach the patient to avoid hilltops, riverbanks, hedges, telephone poles, and trees during a storm with thunder and lightning. The safest shelter in a storm is a closed house; otherwise, tell the patient to seek a closed auto, cave or ditch, or lie on the ground curled up with hands close together.

➡ **ALERT** Tell the patient to call the PCP to report any pain persisting beyond 48 hours or signs or symptoms of infection (fever, redness, increasing pain, swelling, purulent drainage, fever above 101° F [38.3° C]).

Cardiac arrest

ICD-9-CM 427.5

Cardiac arrest — the cessation of heart contractions — suppresses cardiac output. As a result, the brain and all other organs are deprived of a circulating blood supply. This, in turn, leads to multiple organ dysfunction syndrome.

Cardiac arrest leads to irreversible brain damage within 4 to 6 minutes and to death within 10 minutes, depending on the patient's condition, the nature of the arrest, and the elapsed time between onset of symptoms and initiation of cardiopulmonary resuscitation (CPR).

Even after successful CPR, complications may arise from improper resuscitation technique. For instance, chest compressions may worsen myocardial damage if they're performed on a patient who still has a pulse. Regardless of whether it's performed properly, CPR can cause rib or sternum fracture, separation of the ribs from the sternum, pneumothorax, hemothorax, lung contusion, liver or spleen laceration, or fat emboli.

COMMON ARRHYTHMIAS IN CARDIAC ARREST

The arrhythmias most commonly identified during cardiac arrest are ventricular fibrillation, ventricular asystole, and electromechanical dissociation.

Ventricular fibrillation

In this arrhythmia, the ventricular rhythm is rapid and chaotic. The patient has no pulse, heart sounds, or blood pressure. Ventricular fibrillation commonly results from ischemia, characterized by a sudden drop in the amplitude and duration of the action potential (the series of polarization and depolarization) on the electrocardiogram (ECG). The arrhythmia can cause death within 4 minutes.

Ventricular asystole (cardiac standstill)

Electrical activity in the ventricles ceases in this arrhythmia. Myocardial cells aren't depolarized, and action potentials are absent. The heart may suffer extensive damage.

Electromechanical dissociation

In this arrhythmia, a heart rhythm appears on the ECG but with no evidence of effective heart contraction. The patient lacks a palpable pulse. Causes of electromechanical dissociation include massive pulmonary embolism, a malfunctioning prosthetic heart valve, and cardiac tamponade.

Multisystemic organ failure after cardiac arrest may also lead to adult respiratory distress syndrome, disseminated intravascular coagulation, shock, and neurologic deficits.

Causes

Immediate causes of cardiac arrest include ventricular fibrillation, ventricular asystole (cardiac standstill), and electromechanical dissociation. Usually, these problems result from coronary artery disease or its complications.

Ventricular fibrillation and ventricular asystole may result from heart damage caused by a previous myocardial infarction or from toxic doses of sympathomimetic drugs (such as dobutamine and dopamine), antiarrhythmic drugs (such as quinidine and disopyramide), or parasympathomimetic drugs (such as neostigmine and bethanechol). Cocaine abuse has also been linked to cardiac arrest.

Other causes of cardiac arrest include:

- blood loss, lack of oxygen, or too much carbon dioxide in the blood (respiratory failure frequently precedes cardiac arrest, particularly in children)
- vagal stimulation associated with straining, endotracheal intubation, or colonoscopy, which can lead to cardiac arrest by triggering bradycardia
- hypothermia, acidosis, and hypokalemia, which can induce ventricular fibrillation and, in turn, cardiac arrest
- trauma, which can bring on cardiac arrest by causing a severe oxygen deficiency and profound metabolic acidosis
- extreme psychological stress
- arrhythmias, including ectopic heart beats, more than six premature ventricular contractions (PVCs) per minute, three or more successive PVCs, multifocal PVCs, bigeminy, and R-on-T phenomenon. (See *Common arrhythmias in cardiac arrest.*)

Clinical presentation

Cardiac arrest causes an absent or extremely slow pulse (typically less than 40 beats/minute) or a chaotic heart rhythm (ventricular fibrillation). Some patients have no heart rhythm or have a heart rhythm but no pulse (electromechanical dissociation), as shown on electrocardiogram (ECG). Lack of a pulse always indicates cardiac arrest regardless of which heart rhythm appears on the ECG monitor.

Management

Immediate actions

If the patient shows signs or symptoms of cardiac arrest, check his airway, breathing, and circulation. Perform CPR as needed. Inform emergency medical services personnel of pertinent information, including the patient's condition when you first saw him, his medical history, allergies, and the name of the primary care provider (PCP).

Later actions

For symptoms of heart attack (heavy or crushing pressure; pain radiating into the inner part of the arms, back, jaw, neck, or shoulder; nausea and vomiting; shortness of breath; sweating; feeling clammy, weak, or anxious; or feeling of overwhelming doom), activate emergency medical services.

If the patient continues to have dangerous arrhythmias despite antiarrhythmic drug therapy, he may be a candidate for an implantable cardioverter-defibrillator. This small pulse generator is implanted in the patient's chest, and a leadwire (or wires) is positioned transvenously in the endocardium of the right ventricle. The lead senses the heart rate and delivers shocks or antitachycardia pacing to terminate the arrhythmia. The device can be programmed to suit the patient's specific needs. It uses far less energy (up to 37 joules) than an external defibrillator (360 joules).

Referral or consultation

 COLLABORATION Any patient in cardiac arrest requires emergency medical transport to an emergency department. Follow up within 24 hours if cardiac arrest is due to a secondary cause; follow up within 1 week of hospital discharge for cardiac disease.

Patient teaching

 ALERT Tell the patient to call the PCP to report any pain that changes in character or increases in frequency and duration.

Concussion

ICD-9-CM 850.9, with loss of consciousness 850.5, due to any kind of blast/high impact 869.0

A relatively minor brain injury, a concussion may result from a direct blow to the head such as when a person slips on ice and hits his head on the sidewalk, or it may come from an acceleration-deceleration injury, as often occurs in a head-on motor vehicle collision. In this injury, the head is hurled forward and then stops abruptly as it hits the windshield. The brain, however, keeps moving, slapping against the skull and then rebounding against the opposite side. There is no penetrating trauma, but a transient loss of consciousness of at least a few seconds may have occurred.

Most patients recover from concussion within 48 hours and don't suffer lasting damage. Patients may complain of memory loss, persistent headaches, insomnia, and dizziness that may (uncommonly) last for months after injury. However, there may be some intracranial bleeding that can lead to permanent injury or death if not treated promptly. Increased intracranial pressure (ICP more than 15 mm Hg) is an ominous sign. If uncorrected, increased ICP leads to acute vasodilatation, loss of consciousness, decerebrate posturing, and high risk of mortality.

Repeated concussions have a cumulative effect on the brain and can result in permanent brain damage.

Causes

Usually, a concussion results from a direct blow to the head. The shock wave from an explosion can also cause concussion.

Clinical presentation

The patient history may reveal confusion or disorientation, and a brief loss of consciousness.

Examination may elicit dizziness, nausea and vomiting, severe headache, blurred or double vision, and inability to remember what happened just before or after the injury.

Diagnosis

Concussion differs from more serious head injuries by the following criteria: no loss of consciousness at the time of the injury, no nausea or vomiting, no change in mental status from the time of incident until the time seen, and no focal neurologic deficit. The patient may have minimal to moderate headache.

For up to 1 year after a concussion, some patients experience delayed effects, or *postconcussion syndrome.* Signs and symptoms include lack of usual energy, double vision, memory loss, irritability, emotional lability, poor concentration reduced libido, loss of inhibitions, difficulty relating to others, intolerance to noise, easy intoxication by alcohol, and dizziness, giddiness, or light-headedness. Usually, postconcussion effects subside over time.

Management

Any finding that doesn't fit the definition of concussion should be referred to a doctor. *Subacute subdural hematoma* takes 24 hours to 2 weeks for symptoms to develop; patients at high risk are the elderly and those with alcohol-induced brain atrophy. *Chronic subdural hematoma* is detected more than 2 weeks after the injury and results from liquefaction of the hematoma.

After any head injury, determine whether the patient is alert. If the patient is awake and alert, assess orientation. The Glasgow Coma Scale quickly ascertains neurologic status. (See *Using the Glasgow Coma Scale,* page 288.)

Try to determine if loss of consciousness occurred at any time during or after the accident. If so, the patient may undergo a computed tomography scan to determine the extent of injury.

Monitor vital signs every 5 minutes until the extent of the injury is known. Increasing blood pressure with decreasing pulse suggests increasing ICP, an ominous sign. (See *Grading sports-related concussions,* page 289.)

A patient with a simple concussion usually can recover at home, as long as someone observes him closely for at least 24 hours; symptoms of intracranial bleeding usually occur within 24 hours. The patient must be observed closely for 2 hours, then every 2 hours for 8 hours, then every 4 to 6 hours for 16 hours. Each time,

USING THE GLASGOW COMA SCALE

The Glasgow Coma Scale provides an easy way to describe the patient's mental status and detect changes. A decreased score may signal an impending neurologic crisis. A score of less than 8 indicates severe neurologic damage.

Test	Score
Eyes open	
Spontaneously	4
To speech	3
To pain	2
No response	1
Best motor response	
Obeys	6
Localizes pain (reaches toward pain to remove cause)	5
Flexion-withdrawal (moves away from pain)	4
Abnormal flexion (decorticate rigidity)	3
Extension (decerebrate rigidity)	2
No response	1
Best verbal response	
Oriented	5
Disoriented	4
Inappropriate words	3
Incomprehensible sounds	2
No response	1

check for change in mental status, bruising below the eyes or behind the ears, severe head pain, or dizziness.

Follow up within 24 hours.

Referral or consultation

 COLLABORATION Patients with loss of consciousness, persistent vomiting, or changed neurologic status (such as in vision or personality) should be taken to the emergency department. For a Glasgow Coma score below 6, elevate the head 30 degrees and give mannitol I.V. to decrease ICP. Inform emergency medical services personnel of pertinent information, including the patient's condition when you first saw him, his medical history, any allergies, and the name of the primary care provider (PCP).

Patient teaching

• Advise the patient to eat lightly, especially if nausea or vomiting occurs.

Occasional vomiting is common and nausea usually subsides in a few days. Aggressive evaluation is needed if the patient vomits more than three times in 24 hours after trauma.

• Advise the patient to avoid taking any pain medications for 2 hours after injury. If pain is severe enough to require it, the patient needs to be evaluated. After 2 hours, the patient may take acetaminophen for a headache. To avoid the risk of GI bleeding, don't give aspirin.

• Warn the patient not to drink alcohol for at least 24 hours.

ALERT Tell the family to call the PCP to report any marked changes in behavior, seizure activity, clear fluid leaking from ear or nose, bruising below the eyes or behind the ears, severe head pain (child inconsolable or extremely restless for more than 10 minutes at a time), vomiting more than three times in 24 hours, difficulty waking, confusion, or difficulty walking or

GRADING SPORTS-RELATED CONCUSSIONS

Concussion grades	Clinical presentation	Immediate actions	Least time before returning to sport
Grade 1	No loss of consciousness; mental status change < 15 minutes	Examined on scene by first responder; recheck every 5 minutes for 15 minutes. Second Grade 1 on same day: remove from activity.	Grade 1 once within previous 24 hours: 15 minutes Grade 1 twice in same day: 1 week
Grade 2	No loss of consciousness, mental status change > 15 minutes	Remove from activity; monitor frequently; additional testing as indicated.	Grade 2: 1 week Grade 1, then Grade 2 on same day: 2 weeks
Grade 3	Loss of consciousness or seizure	Emergency medical services transport to emergency department	Brief loss of consciousness: 1 week Prolonged loss of consciousness: 2 weeks Second Grade 3 in lifetime: 1 month

talking in the initial 48 hours after the trauma. After 48 hours, worsening symptoms of postconcussion syndrome should be reported.

Corneal abrasion

ICD-9-CM external 930.9, eyelid 930.1, eyeball 930.8

Often caused by a mechanical or chemical insult, a corneal abrasion is a scratch on the surface epithelium of the cornea. Corneal abrasions are among the most common eye injuries. With treatment, the prognosis is usually good.

Causes

A corneal abrasion usually results from a foreign body, such as a cinder or a piece of dust, dirt, or grit, that becomes embedded under the eyelid. Even if the foreign body is washed out by tears, it may still injure the cornea.

A small piece of metal may become lodged in the eye of a worker who didn't wear eye protection. The metal forms a rust ring on the cornea as well as an abrasion. Corneal abrasions are also common in persons who fall asleep wearing hard contact lenses.

A corneal scratch produced by a fingernail, a piece of paper, or other organic substance may cause a persistent lesion. The epithelium doesn't always heal properly, and a recurrent corneal erosion may develop, with delayed effects more severe than those of the original injury.

Clinical presentation

A history of eye trauma or prolonged wearing of contact lenses, as well as typical symptoms, suggests corneal abrasion. Corneal abrasions typically present with a history of unilateral eye discomfort when blinking, a foreign body sensation and, because the cornea is richly endowed with nerve endings from the trigeminal nerve (cranial nerve V), pain disproportionate to the size of the injury. Examination may reveal photophobia, difficulty keeping the eye open, redness, and increased tearing. A corneal abrasion frequently affects visual acuity, depending on the size and location of the injury.

Diagnosis

When evaluating eye pain, consider a foreign body and keratitis (bacterial, viral, fungal) as well as corneal laceration or perforation.

Staining the cornea with fluorescein stain confirms the diagnosis: The injured area appears yellow-green when examined with a cobalt blue light. Slit-lamp examination discloses the depth of the abrasion.

Examining the eye with a flashlight may reveal a foreign body on the cornea; the eyelid must be everted to check for a foreign body embedded under the lid.

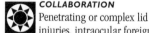 **ALERT** Pain, significantly decreased vision, sluggish pupillary reaction, and a cloudy cornea indicate glaucoma. Pain, decreased vision, sluggish pupillary reaction, but with a dull and swollen iris, suggest iritis. Erythema and edema around the lacrimal duct, combined with mucopurulent discharge on palpation of the lacrimal sac, indicate lacrimal duct obstruction.

Before beginning treatment, test the patient for visual acuity to provide a medical baseline and a legal safeguard.

Management

 COLLABORATION Penetrating or complex lid injuries, intraocular foreign body, significant loss of vision, acute occular pain, or corneal laceration or perforation should be protected by a nonpressure eye shield before the patient is transported for emergency ophthalmologic evaluation. Don't instill antibiotic eyedrops or ointment.

Chemical splashes should be immediately irrigated with tap water while someone calls poison control. If you can't verify a chemical name, contact the poison control center; if you can't verify a specific treatment, irrigate the eye, and then move the patient immediately to an emergency medical facility.

Foreign bodies are initially treated by simply trying to remove them. Attempt removal using a sterile gauze pad moistened with sterile normal saline.

Initial application of a tight pressure patch prevents further corneal irritation when the patient blinks, excluding an abrasion caused by contact lenses. The patch should be worn for 24 to 48 hours. Most corneal abrasions heal in less than 36 hours with a pressure patch.

Pharmacologic treatment options include instilling broad-spectrum antibiotic eyedrops or ointment (gentamicin) in the affected eye four times a day for 2 days to prevent infection or instilling short-acting cycloplegic eyedrops (cyclopentolate) to relieve ciliary spasm. Oral analgesics (acetaminophen) may be used for pain relief.

Follow up daily until healing is complete, focusing on signs of infection. If improvement isn't significant in 24 hours, refer the patient.

Referral or consultation

COLLABORATION Patients with any of the emergency conditions listed above should be referred immediately for ophthalmologic evaluation.

Patient teaching

• Tell the patient with an eye patch to leave the patch in place for 24 to 48 hours. Warn him that wearing a patch alters depth perception and, therefore, advise caution in everyday activities, such as climbing stairs and stepping off a curb.
• Reassure the patient that the corneal epithelium usually heals in 24 to 48 hours.
• Stress the importance of instilling prescribed antibiotic eyedrops as directed because an untreated corneal infection can lead to ulceration and permanent loss of vision. Teach the proper way to instill ophthalmic drugs.
• Emphasize the importance of safety glasses to protect workers' eyes from flying fragments. Also review instructions for wearing and caring for contact lenses.
• Warn the patient not to rub the affected eye.

Corneal ulcers

ICD-9-CM 370.00

A major cause of blindness worldwide, corneal ulcers produce corneal scarring or perforation. They occur in the central or marginal areas of the cornea, vary in shape and size, and may be singular or multiple. Marginal ulcers, caused by a sensitivity to *Staphylococcus aureus,* are the most common form.

Prompt treatment by an ophthalmologist (within hours of onset) can prevent visual impairment.

Causes

Corneal ulcers generally result from bacterial, protozoan, viral, or fungal infections. Common bacterial sources include *Staphylococcus aureus, Pseudomonas aeruginosa, Streptococcus viridans, S. (Diplococcus) pneumoniae,* and *Moraxella liquefaciens*; viral sources, including herpes simplex type 1 and varicella-zoster; common fungal sources include *Candida, Fusarium,* and *Cephalosporium*.

Other causes include trauma, exposure, reactions to bacterial infections, toxins, and allergens. Tuberculoprotein causes a classic phlyctenular keratoconjunctivitis and vitamin A deficiency.

Clinical presentation

Typically, corneal ulceration begins with pain (aggravated by blinking) and photophobia, followed by increased tearing. Eventually, central corneal ulceration produces pronounced visual blurring. The eye may appear injected (red). If a bacterial ulcer is present, purulent discharge is possible.

Diagnosis

A history — of trauma or use of contact lenses — and a flashlight examination that reveals an irregular corneal surface suggest corneal ulcer. Exudate may be present on the cornea, and a hypopyon (accumulation of white cells in the anterior chamber) may appear as a half-moon.

Fluorescein dye, instilled in the conjunctival sac, delineates the outline of the ulcer. Culture and sensitivity testing of corneal scrapings may identify the causative organism and guide antibiotic or antifungal therapy.

Management

A corneal ulcer should never be patched because patching creates the dark, warm, moist environment ideal for bacterial growth. However, it should be protected with a perforated shield.

Because corneal ulcers are quite painful, administer analgesics.

Because an associated iridocyclitis occurs when the cornea is involved, cycloplegic eyedrops are given to reduce ciliary body spasms. If pupil size is not equal at 24-hour check-up, consider the half-life of the cycloplegic drug as a cause.

Watch for signs of secondary glaucoma (transient vision loss and halos around lights).

Follow up within 24 hours.

Referral or consultation

 COLLABORATION Refer as an emergency to an ophthalmologist. Prompt treatment is essential for all forms of corneal ulcer to prevent complications and permanent visual impairment.

Patient teaching

 ALERT Tell the patient to call the primary care provider to report increasing eye pain, fever higher than 101° F (38.3°C), or eye fatigue persisting more than 24 hours.

Foreign body in eye

ICD-9-CM external 930.9, eyelid 930.1, eyeball 930.8

A foreign body lodged in the eye is the most common type of eye injury in primary care. Besides causing pain, it can lead to discomfort, inflammation, and infection. If the foreign body scratches the surface lining of the cornea, a corneal abrasion occurs. If the eye doesn't heal properly, a persistent wound or ulcer can develop, and the cornea may become permanently scarred.

Causes

Typically, the foreign body is a tiny piece of dirt or metal, a cinder, or a bit of dust. Usually, the patient blinks the object into a position along the eyelid, where it can be removed with a clean gauze pad or tissue.

Clinical presentation

A foreign body in the eye can cause mild, unilateral pain as well as redness, tearing, a burning sensation, and photophobia. The patient may report a foreign body sensation; this feeling may persist even after the particle is removed because the eye remains irritated. With a corneal abrasion, the patient is more likely to complain of impaired vision.

Diagnosis

Observation of a foreign body in the eye under light and magnification confirms the diagnosis. Fluorescein stain highlights the ocular foreign body. Also consider the possibility of an intraocular foreign body, corneal abrasion, corneal laceration or perforation, or keratitis (bacterial, viral, or fungal).

Management

Immediate actions

Check the superior and inferior cul-de-sac for foreign bodies. Evert the upper eyelid to enhance visualization (roll the eyelid backward over a smooth object like a pen).

Pharmacologic options include:

- local analgesia (proparacaine) for pain control during removal of the foreign body
- antibiotic ophthalmologic ointment twice daily for 2 to 3 days after removal of the foreign body to prevent infection.

If the patient complains of feeling a foreign body in the eye but the particle isn't visible, help him to rinse the eye under a gentle stream of clean, warm running water while moving the eye in different directions to help flush out the particle.

If the particle remains in the eye after flushing, gently pull the lower eyelid down and examine the inside of the lid. Then ask the patient to look up. If you can see the foreign object on the inside of the lid, remove it with the corner of a moistened sterile gauze pad or a clean cloth or tissue. Never use an instrument such as tweezers or a dry cotton swab to remove a foreign body in the eye. Tweezers could cause injury if they graze the eyeball; dry cotton fibers may stay in the eye, causing irritation.

Depending on the amount of abrasion, patching may be indicated for 24 hours.

If eye irritation continues or the particle is still in the eye, ask the patient to close his eye. Then cover the eye with several gauze pads and tape the pads in place. Rubbing may force a sharp object deeper into the eye or scratch delicate eye tissues. Also, never try to remove an object that is embedded or impaled in the eyeball. Doing so could force the object deeper into the eye, causing further damage. Instead, place a protective shield over the eye. Don't put any pressure on the eyeball. Don't let the patient rub the eye. Keep the patient calm and immediately transport him to an ophthalmologist or emergency department.

Later actions

If the particle is deeply embedded, an ophthalmologist anesthetizes the eye and tries to remove the particle with a foreign body spud, a spadelike device. After removal, antibiotic eyedrops are instilled in the eye every 3 to 4 hours. The patient is advised to wear a pressure patch to prevent further irritation of the cornea during blinking.

 ALERT A tiny piece of metal that becomes lodged in the eye may quickly form a rust ring on the cornea, causing a corneal abrasion. Typical victims of this injury are metal workers who don't wear protective eyewear. To remove a rust ring, the ophthalmologist uses an ophthalmic burr.

Follow up within 24 hours.

Referral or consultation

 COLLABORATION The patient should be referred to an ophthalmologist if he has an intraocular foreign body, significant loss of vision, progressive pain, redness or discharge, acute ocular pain, and corneal laceration or perforation. Don't instill antibiotic eyedrops or ointment, patch the eye with a protective shield, and avoid putting pressure on the eye.

Patient teaching

- Caution the patient not to rub the eye.
- Advise the patient to wear protective glasses.

Hyperthermia

ICD-9-CM of unknown origin 780.6, newborn 778.4

Hyperthermia — an above-normal body temperature — is the body's defense against infection by organisms that can't reproduce at high temperatures. Because normal body temperature varies from person to person, the definition of hyperthermia varies too. Some consider anything above 99° F (37.2° C) a fever; others believe a fever begins at 101° F (38.3° C).

Hyperthermia can lead to multisystemic organ failure and, ultimately, death because of the high and constant metabolic demand it imposes on the tissues.

Causes

Hyperthermia may result from hundreds of illnesses, some of them life-threatening, as well as from injury, immunization, and use of certain drugs.

Clinical presentation

The most important features of hyperthermia are its severity and duration. Most fevers are mild and last a short time; a slight rise or fall in body temperature is rarely significant. But a steep increase, to 104° F (40° C) or higher, may signal a serious condition.

A fever seldom occurs alone. Usually, the patient also feels overheated and generally ill. Accompanying symptoms may help reveal the cause of the fever. For instance, an infection may cause a cough, a sore throat, or an earache. Children can have fevers, even very high ones, without being seriously ill or appearing uncomfortable. But this doesn't mean a fever in a child can be ignored.

Management
Immediate actions
Aggressive evaluation is needed if the patient has a fever accompanied by toxic signs that may indicate serious disorders such as meningitis or pneumonia. These signs may include skin abnormalities (petechiae [purple spots

of blood under the skin], central cyanosis, or pallor), severe headache, severe back pain, nuchal rigidity (very stiff neck), confusion, irritability, abdominal pain, head bobbing, poor muscle tone, coughing up of brown or green sputum, breathing irregularities, and painful urination.

Hyperthermia also requires prompt medical attention if it occurs for no obvious reason; if it occurs in a patient with a serious chronic disease, such as respiratory or heart disease; if it occurs in an infant under age 4 months; if it lasts longer than 5 days (3 days for a child); if it recurs after first abating with treatment; if it's accompanied by signs of dehydration (extreme thirst, dry mouth, lightheadedness, skin tenting [reduced skin turgor], dark urine [fewer than three urinations in 24 hours]); and if fever suddenly rises from slight (99° F [37.2° C]) to high (104° F [40° C]), especially in an infant under age 4 months.

A patient with an extremely high temperature may be restless, agitated, and confused. To prevent him from harming himself, don't leave him unattended.

Depending on the clinical picture, order blood, urine, and sputum cultures, lumbar puncture, computed tomography (CT) scans, and X-rays (to detect encapsulated infections, such as empyemas or abscesses). Aspiration may be done to analyze suspicious areas found on CT scans or X-rays.

To ease discomfort from a fever, suggest that the patient take a tepid bath, remove excessive clothing, reduce room temperature, or take aspirin, acetaminophen, or ibuprofen to reduce the fever.

Children under age 16 should take acetaminophen or ibuprofen—not aspirin—to avoid the risk of Reye's syndrome, a life-threatening condition affecting the brain.

Consider prescribing antibiotics for immunosuppressed patients and those with strong indication of bacterial infection.

Follow up within 24 hours.

Referral or consultation

If you can't evaluate the patient yourself, instruct the patient or caregiver to go to the nearest hospital emergency department.

 COLLABORATION Immediate transport to an emergency department is needed if the patient has a fever accompanied by toxic signs.

Hypothermia

ICD-9-CM accidental 991.6, not associated with low environmental temperature 780.9

Hypothermia occurs when a person's core body temperature drops below 95° F (35° C). Mild hypothermia occurs with a core (rectal) body temperature from 93.2° to 95°F (34° to 35° C).

Moderate to severe hypothermia occurs with temperature below 93.2° F (34° C), the temperature when metabolism slows. The typical victim of hypothermia is a homeless person or a hiker caught in a sudden snowstorm.

Wind and wet weather increase the risk of hypothermia. Unlike frostbite, which affects only a specific body part, hypothermia affects the entire body. Hypothermia can, if not treated promptly, lead to severe infection, pneumonia, arrhythmias, kidney failure, and death.

Patients at high risk for hypothermia include those with heart disease or malnutrition, cigarette smokers, drug or alcohol abusers, young children, the elderly, and those with a history of thyroidectomy (check the neck for a scar).

Other risk factors include wet or inadequate clothing, fatigue, hunger, and inadequate body fat (fat insulates against the cold).

Causes

Hypothermia can result from drinking a large amount of cold fluids, near-drowning in cold water, and prolonged exposure to cold temperatures, such as chilly weather (around 50° F [10° C]), especially when in wet clothing. It can also result from being transfused with a large amount of cold blood or blood products, myxedema coma, and shock.

Clinical presentation

Signs of hypothermia vary with the severity of the condition.

Mild hypothermia

History reveals complaint of feeling cold. Examination reveals shivering and fine muscle tremors, increased pulse and blood pressure, tachypnea, and declining neurologic status (clumsiness, apathy, confusion, slurred speech, forgetfulness).

Moderate to severe hypothermia

Examination reveals violent shivering progressing to muscle rigidity, diaphoresis, cardiac arrhythmias, and decreased level of consciousness (memory loss, stupor), as well as respiratory rate and depth, gag and cough reflex, and pulse rate and blood pressure.

Management

ALERT Resuscitation efforts in hypothermia should continue until the patient is fully rewarmed. This principle is summed up in the slogan, "The patient isn't dead until he's warm and dead." In moderate to severe hypothermia, fluid shifts from the intravascular to the extravascular space. At this stage, cardiac output decreases and cardiac arrhythmias appear. These arrhythmias shouldn't be treated because they often resolve spontaneously with rewarming. However, rough handling of the patient can precipitate deadly arrhythmias.

Immediate actions

 COLLABORATION If the patient has a core body temperature below 93.2° F (34° C), he requires emergency medical transport to the nearest emergency department.

Shake the patient gently, and check airway, breathing, and circulation (ABCs). Perform cardiopulmonary resuscitation (CPR) as needed. Continue CPR until the patient's core (rectal) body temperature has rewarmed to at least 93.2° F (34° C). Place the patient on a cardiac monitor and give warmed 100% oxygen via face mask.

Notify emergency medical services personnel of pertinent information, including the patient's condition when first seen, steps taken and response, medical history, and any allergies.

If ABCs are intact, gently move the patient to a warm place and start gradual rewarming.

To rewarm the patient:
• Remove the patient's wet clothes.
• Dry the patient and wrap in warm blankets.
• Offer warm, noncaffeinated beverages. Warn the patient against drinking alcohol- or caffeine-containing drinks during the acute phase because they may cause arrhythmias.
• Don't warm the patient too quickly; rewarming shock can occur if the outside of the body rewarms faster than the inside.

• Never use dry heat to warm the patient because this can permanently damage body tissues.
• Don't let the patient put his hands or feet on or near a radiator or hot stove.
• Don't immerse the patient's whole body in warm water. This could cause heart problems.
• Don't let the patient smoke because smoking impairs circulation, slowing the warming process.

For minor cold exposure

Cover the patient with warmed blankets or towels, or immerse him in warm water. Wrap a hot-water bottle in a blanket or towel before applying.

In a medical facility, the patient may be warmed internally and externally, with constant monitoring of core body temperature. Rewarming methods include administering heated I.V. fluids; administering warmed, humidified oxygen; gastric lavage (instilling warm fluids through a tube into the GI tract); bladder lavage; pleural lavage; and transfusing warmed blood products.

Follow up within 24 hours, focusing on peripheral vasculature, arrhythmias, and renal function.

Referral or consultation

 COLLABORATION All conditions except minor cold exposure require emergency measures and transport to the nearest emergency department.

Insect bites and stings

ICD-9-CM chigger 133.8, fire ant/ spider/snake/venomous insect 989.5

At the very least, bites from mosquitoes, ticks, spiders, and other insects can be annoying. At worst, they can

HOW TO RECOGNIZE TICKS AND SPIDERS

Knowing how to spot certain ticks and spiders can protect you and those around you from potentially dangerous bites. Use this guide to help you to recognize dangerous insects.

Deer tick

Common throughout the United States, the deer tick is responsible for transmitting Lyme disease. The deer tick matures in stages. Between the larval and adult stage, it's as small as a pencil point. Growing to ⅛" (0.32 cm), the deer tick seeks a host. After it attaches to a host, it swells to five to seven times its original size.

Wood tick

The flat, brown-speckled wood tick is found in woods and fields throughout North America. It attaches to humans and feeds on their blood. The wood tick may inject a poison that can cause acute paralysis or transmit Rocky Mountain spotted fever, a potentially lethal disease.

Brown recluse spider

The brown recluse spider is small and light brown, with three pairs of eyes. The hallmark of a brown recluse spider is a violin-shaped darker area found on the cephalothorax; it's about 1" (2.54 cm) long, including the legs. Found in the south-central part of the United States, it favors dark areas, such as barns and woodsheds, and most commonly bites between April and October. The brown recluse spider injects a poison that causes its victim's blood to clot within 2 to 8 hours after the bite.

Black widow spider

The female black widow spider is glossy and coal-black with a red or orange hourglass mark on its underside; it's ½" (1.27 cm) in length, with legs 1½" (3.81 cm) long. (The male doesn't bite.) Common throughout the United States, especially in warmer climates, the black widow spider is usually found in dark areas, such as outdoor privies and woodsheds. Its venom is toxic to the nerves and muscles of a human victim, causing muscle spasms in the arms and legs, rigidity of stomach muscles, and ascending paralysis that leads to difficulty swallowing and breathing; circulatory collapse may follow.

cause anaphylaxis, respiratory failure, and death. In addition, many insects can transmit diseases.

Causes

Ticks actively seek warm-blooded hosts and feed on their blood. Spiders bite if they're accidentally disturbed. A black widow or brown recluse spider bite can cause an anaphylactic reaction that leads to shock, respiratory arrest, and death. This reaction may result from either a toxin released during the bite or an allergy to the bite. (See "Anaphylaxis," page 278.) Mosquitoes can transmit malaria, wood ticks and dog ticks can transmit Rocky Mountain spotted fever, and deer ticks can transmit Lyme disease. (See *How to recognize ticks and spiders*.)

Clinical presentation

Any insect bite may cause local pain and swelling. Also, an insect's stinger may be left in the skin, or a bite or puncture mark may be visible. Other signs and symptoms of insect bites vary because specific poisons act on specific areas of the body.

Tick bites

Tick bites are painless at first and may cause itching at the site. If the tick isn't removed or the head is left in the body, the site will become irritated and, possibly, infected. Some people experience tick paralysis, which causes weakness, pain in the feet or legs, or respiratory failure. It's frequently unnoticed because the deer tick is only as big as the period at the end of this sentence, and its bite produces no sensation. Within a few days, a bull's-eye rash may appear. Then, over the next few weeks, months, or even years, severe symptoms may occur. (See "Lyme disease" in chapter 5, page 145.)

Spider bites

Black widow spider bites cause an immediate sharp, stinging pain followed by a dull, numbing pain. The bitten area begins to swell, and tiny red bite marks appear. Within 10 to 40 minutes after the bite, stomach muscles become rigid and severe abdominal pain occurs. Both problems subside within 48 hours. Muscle spasms in the arms and legs also occur.

Some people experience a systemic reaction from a black widow spider bite. This reaction causes extreme restlessness, dizziness, sweating or chills, pallor, seizures (especially in children), nausea, vomiting, headache, eyelid swelling, hives, pruritus, and fever.

Bites from brown recluse spiders cause little or no pain at first. However, these bites usually become painful over time. About 2 to 8 hours after the bite, a small, red puncture wound forms a small blister. The center becomes dark and hard 3 to 4 days later. In 2 to 3 weeks, a sore develops. Some people have systemic reactions, which may include fever, chills, nausea, vomiting, fatigue, muscle pain, and pinpoint red spots on the skin.

Scorpion, tarantula, and toxic spider bites

Bites from scorpions and tarantulas may cause severe signs and symptoms, especially pain. Expect to see puncture marks and some redness and swelling at the site. The patient may have muscle pain and cramps in the arms, legs, shoulders, and back. Although symptoms usually subside after 6 to 12 hours, some patients experience life-threatening effects such as circulatory or respiratory failure.

Hymenoptera (bee, wasp, ant) stings

Local reactions to bee, wasp, or ant stings include local edema and are a problem if the reaction involves the mouth or throat (possible respiratory compromise) or the eye (possible long-term injuries, such as cataracts, iris atrophy, and refractive changes).

Toxic reactions are defined as more than nine stings in one episode; they can cause nausea, syncope, diarrhea, edema, involuntary muscle spasms, headache, and seizures. Toxic reaction is differentiated from an anaphylactic response by the absence of urticaria or bronchospasm, increased incidence and severity of diarrhea, and the need for multiple stings to precipitate the reaction.

In anaphylactic response, there may be an inverse relation between the severity of the reaction and the length of time from the initial sting to the time of systemic reaction; less time to react equals a more severe reaction. Delayed reaction is uncommon; it presents with constitutional signs (fever, malaise, headache, urticaria, lymphadenopathy, and polyarthritis) up to 2 weeks after the sting.

Management

Immediate actions

If the patient is in distress, first check his airway, breathing, and circulation. Give cardiopulmonary resuscitation as needed.

 ALERT Anyone bitten by a toxic spider or scorpion needs to receive antivenin. While waiting for antivenin, tie a tight band around the involved extremity between the bite location and the patient's heart. Then apply a cold pack or ice to the bite. The bitten arm or leg should be splinted and kept lower than the patient's heart.

After any insect bite, watch for the following signs and symptoms, which may indicate a systemic reaction from a toxin or an allergic reaction: weakness, extreme restlessness, nausea, vomiting, dizziness, and difficulty breathing (which may signal respiratory failure).

For a tick bite, firmly grasp the tick at its head with tweezers, and then slowly and gently pull the tick out. Don't apply oil or ointment because the tick is more likely to inject into the skin as it suffocates. Don't pull a tick out with your hand; this action could leave the tick's head embedded in the skin. Don't try to remove the tick with a lighted match or cigarette.

Clean the wound with an antiseptic or rubbing alcohol. If the patient or companion is unable to remove the entire tick, including the head, it needs to be removed by a health care provider.

After any spider bite, the patient should receive tetanus immunization. For black widow bites, *Latrodectus mactans* antivenin should be given when symptomatic treatment is unsuccessful. The manufacturer recommends the use of a skeletal muscle relaxant as well. Skin testing must be performed before administration to check for possible anaphylactic response to antivenin. For brown recluse bites, give systemic steroids (methylprednisolone I.V. followed by oral prednisone for 5 days). Acute monitoring, including laboratory tests and urine output, is needed to detect renal failure that may require dialysis.

For severe local or toxic hymenoptera stings, consider short-term oral steroid use (prednisone 60 mg orally for 5 days) and oral antihistamines (diphenhydramine) to decrease inflammatory response.

Treatment for less severe insect or spider bites depends on which species inflicted the bite. A mild reaction is no cause for alarm and can be treated conservatively with cold compresses and acetaminophen. To relieve minor discomfort from an insect bite, apply ice or ice water to the bite. This stops the swelling, decreases pain, and slows absorption of any toxin. Or, you can apply a paste of baking soda and water or a cloth dampened with aloe vera juice.

Later actions

A patient with symptoms of Lyme disease may receive an antibiotic. Typically, adults receive oral tetracycline four times per day and children receive oral amoxicillin three times per day for 10 to 21 days. When given in the early stages of Lyme disease, these drugs can minimize later complications. In later stages, high-dose antibiotics (penicillin 20 million units I.V. for 2 to 3 weeks or ceftriaxone 2 g I.V. for 2 weeks) are indicated. See "Lyme disease" in chapter 5, page 145.

 SPECIAL POPULATIONS Children react more strongly to toxins from insect, scorpion, tick, and spider bites because they're smaller than adults. Such a bite in a child is considered a medical emergency.

Follow up with an office visit within 1 week of discharge from the hospital, or within 2 days if emergency treatment only was required. Consider providing an emergency anaphylaxis kit, such as EpiPen or Ana-Kit, as well as medical identification jewelry.

Referral or consultation

 COLLABORATION If the patient has symptoms of a systemic reaction or involvement of three or more body systems, he requires immediate transport to the nearest emergency department. Notify emergency medical services personnel of pertinent information, including the patient's condition when first bitten, duration between bite and arrival of emergency transport, his medical history, and any allergies.

Mammal bites

ICD-9-CM by site (with tendon involvement, add suffix .2): arm 884, ear 872, buttock 877, leg 891, face 873.4, foot 892, lip 873.43

Although seldom fatal, bites from animals or humans can cause injuries ranging from bruises and superficial scratches to severe crush injuries, deep puncture wounds, tissue loss, and severe damage to blood vessels. In the United States, 60% to 90% of animal bites come from dogs, about 10% come from cats, and the third most common bites are from humans. Surprisingly, human bites are the most to be feared due to the great variety of infectious bacteria and viruses normally present in the oral cavity.

A dog bite may cause muscle, tendon, and nerve damage; dislocation of involved joints; and crush injuries. Cat bites usually aren't as serious. Cats' sharp teeth, however, can cause deep puncture wounds that damage muscles, tendons, and bones; because these tissues have a limited blood supply, the risk of infection is 30% to 50% greater than with dog bites.

Infection is more likely if the wound isn't tended promptly, if there is a crush injury, or if the hand is involved. Clenched-fist injuries are the most serious because damaged joint capsules increase the risk of developing osteomyelitis and septic arthritis.

Unfortunately, many animals — usually wild ones — carry the rabies virus in their saliva and can transmit it by biting or by licking an open wound. Rabies is rare in the United States, but it's always fatal unless treated. The risk of getting rabies from a dog is low but possible. Bats, skunks, and raccoons cause nearly all cases of rabies in the United States.

Human bites can infect other humans with diseases, such as herpes simplex virus, cytomegalovirus, syphilis, tuberculosis and, possibly, acquired immunodeficiency syndrome.

Causes

Animal bites commonly occur when a sick or injured animal is trying to protect itself or when an animal is protecting its food, territory, or young. Human bites most often result from fights among school-age children and young adults.

Clinical presentation

A dog bite may cause bleeding, pain, tenderness, swelling, and decreased sensation at the injury site. A large dog usually inflicts a more severe wound than a smaller dog. A cat bite may cause small, deep puncture wounds.

A human bite may induce bleeding, which may be scant or profuse.

If the bite results in a puncture wound or a tear, bleeding may occur immediately, with bruising and swelling appearing later.

Management

Immediate actions

If the bite wound isn't bleeding heavily (as with a puncture wound), wash it vigorously with soap and water for 5 to 10 minutes. Let it bleed a bit to help flush out pathogens. A syringe and catheter may be used to create a high-pressure water stream to clean wounds.

 ALERT Don't scrub a bite wound; you could bruise the tissue. Also, don't tape the wound or seal it in any way — doing so increases the risk of infection. Apply an ice pack to the wound site for 20 minutes to decrease edema and pain.

Pharmacologic treatment options include:

• over-the-counter analgesics (acetaminophen, ibuprofen) for local pain.

• tetanus prophylaxis: 0.5 ml of tetanus toxoid I.M. for patients who have been immunized in the past but haven't had a booster within the past 5 years; 0.5 ml of tetanus toxoid and tetanus immune globulin for patients who haven't had an initial immunization series.

• rabies prophylaxis, if rabies is considered possible. It should be given without delay; consult a doctor before starting therapy. (See *Guide to postexposure rabies prophylaxis,* page 302.)

• antibiotics to nullify infection, as indicated.

Later actions

Animal bites. If the puncture wounds are simple and don't involve the hands, no other treatment is necessary.

Moderate to severe wounds should be debrided, and the patient should be given penicillin orally four times per day, for 3 to 5 days. If no signs or symptoms of infection appear after 2 days, the wound may be closed with sutures or tape strips.

Human bites. Obtain wound cultures to rule out gram-negative organisms.

The patient should receive penicillin and a beta-lactamase-resistant penicillin, such as amoxicillin. Wound closure should be delayed for 2 days; the wound should then be closed only if no infection is evident.

Splint clenched-fist injuries and elevate; use X-ray to rule out fractures.

Follow up within 2 to 3 days.

Referral or consultation

 COLLABORATION Collaborate with the doctor for all bites in which rabies is suspected. Refer clenched-fist injuries to a plastic surgeon or hand surgeon. Refer facial wounds to a plastic surgeon.

Patient teaching

• Advise anyone who has witnessed an animal bite to tell the authorities where the incident occurred and the animal owner's name, if possible. If the animal was wild, tell them the animal's location at the time of the bite. Authorities will try to capture the animal and then confine it for 10 days of observation. If it appears rabid, it will be killed and its brain tissue tested for rabies.

• Tell the patient that symptoms of infection usually appear after 24 hours. At least once daily, observe for signs of infection (fever higher than 101° F [38.3° C], redness, increased swelling, red streaks in the skin, or cloudy, yellow, or green drainage) or a lump in the wound that grows.

GUIDE TO POSTEXPOSURE RABIES PROPHYLAXIS

Decisions about rabies treatment must consider the details of the exposure, the animal's species and vaccination status, and the prevalence of rabies in the region. The wound should be thoroughly cleaned with soap and water. All bites by an animal of questionable health or vaccination status require prompt evaluation. The table below provides general guidelines for the next actions to take. Note that all three types of rabies vaccines are considered equally safe and effective by the Food and Drug Administration (FDA).

Animal species	Condition of animal at time of attack	Treatment of exposed human
Wild: Skunk Raccoon Bat Other carnivores	Considered rabid unless proven negative (the animal should be killed and the head tested immediately; observation not recommended)	Rabies immune globulin, human (RIG)* and human diploid cell vaccine (HDCV) or rabies vaccine, adsorbed (RVA**)
Domestic: Cat Dog	Healthy and available: 10 days of isolation and observation	None
	Unknown (escaped)	Consult public health officials and a doctor; if treatment is indicated, give RIG* and HDCV or RVA
Other: Livestock Gnawing animals (such as hamsters, rabbits, and beavers)	Rabies suspected or known	RIG* and HDCV or RVA** Consider individually

*RIG should be administered at the beginning of treatment. Administer 20 IU/kg I.M. This product isn't FDA approved for intradermal use.

**HDCV or RVA are equally effective. Administer 1 ml of vaccine I.M. on days 0, 3, 14, and 28. If using HDCV, divide the dose in half, giving one-half I.M. and one-half infiltrated thoroughly around the wound. HDCV is the only rabies vaccine approved by the FDA for intradermal use.

Adapted with permission from Goroll, A., et al. *Primary Care Medicine: Office Evaluation and Management of the Adult Patient*, 2nd ed. Philadelphia: Lippincott Williams & Wilkins, 1987.

ALERT Tell the patient to call the primary care provider to report any signs of infection.

Open trauma wounds
ICD-9-CM 879.8

Open trauma wounds (abrasions, avulsions, crush wounds, lacerations, missile injuries, and punctures) are injuries that commonly result from home, work, or motor vehicle accidents and from acts of violence.

Clinical presentation

In all open wounds, assess the extent of injury, vital signs, level of consciousness (LOC), obvious skeletal damage, local neurologic deficits, and general patient condition. Obtain an accurate history of the injury from the patient and witnesses, including such details as mechanism and time of injury, LOC, and any treatment provided. If the injury involved a weapon, notify the police as mandated by law.

Also assess for peripheral nerve damage — a common complication in lacerations and other open trauma wounds — as well as for fractures and dislocations. Signs of peripheral nerve damage vary with wound location as follows:
• radial nerve: weak forearm dorsiflexion, inability to extend thumb in a hitchhiker's sign
• median nerve: numbness in the tip of the index finger; inability to place the forearm in a prone position; weak forearm, thumb, and index finger flexion
• ulnar nerve: numbness in the tip of the little finger, clawing of hand
• peroneal nerve: footdrop, inability to extend the foot or big toe
• sciatic and tibial nerves: paralysis of ankles and toes, footdrop, weakness in leg, numbness in sole.

Management

Stop bleeding by applying direct pressure on the wound. If the wound is on an extremity, elevate it if possible, and apply pressure to pulse points proximal to the wound. Don't apply a tourniquet unless you must risk loss of the limb to save the patient's life; it may cause tissue damage that requires amputation.

Increased respirations, decreasing LOC, thirst, and cool, clammy skin all indicate blood loss and shock, and emergency medical services should be activated.

For all types of open wounds, follow up in 2 to 3 days.

Abrasions

Abrasions are open surface wounds of the epidermis and possibly the dermis, resulting from friction; nerve endings are exposed. Abrasions present as scratches, reddish welts, or bruises, accompanied by pain and a history of friction injury.

Obtain a history to distinguish the injury from a second-degree burn.

Clean the wound gently with a topical germicide, and irrigate it. Avoid vigorous scrubbing of abrasions, which increases tissue damage.

Remove all imbedded foreign objects. Apply a local anesthetic (lidocaine) if cleaning is painful.

Apply a light, water-soluble antibiotic ointment (bacitracin) to prevent infection.

If the wound is severe, apply a loose protective dressing that allows air to circulate.

If appropriate, give tetanus prophylaxis: 0.5 ml of tetanus toxoid I.M. for patients who have been immunized in the past but haven't had a booster within the past 5 years, or 0.5 ml of tetanus toxoid and tetanus immune globulin for patients who haven't had an initial immunization series.

Puncture wounds

Simple puncture wounds of extremities are small-entry wounds that aren't likely to involve damage to underlying structures or have any retained foreign objects. They commonly have ragged edges, occur on the face or fingers, and may be caused by a human or animal bite. If you suspect damage to underlying structures or the presence of a foreign object, immediately refer the patient to an emergency department.

Check the patient history for bleeding tendencies and use of anti-coagulants, and check the description of the injury, including force and depth of entry.

ALERT Don't remove impaling objects before transporting the patient to the emergency department. If an eye is involved, call an ophthalmologist immediately.

Thoroughly clean the injured area with soap and water. Irrigate all minor wounds with saline solution after removing any foreign object. Apply a dry, sterile dressing.

Provide tetanus prophylaxis: 0.5 ml of tetanus toxoid I.M. in patients who have been immunized in the past but haven't had a booster within the past 5 years, or 0.5 ml of tetanus toxoid and tetanus immune globulin in patients who haven't had an initial immunization series.

Lacerations

Lacerations are open wounds resulting from penetration by a sharp object or from a severe blow with a blunt object.

Apply pressure and elevate the injured extremity to control bleeding. Irrigate with saline solution. Debride necrotic margins and close the wound using strips of tape or sutures unless contamination is likely.

Grossly contaminated lacerations or lacerations over 8 hours old. Order a broad-spectrum antibiotic (cephalexin) for at least a 5-day course. Don't close the wound, but do apply a sterile dressing and splint. After 5 to 7 days, close the wound with sutures or tape strips if it appears uninfected and shows healthy granulated tissue.

All other lacerations. Check the patient history for bleeding tendencies and anticoagulant use. Determine the approximate time of the injury and estimate the amount of blood lost. Assess for neuromuscular, tendon, and circulatory damage.

Give tetanus prophylaxis: 0.5 ml of tetanus toxoid I.M. in patients who have been immunized in the past but haven't had a booster within the past 5 years, or 0.5 ml of tetanus toxoid and tetanus immune globulin in patients who haven't had an initial immunization series.

Stress the need for follow-up and suture removal.

ALERT If sutures become infected, culture the wound and scrub with surgical soap preparation. Remove some or all sutures, and give a broad-spectrum antibiotic such as cephalexin. Instruct the patient to soak the wound in warm, soapy water for 15 minutes three times a day and to return for a follow-up visit every 2 to 3 days until the wound heals. If the injury is the result of foul play, report it to the authorities as required by law.

Referral or consultation

COLLABORATION Many open wounds require emergency medical transport to the emergency department, including any avulsion injury, crush injury, deep puncture wound, a wound that may contain a retained object, one in which underlying structures may be damaged, a wound with ragged edges, or a missile injury such as a gunshot wound. Inform emergency medical services personnel of pertinent information, including the patient's condition when you first saw him, his medical history, allergies, and the name of the primary care provider.

All lacerations that are gaping or are more than ¼″ (0.64 cm) long involving the face or areas of possible functional disability, such as the elbow or hand, need to be seen by a doctor or a plastic surgeon in the emergency department.

Patient teaching

• For puncture wounds, instruct the patient to apply warm soaks daily and to report any signs or symptoms of infection.
• For lacerations, instruct the patient to elevate the injured extremity for 24 hours after injury to reduce edema. Tell him to keep the dressing clean and dry and to report any signs or symptoms of infection.

Poisoning

ICD-9-CM due to botulinum 005.1, Salmonella 003.9, Staphylococcus 005.0, Streptococcus 005.8, noxious or naturally toxic foods 988.0, acute/bacterial/disease/infected food 005.9 (more specific code may be required)

Poisoning may involve a variety of substances. In most cases, the poisonous substance is ingested. With an ingested poison, the main concern is the possibility of systemic effects. Poisoning can result in organ failure or death, depending on the substance and the extent of exposure. Most accidental poisonings involving children under age 6 are harmless because they have ingested nontoxic substances or toxic substances in amounts so minute that they're harmless. Most toxic substances are bad tasting, and the child usually spits them out. One exception to be aware of is antifreeze, which tastes sweet. Most poisoning episodes can be managed in primary care settings.

Ingested poisons fall into three general categories:
• corrosive (caustic) substances, such as household bleaches, metal polishes, antirust solutions, paint and varnish removers, drain cleaners, refrigerants, fertilizers, and photographic chemicals

• petroleum-based substances, such as floor polish and wax, furniture polish and wax, gasoline, kerosene, and lighter fluid
• substances that are neither corrosive nor petroleum-based. Most accidental poisons are of this type.

Causes

Poisonings can be accidental or purposeful (as in a suicide attempt). Children are the typical victims of accidental poisoning because of their natural curiosity.

The patient history must be focused and specific but nonjudgmental because purposeful poisonings are cries for help and caregivers of accident victims usually feel guilty or distraught.

 ALERT The patient who is suspected of having tried purposeful poisoning should be closely watched and requires emergency psychiatric evaluation.

Clinical presentation

Signs and symptoms of poisoning vary with the type and amount of poison swallowed. Often, the ingestion is suspected soon after it happens, and signs and symptoms will be absent. Also, many substances will never produce signs and symptoms because they are of low toxicity.

History may reveal nausea and vomiting, stomach cramps, headache, weakness, and burning sensations in the mouth, throat, or stomach.

Examination may reveal respiratory changes or difficulty breathing; diarrhea, possibly with stomach cramps; excessively dilated or constricted ("pinhole") pupils; a dull, masklike facial expression; facial twitching; drooling or excessive salivation; diaphoresis; an altered state of consciousness, delirium, or mental disturbances; changes in skin color,

WHAT THE PATIENT'S BREATH MAY REVEAL

Some swallowed poisons affect the patient's breath, as described in this table. If you suspect your patient has been poisoned, smell his breath and report any peculiar breath odor to the primary care provider or emergency medical services personnel.

Odor	Possible poison
Alcohol-like	Alcohol
Bitter almonds	Cyanide
Garliclike	Phosphorus, arsenic
Gasoline-like	Petroleum-like products
Pearlike	Chloral hydrate
Shoe polish-like	Nitrobenzene
Stale tobacco	Nicotine
Sweet	Acetone
Violets	Turpentine

particularly around the lips or fingernails; abnormally fast or slow pulse; coughing; abdominal gas; muscle spasms; seizures; complete or partial paralysis; loss of voluntary muscle control; clumsiness; burned or damaged skin; unusual breath odor; change in urine or stool color; and vision or hearing problems.

If such signs or symptoms are present but no one witnessed the poisoning, instruct someone at the site to check for telltale signs that a poisoning has occurred — an open medicine or household chemical container; spilled liquid, powder, or pills; liquid, powder, or pills in the patient's mouth or on the teeth; stains on the patient's clothing; burns or swelling on the hands or mouth; or a peculiar odor on the patient's breath, body, or clothes. (See *What the patient's breath may reveal.*)

Management

Immediate actions

If the patient shows signs or symptoms of poisoning, shake him gently and then check his airway, breathing, and circulation (ABCs). Administer cardiopulmonary resuscitation as needed.

Check vital signs every 5 minutes, apply pulse oximetry, and provide oxygen via facemask until the nature of the poison is known.

 COLLABORATION Call the poison control center immediately. Have the following information ready when you call:
• the patient's age and weight
• the name of the poison and its ingredients (or if it's a plant, the type of plant) and the amount of poison the patient has swallowed, if you know
• the time the poisoning occurred
• the patient's signs and symptoms
• any medical condition the patient suffers from — for instance, diabetes mellitus, high blood pressure, heart disease, or epilepsy — and what medications, if any, the patient takes regularly. Follow the instructions of the poison control center exactly.

WHEN NOT TO INDUCE VOMITING

Never induce vomiting in someone who has swallowed a corrosive or petroleum-like substance. Vomiting could cause further damage or lead to other complications. For example, an acidic or alkaline substance burns the mouth and throat when swallowed and can cause more burning if vomited. A petroleum-like product gives off fumes that can cause severe pneumonia if inhaled into the lungs during vomiting.

Also, never induce vomiting in a patient who:
- is unconscious or losing consciousness
- is having or has just had a seizure
- complains of pain or a burning sensation in the mouth or throat
- has a serious heart condition (the strain of vomiting could aggravate the condition).

Aiding a conscious patient

If ABCs are present, maintain the airway by suctioning secretions, performing aspiration precautions, and placing an oral airway if needed.

If the patient is experiencing a seizure, take appropriate steps. (See "Seizure," page 310.)

Immediately contact the poison control center for any suspected ingestion of a nonfood. The poison control center has information on every available drug, household products, plants, and foods that can be dangerous. (Also see "Drug overdoses" in chapter 10, page 379.)

Giving ipecac syrup

Vomiting isn't induced in certain circumstances. (See *When not to induce vomiting.*)

If the patient doesn't vomit after you've given ipecac syrup twice, call the poison control center for further instructions. If the patient must be taken to a hospital emergency department immediately, send the following materials with him:
- a container of the patient's vomitus. It can be tested to determine the nature of the poison. Also notify emergency medical services personnel if the patient has vomited undigested tablets; if possible, estimate how many tablets the patient took by inspecting the vomitus.

- the poison container and any of its remaining contents to help identify the poison and estimate how much the patient swallowed. Send enough of a poisonous plant to allow accurate identification — for example, an entire mushroom or a branch with leaves, flowers, and berries.

Referral or consultation

 COLLABORATION Refer the patient to the emergency department when indicated by the poison control center or for symptoms of concern. Notify emergency medical services personnel of data given to the poison control center, plus psychiatric history, pertinent social history, current and past medication usage, and prior hospitalizations. Initiate emergency psychiatric consultation for suspected purposeful poisoning.

Patient teaching

 ALERT Instruct parents to childproof their homes by keeping all medicines in safety-cap bottles; locking away all medicines and toxins such as cleaning supplies, drain-cleaners, paints and thinners, auto products, and garden sprays; and labeling all containers and storing only edible substances in food and drink containers. Ipecac syrup should always be available for emergencies.

Respiratory arrest

ICD-9-CM 799.1

Respiratory arrest occurs when a person stops breathing. This life-threatening emergency prevents body organs from getting the blood and oxygen they need to function.

 ALERT Without oxygen, brain cells start to die within 4 to 6 minutes; irreversible brain damage and death follow quickly. Initiating artificial respiration within a few minutes increases the chances for survival.

Causes

A blocked airway, depression of the respiratory center, and cardiac arrest are among the most common causes of respiratory arrest.

Blocked airway
In a person who has lost consciousness, breathing may stop as the muscles slacken and the base of the tongue falls backward, cutting off the airway. In a conscious person, a blocked airway can come from choking on food, swelling or spasms of the throat, or airway injury.

Depression of the respiratory center
The brain controls breathing through the respiratory center in the base of the brain. If a condition such as a stroke, head injury, or an overdose of certain drugs such as narcotics depresses the respiratory center, breathing slows and may even stop completely. In addition, electric shock can stun the respiratory center, halting breathing at least temporarily.

Cardiac arrest
When the heart stops beating—for example, from a massive myocardial infarction—the brain and other organs lose their blood supply and cease functioning. This prevents the respiratory center from sending signals to the pulmonary system telling it to keep breathing. About 1 minute after the heart stops beating, breathing ceases.

Clinical presentation

The hallmark of respiratory arrest is absence of breathing. If you come upon someone who seems to be unconscious, look, listen, and feel for signs of breathing, taking no more than 5 seconds. If you don't see the chest move or hear or feel the flow of air, assume the patient isn't breathing.

You may also notice other indications of respiratory arrest such as cyanosis. In a light-skinned person, look for a dusky or bluish tinge to the skin and mucous membranes. In a dark-skinned person, check for ashen gray oral mucous membranes and lips.

Management

Immediate actions
For an unconscious patient, check airway, breathing, and circulation and begin cardiopulmonary resuscitation as needed.

Although you'll usually use mouth-to-mouth resuscitation when administering rescue breaths, this method isn't right for everyone. You may need to assist these patients differently, as described below.

Giving mouth-to-nose resuscitation:
You'll need to give mouth-to-nose resuscitation if the victim is an infant, you can't get the patient's mouth

PROTECTION IN A POCKET MASK

Most emergency medical personnel and other professional rescuers carry a pocket mask. By diverting the patient's exhaled air away from the rescuer's mouth during artificial respiration, this device eliminates direct contact with the patient's mouth or nose and greatly reduces the risk of contact with secretions.

Other advantages

Besides virtually eliminating the risk of catching a disease during artificial respiration, the pocket mask has other advantages:

• If appropriately equipped, the mask can be connected to an oxygen cylinder. This allows delivery of a high flow of oxygen to help support body tissues as the rescue effort continues.
• The mask can be strapped to the face and used as a face mask to deliver oxygen when the patient resumes breathing.

How to use the mask

Fit the mask over the patient's nose and mouth, clamp it to his face, and exhale into it until the patient's chest rises.

open, the patient's mouth has been badly injured, or you can't create an effective seal around the person's mouth — for example, because of loose dentures or lack of teeth.

To give mouth-to-nose resuscitation, first tilt the patient's head back by pressing one hand on the forehead. Using your other hand, lift his lower jaw and close his mouth. Take a deep breath, and then seal your mouth around the patient's nose. Exhale until you see his chest rise, and then remove your mouth from the patient's nose. If possible, open his mouth to let the air out.

Giving mouth-to-stoma resuscitation:

A patient who has had his larynx removed breathes through a stoma in the front of the neck; mouth-to-mouth or mouth-to-nose resuscitation won't be effective because the air won't reach the lower airway. Instead, you must deliver breaths directly into the stoma.

To do this, uncover the stoma. Remove any clothing and jewelry covering the stoma, and clear any foreign matter from the stoma. If the patient has a breathing tube, make sure it

isn't clogged. If the tube is clear, leave it in place; otherwise, remove it.

Next, take a deep breath. Then seal your mouth over the stoma. Blow into the stoma the same way you would to give breaths at the mouth.

Although some people are afraid of catching acquired immunodeficiency syndrome (AIDS) when giving mouth-to-mouth resuscitation, only a small percentage of people with AIDS carry human immunodeficiency virus (HIV) in their saliva. There are no documented cases in which HIV has been transmitted this way— not even among rescuers who have given mouth-to-mouth respiration to people with AIDS.

Physicians estimate that the chance of becoming infected with HIV while giving mouth-to-mouth resuscitation is extremely small. To help eliminate even this tiny risk, many professionals use a pocket mask during resuscitation. (See *Protection in a pocket mask*.)

Referral or consultation

 COLLABORATION All patients with respiratory arrest need to be evaluated in the emergency department. Activate emergency medical services. Inform emergency medical services personnel of pertinent information, including the patient's condition when you first saw him, his medical history, allergies, and the name of the primary care provider.

Seizure

ICD-9-CM 780.39, atonic 345, febrile 780.31, repetitive 780.39

A seizure is a sudden episode of uncontrolled electrical discharge along the neurons of the brain causing abnormal neurologic functioning. It may result in respiratory arrest from secretions blocking the airway, status epilepticus, head or spinal injuries, bruises, Todd's paralysis and, rarely, cardiac arrest. (See *How a seizure develops*.)

Seizures may be partial (stemming from abnormal electrical activity in a specific brain region) or generalized (caused by abnormal electrical activity throughout the brain). The most severe type of seizure, generalized tonic-clonic (grand mal) seizure, reflects the paroxysmal, uncontrolled discharge of neurons, leading to neurologic dysfunction. A generalized tonic-clonic seizure can strike when the patient is awake and active or when he's sleeping.

Other types of generalized seizures include myoclonic, clonic, tonic, atonic, akinetic, and absence seizures. Types of partial seizures include simple partial and complex partial.

Causes

A seizure can occur for no known reason (called idiopathic or primary epilepsy). In children, fever sometimes brings on generalized seizures. Sometimes, however, the underlying cause is a life-threatening condition,

such as arsenic poisoning, brain abscess, lead poisoning, severe pre-eclampsia, myxedema coma, meningitis, electrolyte abnormalities, hypoglycemia, cerebral hemorrhage, or Reye's syndrome.

Other conditions that may precipitate a seizure include reaction to the contrast agents used in radiologic tests, arteriovenous malformation, brain tumor, cerebral aneurysm rupture, cerebrovascular accident (stroke), chronic renal failure, hepatic encephalopathy, hypoparathyroidism, hypoxic encephalopathy, inborn errors of metabolism, intermittent acute porphyria, multiple sclerosis, neurofibromatosis, trauma, sarcoidosis, Sturge-Weber syndrome, infection or brain abscess, ingestion of toxins (mercury or lead), and metabolic abnormalities, including hypoglycemia or hyperglycemia.

To identify common causes of seizures, use this mnemonic device: WITH LA COPS — *W*ithdrawal from alcohol or barbiturates; *I*soniazid; *T*heophylline and tricyclic antidepressants; *H*ypoglycemia and hypoxia; *L*ead, local anesthetics, and lithium; *A*nticholinergics, aminophylline, alprostadil, amphetamines, and analgesics (meperidine and propoxyphene); *C*holinergics, camphor, carbon monoxide, cimetidine, and chloroacetophenone (tear gas); *O*rganophosphates; *P*henothiazines, penicillins, and phencyclidine; and *S*ympathomimetics, salicylates, and strychnine.

Clinical presentation

Assessment findings depend on the type of seizure and may vary with the underlying cause.

Status epilepticus

Status epilepticus may occur as one prolonged seizure or as many consecutive seizures without the patient ful-

HOW A SEIZURE DEVELOPS

A seizure results from a disturbance in the depolarization-repolarization cycle of neurons, caused by the following sequence of events:

• The glial cell fails to keep the extra-cellular potassium level down.
• At the dendrite, the resulting potassium leakage leads to abnormal excitability.
• In the nerve cell body, abnormal membrane permeability leads to a defect in the pumping mechanism, causing depolarization.
• At the synapse, repetitive after-discharge stimulation causes abnormal "reverse activation."

ly recovering in between. It's most commonly triggered by abrupt discontinuation of anticonvulsant drugs. If the seizure is generalized, it can threaten the patient's life by jeopardizing cardiopulmonary function. Status epilepticus can also cause brain damage.

Generalized tonic-clonic seizure

Just before onset of a tonic-clonic seizure, the patient may experience mood changes along with an aura (smelling, tasting, feeling, hearing, or seeing peculiar things). As seizure activity spreads throughout the brain, the patient loses consciousness and falls to the ground. His body stiffens and then undergoes rapid, synchronous muscle jerking and hyperventilation. The seizure usually stops after 2 to 5 minutes, when abnormal conduction of neurons stops.

Myoclonic seizure

During a myoclonic seizure, the patient experiences jerking of one or more muscle groups, which lasts several seconds.

Atonic seizure

Also called a drop attack, an atonic seizure causes muscle jerking followed by muscle slackening.

Akinetic seizure

The patient experiencing an akinetic seizure has a brief, complete loss of muscle tone and consciousness and then falls to the ground, possibly suffering a head injury.

Absence seizure

Formerly called petit mal seizure, an absence seizure causes the patient to stop all activity and stare into space, usually for less than 15 seconds. During this time, he isn't aware of his surroundings. Others may notice nothing unusual about his behavior, although over time an observer may notice the staring episodes. Absence seizures are most common in children.

Simple partial seizure

The patient with a simple partial seizure may display odd movements in one part of the body or unusual movements that spread in an orderly fashion to surrounding body parts. Some patients also have tingling or numbness of a body part; however, mental status remains relatively normal.

Complex partial seizure

With a complex partial seizure, the patient usually has an aura and then loses consciousness. He may also experience a twilight state, with time seeming to stand still, or may experience déjà vu. Some patients laugh in-

THERAPEUTIC MANAGEMENT GUIDELINES: STATUS EPILEPTICUS

Status epilepticus is defined as a period of continuous seizure activity lasting longer than 30 minutes or as the occurrence of two or more successive seizures without return of consciousness between them. The diagram on these pages illustrates recommended treatment options for status epilepticus in adults.

Within 5 minutes of onset	6 to 9 minutes after onset	10 to 20 minutes after onset
• Diagnose status epilepticus by observing continuous seizure activity. • Provide life support measures. • Monitor blood pressure (BP), temperature, respiratory function, pulse oximetry, and electrocardiogram (ECG) changes. • Test venous blood for complete blood count and levels of glucose, electrolytes, toxins, and anticonvulsants. • Obtain sample for arterial blood gases to assess oxygenation.	• Administer thiamine 100 mg I.V. • After thiamine, give 50 ml of dextrose 50% solution I.V. piggyback if patient is hypoglycemic or if blood glucose level isn't known. • Monitor BP, temperature, respiratory function, pulse oximetry, and ECG.	• Administer lorazepam 0.1 mg/kg I.V. at 2 mg/min. • Alternatively, administer diazepam 0.2 mg/kg at 5 mg/min. Repeat diazepam if seizures don't stop within 5 minutes. • If diazepam is used to stop the seizures, phenytoin should be administered next to prevent recurrent status epilepticus.

Based on recommendations of the Epilepsy Foundation of America's Working Group on Status Epilepticus. ("Treatment of Convulsive Status Epilepticus," JAMA 270: 854-59, 1993.)

appropriately. If the temporal lobe is the site of the abnormal brain activity, the patient will display automatisms, which are involuntary repetitive movements, such as chewing, lip-smacking, facial grimacing, or rubbing his clothes.

 ALERT Other conditions that laypersons may interpret as seizures are migraine headaches, narcolepsy, panic attacks, and muscle twitches. History should focus on details observed during the episode.

Management

Immediate actions

The top priority in this medical emergency is to keep the patient from harm and to observe him during the seizure. Your observations will help determine what type of seizure the patient has had and which brain area was involved. (See *Therapeutic management guidelines: Status epilepticus.*)

If you're with a patient who experiences an aura, help him into bed or onto the floor, and then place a pil-

21 to 60 minutes after onset	**More than 60 minutes after onset**	
• Administer phenytoin 15 to 20 mg/kg I.V. at a rate not to exceed 50 mg/min by I.V. bolus or I.V. piggyback in normal saline solution. Final concentration should not exceed 5 mg/ml. Flush catheter with saline before and after administration. • Or, administer fosphenytoin 15 to 20 mg PE (phenytoin sodium equivalent)/kg I.V. at a rate not to exceed 150 mg PE/min by I.V. bolus or I.V. piggyback in normal saline solution or dextrose 5% in water. • Monitor for changes in ECG, BP, and respiratory function. If changes occur, decrease infusion rate.	• If status epilepticus doesn't stop with phenytoin 20 mg/kg, administer additional doses of phenytoin 5 mg/kg I.V. to maximum cumulative dose of 30 mg/kg. • If status epilepticus persists, administer phenobarbital 20 mg/kg I.V. at 60 mg/min. Monitor BP and respiratory function.	If status epilepticus persists: • Obtain neurologic consultation. • Consider initiating barbiturate-induced coma using phenobarbital or pentobarbital I.V. • Monitor vital signs continuously. • Provide ventilatory assistance and vasopressors as needed.

low, blanket, or other soft material under his head. Loosen his clothing, and move any sharp or hard objects out of the way.

During a seizure, stay with the patient and be ready to intervene in case airway obstruction or other complications occur. If possible, have another person obtain appropriate equipment (soft pillow and blanket, for example) and activate emergency medical services. Note the time of seizure onset.

Don't try to restrain the patient or restrict his movements during a seizure. The force of the patient's movements can cause a fracture.

If a patient seems to be in the beginning of the tonic phase of a tonic-clonic seizure (marked by muscle contraction and stiffening of the body), insert an oral airway into his mouth, if available, so his tongue won't block his airway.

ALERT If an oral airway isn't available, don't try to hold the patient's mouth open or place your hands inside his mouth because you may be injured. When his jaw becomes rigid, don't try to force an oral airway (or any other hard object) into place because this may cause further injury, such as broken teeth.

To allow secretions to drain, turn the patient onto his side during the seizure (or during the clonic phase of a generalized tonic-clonic seizure, when respirations resume). If respirations don't return, check the patient's airway for an obstruction. Then check breathing and circulation, and begin cardiopulmonary resuscitation as needed.

Caring for the patient after the seizure

Protect the patient by providing a safe area where he can rest. When he awakens, reassure and reorient him. Assess his vital signs and neurologic status. Then record the following information:

• time the seizure started and stopped
• what happened just before the seizure (such as an aura or a strange mood)
• where the seizure began (what part of the body, what side)
• what happened during the seizure (for example, what type of muscle movements the patient made and whether he lost consciousness or fell down, made noises, drooled, lost bowel or bladder control, stopped breathing, frothed at the mouth, or made repetitive movements)
• what happened after the seizure (for instance, whether the patient was confused or groggy, fell asleep, complained of a headache, remembered having had the seizure, and experienced any residual weakness).

If the patient is known to have diabetes mellitus, obtain a blood glucose level and administer 50 ml of dextrose 50% in water by I.V. push as indicated.

A 100-mg bolus of thiamine may be given to a known alcoholic to stop the seizures if alcohol ingestion is suspected. Aggressive examination is needed because it's possible that the patient doesn't remember the trauma or didn't note it while intoxicated. All patients with seizures caused by alcohol withdrawal require hospitalization for treatment.

If the seizure is prolonged and the patient shows signs of oxygen deprivation, resuscitation measures must begin immediately. Rarely, a patient may require endotracheal intubation. Permanent neurologic damage can occur within 1 hour of uncontrolled seizure activity.

Later actions

When the seizure stops or is under control, determine and treat the underlying cause. Extensive evaluation, including magnetic resonance imaging (MRI), is indicated for any adult with his first seizure. MRI is the preferred procedure because it's best for detecting subtle changes; if this isn't available, a computed tomography scan with and without contrast may be used.

Follow-up depends on the etiology of the seizure and is needed for recurrent seizures.

Referral or consultation

 COLLABORATION Status epilepticus is a medical emergency. Call for emergency medical services and report pertinent information, including the patient's condition when you first saw him, his medical history, allergies, and the name of the primary care provider.

Refer the patient to a neurologist or neurosurgeon if any condition in addition to epilepsy is considered.

WHAT HAPPENS IN SHOCK

Normally, blood vessels open or close to control the amount of blood flowing to various parts of the body. In shock, however, blood flow regulation goes awry, and the mechanisms that the body uses to compensate can't keep up with the problem. The result is that body tissues and organs don't get enough blood and oxygen.

Causes
Shock can result from:
• massive blood loss
• blood vessels that open but can't be filled because of a relative shortage of blood
• inability of the heart to pump and circulate enough blood.

Consequences
Without sufficient blood flow to provide oxygen to body organs, cells begin to die. Brain cells in particular can't withstand an oxygen shortage for long without sustaining damage.

Patient teaching

• Most patients experience a period of decreased mental functioning when a seizure ends. Reassure the patient in a calm, confident tone of voice that this is normal and will soon resolve.

The following management regimen is important because up to 70% of patients with a first seizure have another within 1 year. Instruct caregivers to take the following precautions to help prevent injury during a seizure:
• Keep soft pillows and blankets handy.
• Pad sharp edges and hard surfaces of the bed with towels or blankets secured by large safety pins. Cover safety pins with masking or adhesive tape to prevent them from opening.
• Don't take an oral temperature with a glass thermometer because it can shatter during a seizure. Take a rectal or axillary temperature with a glass thermometer because it can shatter during a seizure. Take a rectal or axillary temperature instead.
• Make sure the patient knows to get into bed immediately and call for help if he experiences an aura because this frequently heralds onset of a seizure.

Shock

ICD-9-CM 785.50

Shock is a state of impaired circulation that reduces the flow of blood and oxygen to body cells. The body tries to compensate for these shortages through a series of complex responses. Unless treated promptly, these compensatory mechanisms quickly fail and death occurs. (See *What happens in shock.*)

Causes

Shock can take the form of hypovolemic, cardiogenic, septic, or anaphylactic shock.

Hypovolemic shock occurs when an illness or injury leads to massive blood or fluid loss. Conditions capable of causing massive blood loss include motor vehicle accidents, excessive vomiting or diarrhea, trauma wounds (such as from a knife or gunshot), and burns.

Cardiogenic shock is a condition of diminished cardiac output that severely impairs tissue perfusion. Myocardial infarction (MI) is the most common cause of cardiogenic shock. Other precipitating conditions include myocardial ischemia, papillary muscle dysfunction, and end-stage cardiomyopathy.

Septic shock results from widespread infection, usually gram-negative bacteria, which may begin from a minor infection. Toxic substances are released from certain bacteria in the bloodstream, leading to massive infection. Septic shock usually follows signs and symptoms of severe infection. Diseases and conditions that predispose a patient to septic shock include age extremes (the very young and the elderly), diabetes mellitus, liver disease, invasive procedures (for example, insertion of a catheter), and immune suppression, such as from acquired immunodeficiency syndrome or drug therapy for cancer.

Anaphylactic shock is a severe allergic reaction that may bring on vascular collapse. It results from exposure to sensitizing drugs or other substances, such as serums, vaccines, enzymes, hormones, penicillin and other antibiotics, local anesthetics, salicylates, diagnostic chemicals (such as radiographic contrast dye), foods (such as legumes, nuts, berries, seafood, and egg albumin), sulfite-containing food additives, and insect venom (honeybees, wasps, hornets, yellow jackets, fire ants, mosquitoes, and certain spiders). See "Anaphylaxis," page 278.

Neurogenic shock results from neurologic or psychiatric factors. Examples include spinal cord injury, pain, fright, gastric dilation, and vasodilator drugs.

Clinical presentation

Early signs and symptoms common to all types of shock include anxiety, restlessness, or agitation; possibly a fast, weak pulse; rapid breathing; decreased urine output; cool, pale, clammy skin; and possible thirst.

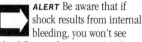 **ALERT** Be aware that if shock results from internal bleeding, you won't see blood flowing from a wound, but you may notice other telltale symptoms. For instance, internal bleeding may cause coffee-ground vomitus, vomiting of bright red blood, or black or bright red stools. Suspect internal bleeding in any patient who has suffered a hard blow, has fallen, has been in an accident, has a stomach ulcer, or is a heavy drinker.

If shock progresses, the patient may show signs and symptoms of decreased blood flow to the brain, such as confusion, sluggishness, or lethargy. Also look for decreasing blood pressure, a weak and thready pulse, shortness of breath, wheezing, cyanotic or pale skin (pale mucous membranes in a dark-skinned patient), cold or clammy skin, edema, nausea, vomiting, enlarged pupils, and orthostatic changes in vital signs.

In late stages of shock, the patient may become unresponsive and severely hypotensive, with an extremely slow, weak-to-absent pulse; rapid breathing or slow, shallow breathing; severely decreased urine output; and cold, mottled, ashen, or cyanotic skin.

Management

The first priority is to treat or remove the underlying cause.

Immediate actions

If you suspect a patient is in shock, immediately activate emergency medical services. Assess airway, breathing, and circulation, and start cardiopulmonary resuscitation as indicated.

If the patient takes one or more drugs such as epinephrine for a severe allergic reaction, help him to take it. Unless you suspect a neck or spine injury, keep the patient lying down, preferably flat on his back. If injuries don't restrict his movement, elevate his feet 12″ to 18″ (30.5 to 45.5 cm). This will promote blood flow to his head and the central organs. If this position causes pain or difficulty breathing, lower the patient's feet. Don't place the patient on his back, however, if he has trouble breathing or symptoms of an MI. Instead, raise him to a half-sitting position to ease his breathing.

If vomiting seems likely or if the patient has suffered a jaw or mouth injury, place him on his side so fluids can drain out of his mouth.

Never move the patient if you suspect a head or neck injury unless his life is in immediate danger from a fire, an explosion, or some other threat. If the patient has a head injury but not a neck injury, raise his head slightly.

If the patient is bleeding, try to stop the bleeding. If you suspect the patient has a broken bone, splint it. (See "Splinting and taping" in chapter 8, page 355.)

Keep the patient warm and comfortable by wrapping him in blankets or other available materials. Be sure to cover his head, neck, and hands. If he's lying on cold, damp ground, put blankets underneath him if you can safely do so unless he has a neck injury. (However, be sure not to make him too warm.) Loosen any tight clothing at the patient's neck, chest, or waist that might restrict his breathing or circulation.

Until the emergency medical services personnel arrive, monitor the patient's pulse at regular intervals and continue to watch for changes in mental status. For instance, as shock worsens, the patient may become confused or sluggish.

If you know the patient is diabetic and he seems alert enough to swallow, give him a small amount of sugar, orange juice, cake icing, milk, candy, or other sugary food to counteract low blood sugar.

Don't give fluids if emergency medical services personnel are en route or if the patient is unconscious, vomiting, or having seizures. Also withhold fluids if you think the patient has a stomach wound, a brain injury, or rectal bleeding.

If the patient is at a medical facility, follow these steps:
• Place the patient in Trendelenburg's position.
• Give oxygen.
• Treat severe pain.
• Obtain blood samples for laboratory tests and arterial blood gas analysis.
• Check urine flow.
• Monitor carotid venous pressure.
• Replace volume with crystalloid solutions and colloid solutions.
• Consider using vasoactive drugs, such as dopamine and dobutamine; corticosteroids such as methylprednisolone; diuretics such as furosemide; and heparin.
• Treat cardiac disorders.

Referral or consultation

 COLLABORATION All patients in shock require evaluation at an emergency department. Inform emergency medical services personnel of pertinent information, including the patient's condition when you first saw him, his medical history, allergies, and the name of the primary care provider.

Sprains and strains

ICD-9-CM 848.9

A sprain is a complete or incomplete tear in the supporting ligaments surrounding a joint that usually follows a sharp twist. A strain is an injury to a muscle or tendinous attachment. Both injuries usually heal without surgical repair.

Clinical presentation

In assessing these injuries, it's important to err on the side of caution; pain over a bone is considered a fracture until proven otherwise. A sprain causes local pain (especially during joint movement), swelling, loss of mobility (which may not occur until several hours after the injury), and a black-and-blue discoloration from blood extravasating into surrounding tissues. A sprained ankle is the most common joint injury.

A sprain causes maximal pain when the ligament is stretched. For example, inversion and plantar flexion of the foot commonly causes pain in a sprained ankle, whereas eversion and plantar flexion are relatively painless.

A strain may be acute, resulting from vigorous muscle overuse or overstress, or chronic, resulting from repeated overuse. An acute strain causes a sharp, transient pain (the patient may report hearing a "snapping noise") and rapid swelling. When severe pain subsides, the muscle is tender; after several days, ecchymoses appear. A chronic strain causes stiffness, soreness, and generalized tenderness several hours after the injury.

In sprain or strain, history usually reveals a recent injury or chronic overuse.

The patient history and examination may reveal more serious injuries, such as inability to bear any weight due to pain, joint instability, tenderness localized to a particular bone, increasing pain or edema, or signs of vascular compromise (pallor or cyanosis, paresthesia, "pins and needles" sensation, inability to move the joint).

Sprains are graded based on their severity, as follows:
• *Grade I:* partial or complete tear of the ligament, causing local tenderness, minimal edema; usually able to bear weight. Treatment is usually symptomatic with elastic compression support to control edema. Intermittent removal of immobilization, with active range-of-motion (ROM) exercises, progresses as tolerated. Strengthening exercises start at 2 to 3 weeks, depending on patient tolerance.
• *Grade II:* partial or complete tear of ligaments, causing painful weight bearing and minimal ligament function during examination. Treatment is the same as for Grade I, plus immobilization and nonweight bearing with an air splint or cast; treatment may switch to hinged-joint immobilization at 2 weeks.
• *Grade III:* Ligamentous laxity, instability, and complete interruption in alignment causing inability to bear weight and, often, obvious deformity. After evaluation by an orthopedic surgeon, treatment usually consists of a cast worn for 3 weeks. After 3 weeks, physical therapy, including ROM exercises, strengthening exercises, and proprioception training, begins. However, the orthopedic surgeon may cast for up to 6 weeks or perform surgical repair.

Diagnosis

A history of recent injury or chronic overuse, clinical findings, and an X-ray to rule out fractures establish the diagnosis.

ALERT If there is pain within 2″ (5.1 cm) proximal or distal to the joint plus bone tenderness within 2½″ (6.35 cm) of the bone, X-rays are required to check for fracture. Orthopedic referral is needed for any patient who's unable to bear any weight on the affected extremity from immediately after the trauma until the time of examination. All new bony abnormalities, regardless of size, require urgent orthopedic referral. If such a referral is unavailable, refer the patient to the emergency department.

Management

Treatment of sprains consists of controlling pain and swelling plus immobilizing the injured joint to prevent further injury and allow healing. Immediately after the injury, use RICE therapy (rest, ice, compression, elevation). Apply an elastic bandage wrap or, if the sprain is severe, a soft cast or splint. The goal is pain-free full range of motion. Codeine or another analgesic may be necessary if the injury is severe.

Chronic strains usually don't need treatment, but heat application, nonsteroidal anti-inflammatory drugs such as ibuprofen, or an analgesic-muscle relaxant such as cyclobenzaprine can relieve discomfort.

Control swelling by resting as much as possible and intermittently applying ice for 12 to 48 hours. To prevent frostbite, place a towel between the ice pack and the skin, leaving it in place for no more than 20 minutes at a time.

Immobilize the joint, and control swelling by using an elastic bandage as directed. Teach the patient to reapply it by wrapping from below to above the injury, forming a figure eight. For a sprained ankle, apply the bandage from the toes to midcalf. Tell the patient to remove the bandage before going to sleep and to loosen it if it causes the limb to become pale, numb, or painful.

Position the limb with the affected joint elevated above the level of the heart as much as possible for 2 to 3 days; pillows can be used for elevation during sleep.

Patients with sprains or strains are usually treated on an outpatient basis, so provide gait training and verify proper technique with crutches to reduce the risk of permanent axillary nerve damage and falls.

After 48 hours, a heating pad set at WARM replaces the ice packs, using the same schedule for pain relief and to enhance resorption of edema.

Call the primary care provider if pain worsens or persists; a later X-ray may reveal a fracture that wasn't originally visible.

Follow up within 1 week and then as needed if the patient is greatly improved. Refer to an orthopedist in 2 weeks if little improvement is noted.

Referral or consultation

 COLLABORATION Urgent orthopedic or emergency department evaluation is needed for Grade III sprains or strains (obvious deformity, inability to bear any weight on the joint, or joint instability). See *Muscle-tendon ruptures,* page 320.

Patient teaching

• Inform the patient that an immobilized sprain usually heals in 4 to 6 weeks, after which the patient can gradually resume normal activities. Occasionally, however, torn ligaments don't heal properly and cause recurrent dislocation, requiring surgical repair.
• Athletes may tape their wrists and ankles before sports activities to prevent injury.

MUSCLE-TENDON RUPTURES

Perhaps the most serious muscle-tendon injury is a rupture of the muscle-tendon junction. This type of rupture may occur at any such junction, but it's most common at the Achilles tendon, which extends from the posterior calf muscle to the foot. An Achilles tendon rupture produces a sudden, sharp pain and, until swelling begins, a palpable defect. Such a rupture typically occurs in men between ages 35 and 40, especially during physical activities, such as jogging or tennis.

To distinguish an Achilles tendon rupture from other ankle injuries, the primary care provider (PCP) performs this simple test: With the patient prone and his feet hanging off the foot of the table, the PCP squeezes the calf muscle. If this causes plantar flexion, the tendon is intact; if it causes ankle dorsiflexion, it's partially intact; if there is no flexion of any kind, the tendon is ruptured.

An Achilles tendon rupture usually requires surgical repair, followed first by a long leg cast for 4 weeks and then by a short cast for an additional 4 weeks.

• Avoid excessive physical stress, and wear appropriate gear for activity. Be aware of the risks associated with specific activities (for example, sports).
• Emphasize rationale for appropriate conditioning, warm-up, and cool-down exercises.

Subconjunctival hemorrhage

ICD-9-CM 372.72

Subconjunctival hemorrhage is a local blood vessel rupture that causes a flat, bright-red hemorrhage under the conjunctiva. It is a self-limited, benign condition that clears within 3 weeks.

Causes

Subconjunctival hemorrhage may result from minor trauma or from a Valsalva maneuver, such as coughing, sneezing, vomiting, or attempting to defecate.

Clinical presentation

The condition is asymptomatic, except for startling appearance. Consider conjunctivitis if any symptoms are present.

Management

This condition resolves spontaneously within 3 weeks. Aggressive evaluation is needed to locate other sites of bleeding. Hematology (prothrombin time/partial thromboplastin time/International Normalizing Ratio) is required if the patient is taking anticoagulants.

Follow up for any new or worsening symptoms.

Referral or consultation

 COLLABORATION Refer the patient to an ophthalmologist if blood appeared after trauma to the area or if there are persistent recurrences, pain, blurring or vision loss, any discharge, blood in the pupil or iris, or if the hemorrhage covers more than 25% of the sclera.

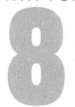

CHAPTER

8

Primary care procedures

Performing them
with confidence

Key procedures

Abscess incision and drainage

CPT code: 10060 I&D of abscess; 10080 I&D of pilonidal cyst, simple; 10081 I&D of pilonidal cyst, complicated; 10140 I&D of hematoma or seroma, or fluid collection

An abscess is a local collection of pus in a cavity formed by the breakdown of tissue and surrounded by inflamed tissue. Abscesses typically result from *Staphylococcus aureus* or a streptococcal infection. Males and children have a higher incidence of abscess formation.

Specific types of abscesses include furuncles, paronychia, pilonidal cysts, and perianal cysts. Furuncles, or boils, occur in hair follicles or sweat glands. Paronychia progress from cellulitis to abscesses over time and involve one or more fingernails or toenails. Pilonidal cysts result from ingrown hairs close to the anus and may have sinus openings. Perianal cysts typically result from a rectal fistula.

Equipment

ALERT Informed consent is required.

Antiseptic skin cleaner (such as povidone-iodine) ✧ topical anesthetic (such as ethyl chloride or a tissue freezing kit) ✧ 1% to 2% lidocaine with or without epinephrine or 50 mg/ml diphenhydramine (Benadryl) ✧ 3- to 10-ml syringe ✧ 25G to 30G ½″ needle ✧ 16G to 18G needle ✧ 4″ × 4″ sterile gauze pads ✧ #11 scalpel ✧ sterile drape ✧ sterile latex gloves (unless patient is allergic to latex) ✧ sterile curved hemostats ✧ iodoform gauze ✧ culture swab ✧ sterile scissors ✧ tape ✧ protective eyewear if abscess contents appear under pressure

Essential steps

• Position the patient comfortably with the abscess exposed.
• Clean the site and surrounding area with antiseptic skin cleaner.
• Apply the sterile drape, and put on sterile gloves.
• Anesthetize the area by freezing the surface with topical anesthetic or injecting the perimeter with lidocaine solution.
• With the scalpel, make an incision deep and wide enough to allow purulent material to drain easily and to prevent premature closure.
• Insert the culture swab deep into the wound to collect material for culturing. Alternatively, use a 16G or an 18G needle and syringe to withdraw fluid for culturing before incising.
• Use curved hemostats to explore the cavity and break down membranes leading to other fluid-filled compartments.
• After expressing all purulent material, pack the cavity with iodoform gauze, leaving at least ¼″ (0.6 cm) of gauze extending outside the wound.
• Dress the wound with sterile gauze.

Drugs

• Administer broad-spectrum antibiotic prophylaxis, such as cephalexin 500 mg three times as day, or cefadroxil 500 mg twice a day.
• Give a narcotic analgesic the first day, such as Tylenol #3 1 to 2 tablets every 4 hours, as needed.
• After day 1, administer a nonsteroidal anti-inflammatory drug (NSAID) such as ibuprofen.

Complications

Recurrence, cellulitis, gangrene, pain, scarring

Special considerations

• Don't inject lidocaine into the abscess because lidocaine loses its effectiveness in an acidic environment.
• Biopsy breast abscesses, excluding subareolar abscesses.
• For paronychia under the nail, use a hot paper clip or needle to bore through the nail and facilitate drainage. Partial removal of the nail may be necessary.
• For a pilonidal cyst, position the patient in the left lateral or lithotomy position. Probe the sinus tracts with a cotton-tipped applicator. If the abscess is more than 5 mm deep, refer the patient to a surgeon. If it's less than 5 mm deep, perform elliptical excision for pilonidal sinus. (See "Elliptical excision," page 338.)

Patient teaching

• Tell the patient to return for follow-up in 2 days.
• Tell the patient with a pilonidal cyst to take a sitz bath four times a day. Tell him to clean and irrigate the area with a flexible shower hose or water from a squeeze bottle and to leave the wound open to air to promote drainage and healing. Explain that the wound must heal from the inside outward, which can take up to 3 months.

 ALERT Tell the patient to call the primary care provider for signs of infection (increasing redness, swelling, pain, and warmth; cloudy yellow, green, or brown drainage; opening of wound; foul odor; a red streak from the wound area; or fever).

Anesthesia: Topical and local

CPT code: 01460 anesthesia for all integumentary system procedures involving lower leg, ankle, and foot; 01800 anesthesia for all integumentary system procedures involving forearm, wrist, and hand; 64450 introduction/injection of anesthetic agent for nerve block

Anesthesia causes loss of sensation, permitting surgical repair (such as incision and drainage), laceration repair, biopsy, foreign-body removal, and dislocation reduction. It's indicated for any procedure that causes pain that an anesthetic could eliminate and is contraindicated in patients who are allergic to a specific anesthetic. Factors that affect the type, amount, and duration of anesthetic needed include local blood supply, presence of infection, effects of certain chronic diseases, size of the affected area, and diameter and conduction of nerve fibers as well as psychological factors, such as anxiety and pain threshold.

Equipment and preparation

 ALERT Informed consent is required.

Topical, open wound less than 5 cm long

Tetracaine 2.5 mg with epinephrine 1:1,000, 2.5 ml, and cocaine 0.59G (TAC solution) diluted with sterile water to 5 ml

Topical, intact skin

Eutectic mixture of local anesthetic (EMLA)

ALERT Penetration occurs more quickly in diseased tissue, and effect penetrates less than 5 mm. EMLA is contraindicated for mucous membranes and genitalia.

Topical, intact skin, procedure lasting less than 3 seconds

Ice or ethyl chloride

Local

Medication appropriate for location and size of area requiring numbing ✧ antiseptic skin cleaner such as povidone-iodine solution (Betadine) ✧ clean latex gloves (unless patient is allergic to latex) ✧ appropriate-sized syringe for site ✧ 25G to 30G ½″ to 1″ needle ✧ anesthetic without a vasoconstrictor for poorly vascularized or infected areas or immunocompromised patients (optional addition of sodium bicarbonate 1 mg/ml:10 ml of a 1% concentration of anesthetic to significantly reduce initial burning sensation) ✧ anesthetic with a vasoconstrictor such as epinephrine for a clean wound in a highly vascular area (to reduce bleeding and systemic absorption) ✧ 4″ × 4″ sterile gauze pads

ALERT A vasoconstrictor is contraindicated for use in extremities (digits, nose, ear, penis); in patients with vascular disorders, diabetes, or thyrotoxicosis; and in areas with compromised blood flow (such as a skin flap).

Perform a complete neurologic examination of the affected area before the procedure, and document your findings in the medical record and consent form. Have the patient sign next to the description of the preprocedure abnormality. Check for allergies, particularly to iodine and latex.

Essential steps

Topical, open wound less than 5 cm long

• Remove visible debris.
• Fill the wound with TAC solution, or apply cotton balls soaked with TAC for 10 minutes.
• Monitor for systemic absorption and toxicity.

Topical, intact skin

• Remove oils from skin with soap, acetone, or alcohol.
• Apply EMLA and an occlusive dressing for 1 to 2 hours.

Topical, intact skin, procedure lasting less than 3 seconds

• Rub the skin firmly with ice for 10 seconds, or spray with ethyl chloride for no longer than 2 seconds (to reduce risk of blistering).

Local

• Position the patient with the affected area exposed.
• Put on gloves.
• Clean site and surrounding area with povidone-iodine solution.
• Identify the appropriate injection site. For digital anesthesia, use anterior and posterior web spaces of digit, close to the bone.
• Insert the needle at a 45-degree angle.
• Ask the patient if he notices any change in sensation. If he reports pain, indicating direct contact with the nerve, withdraw the needle 1 mm.
• Aspirate to make sure there's no blood return. If there is, the needle is in a blood vessel. Withdraw the needle slightly and reinsert in another area.
• Inject 1 to 2 ml of lidocaine while partially withdrawing the needle. Then redirect the needle across the surface, advance it, and inject another 0.5 ml while withdrawing the needle. This method distributes the anesthetic uniformly, providing the optimal effect.
• Massage the area gently. Maximum effect should occur in 5 to 15 minutes.

Complications

Ice or ethyl chloride: blistering from excessive freezing; TAC solution: mental status changes, seizures, arrhythmia, vomiting, flushing, urticaria; local: allergic reaction, anaphylaxis, ischemia, mental status changes, arrhythmia (from systemic absorption)

Special considerations

• TAC solution causes a positive urine cocaine screen for 72 hours.
• The duration of EMLA is 2 hours after removal of the dressing.
• Ice or ethyl chloride is useful for such procedures as skin tag clipping and before injecting a local anesthetic.
• Topical anesthesia is indicated for nosebleeds and eye injuries and before painful procedures on mucous membranes.
• Topical lidocaine and cocaine (a vasoconstrictor) start working in under 5 minutes. A dose of 1 to 2 drops of tetracaine (0.5%) is indicated before examination of an eye injury and has an onset of action of 5 to 8 minutes. These drugs readily penetrate mucous membranes. Topical phenylephrine (0.005%) can also cause vasoconstriction. Most topical anesthetics have a duration of action of 30 to 45 minutes.
• Duration of anesthetic for nerve block is 30 minutes to 1 hour; duration increases if a vasoconstrictor (such as epinephrine) is also used.

Patient teaching

Tell the patient that full sensation usually returns within 2 hours.

 ALERT Tell the patient to call the primary care provider for changes in sensation for more than 2 hours or signs of infection (increasing redness, swelling, pain, and warmth; cloudy yellow, green, or brown drainage; opening of wound; foul odor; red streak from wound area; or fever).

Corneal abrasion treatment

CPT code: 65205 removal of foreign body, external eye, conjunctival, superficial; 65210 removal of foreign body, external eye, conjunctival, embedded; 65220 removal of foreign body, external eye, conjunctival, corneal without slit lamp; 99070 eye tray: Supplies and material provided by doctor over and above what is usually included in office visit. ICD-9: 918.1

Injury to the covering of the cornea results in a corneal abrasion. The cornea has five layers: the epithelium (outer), Bowman's layer, stroma (middle), Descemet's layer, and endothelium (inner). The abrasion can result from chemical or mechanical injury (trauma), typically a contact lens or other foreign body in the eye. Injury limited to the epithelium heals without scarring; if the injury extends to Bowman's layer, scar tissue may form. Signs and symptoms include pain, the feeling that there is something in the eye, photophobia, tearing, blurred vision, and blepharospasm; the conjunctiva may also appear red from vascular response to the injury.

Equipment

Snellen chart ✧ topical ophthalmic anesthetic (such as 0.5% proparacaine or 0.4% benoxinate, unless the patient is allergic to ester anesthetics) ✧ sterile fluorescein sodium strips ✧ sterile cotton-tipped applicators ✧ bright white light source (penlight) ✧ Wood's light or other source of cobalt-blue light ✧ 8- to 10-power magnification (magnifying glass, ophthalmoscope on the +20 to +40 diopter setting) ✧ isotonic irrigant (sterile saline or other eye irrigation solution, such as Dacriose) ✧ sterile eye patches and 1″ paper tape ✧ cycloplegic drops for severe pain, such as 1 drop of 1% cyclopentolate HCl (2% for heavily pigmented eyes), repeated in 5 minutes if needed. (Note that the drug's effects peak in about 45 minutes and have a duration of up to a day, so pupils may be unequal on follow-up examination.)

ALERT *Don't* use fluorescein solution in place of fluorescein sodium strips. Use of fluorescein solution increases the risk of infection.

Essential steps

• Obtain a history of allergies, injury, and contact lens use and protective eyewear use.
• Perform vision screening.
• Examine the patient's pupillary reflex, extraocular movements, anterior and posterior chambers, and fundi.
• Have the patient remove contact lenses.
• Wash your hands and follow standard precautions.
• Inspect the eye and eyelid for erythema, drainage, and foreign objects.
• Place the patient in the supine position, with his head turned laterally to the affected side.
• Irrigate the eye copiously with ophthalmic irrigant.
• Tell the patient that the anesthetic causes a burning sensation at first. Then open the affected eye and instill 1 to 2 drops of ophthalmic anesthetic solution.
• Inspect the eye using the penlight and compare it with the unaffected eye. The sclera should appear intact, the anterior chamber free of mucus or blood, the iris normal in size and shape, the pupil normal in size and shape, and the pupils equally reactive to light. If the eye deviates from those findings, refer the patient to an ophthalmologist.

• Evert the upper lid by placing a cotton-tipped applicator on the upper lid, grasping the lashes, and turning the lid inside out over the applicator to expose the posterior surface of the upper lid. If available, use eyelid retractors to expose the conjunctiva.
• Examine for signs of trauma, foreign bodies, infection, sty, or inverted eyelash. (For foreign bodies, see "Removal of foreign body from the eye," page 349.)
• Moisten a fluorescein strip with 1 to 2 drops of sterile normal saline solution; you may use the patient's own tears instead. Don't use too much solution or too much staining will occur, making it difficult to identify a defect.
• Retract the lower lid and touch the fluorescein strip to the conjunctiva.
• Instruct the patient to blink to distribute the stain.
• Use Wood's light to examine the entire cornea and to identify areas of bright green concentrated fluorescence on the conjunctiva. The fluorescence indicates the location of the abrasion.
• If you don't find a defect or if you note vertical streaking on the cornea, suspect a foreign body embedded on the conjunctiva of the eyelid, and examine the entire conjunctiva.

ALERT If you still can't find the cause of the patient's signs and symptoms, refer him to an ophthalmologist.

• Gently rinse the eye with sterile saline solution to flush stain from the conjunctiva.
• Consider administering cycloplegic drops for severe pain. Instill antibiotic ointment for prophylaxis against infection. Don't administer more anesthetic because it could decrease the rate of healing, resulting in scarring.
• Encourage the patient to keep the eye closed (to reduce discomfort) and to avoid rubbing it.

• Consider covering the affected eye with an eye patch to promote patient comfort. Have the patient close both eyes and firmly tape two eye patches (the first patch folded in half) over the affected eye. Eye patches are contraindicated in young patients because of the risk of permanent effects on vision.
• Prescribe cycloplegic ophthalmic solution for pain control.
• Administer ophthalmic antibiotics for prophylaxis, such as tobramycin ointment 0.3%, ¼″ to ½″ (0.6 to 1.3 cm) given four times per day for 3 days, or sulfacetamide ointment 10%, ½″ to 1″ (2.5 cm) given four times per day and at bedtime for 3 days.
• Administer tetanus toxoid if the patient hasn't received immunization within the past 5 years.
• Schedule a return office visit in 24 hours for reevaluation and for removal of the eye patch, if applicable.
• Document the size and location of all abrasions. Illustrations can help, but be careful that the illustration doesn't seem to magnify the size of the lesion. During subsequent examinations, document the degree of healing.

Complications

Infection, scarring, permanent visual impairment, uveitis, conjunctivitis

Special considerations

 COLLABORATION For acute vision loss, a herpes lesion, an intraocular foreign body, blunt or sharp trauma to the eye, corneal infection, deterioration of vision or acute vision loss, chemical burns (after immediate copious irrigation for 15 minutes with tap water from a shower or hose), a metallic foreign body, possibly globe penetration (signs include hyphema, lens opacity, and pupil irregularity), non-

compliance (for instance, a child who may need sedation), a foreign body that can't be irrigated out, or an abrasion that's not healing well within 24 hours or completely healed within 48 hours, refer the patient immediately to an ophthalmologist. Also refer the patient for dendritic, large, or centrally located defects found on fluorescein examination as well as for signs of infection.
• Look carefully for a foreign body in the cul-de-sac if you note a pattern of multiple vertical lines during conjunctival staining.
• Perform Seidel's test if you suspect leakage of intraocular fluid. To do so, place a fluorescein strip directly over the site and look for a flow of green liquid.
• Don't patch the eye in a patient with only a small peripheral defect (less than 5 mm), in children, and in cases of suspected infection.
• Don't use topical corticosteroids; they may interfere with healing.
• If appropriate, encourage the patient to use protective eyewear at work and during recreational activities.
• Use a slit lamp for eye examination only if you're skilled in the technique.

Patient teaching

• Tell the patient that he must monitor his progress everyday until his eye is completely healed to catch such complications as infection at an early, treatable stage.
• Tell him not to rub his eyes; doing so could disrupt new layers of epithelial granulation and delay healing.
• Tell the patient who isn't wearing an eye patch to rest his eye, especially if he's a child or has a history of amblyopia.

 ALERT Tell the patient to call the primary care provider for symptoms that persist or recur, acute changes in vision, and signs of infection (rapidly increasing redness, swelling, pain, and warmth; cloudy appearance of the eye; yellow, green, or brown drainage; or fever).

Cryotherapy

CPT code: 57511 cryocautery of cervix, initial or repeat

Used to treat cervical intraepithelial neoplasia (CIN), cryotherapy uses freezing temperatures to destroy the outermost layer of cervical cells. Temperatures of 4° F (−20° C) or less for 1 minute or more kill the cancerous cervical cells. To perform the procedure, a probe that uses a refrigerant such as nitrous oxide to reach temperatures as low as −103° F (−75° C) is placed on the tissue. Repeated cycles of freezing and thawing produce more tissue destruction than one freezing treatment that lasts an equal amount of time, provided that each freezing cycle produces the maximum effect. Smaller lesions may require only one treatment, but larger lesions may require multiple freeze cycles, and persistent disease may require retreatment.

Cryotherapy is appropriate if the entire extent of the lesion is visible, CIN was diagnosed on biopsy, the patient has a normal endocervical canal and no dysplasia noted on endocervical curettage, and colposcopy, cytology, and histology findings are correlated.

General contraindications include a history of hypersensitivity or adverse reactions. Specific contraindications for cervical cryosurgery include invasive cancer, high-grade dysplasia, pregnancy, lack of correlation between a Papanicolaou (Pap) test or colposcopic impression and biopsies, inability to see entire lesion, a lesion extending beyond the reach of the probe, sexually transmitted disease, and the expected onset of menses within the next week. The procedure should be used cautiously in patients with collagen disorders, ulcerative colitis, glomerulonephritis, or high cryoglobulin levels (abnormal proteins that dissolve at body temperature but precipitate when cooled). The procedure also poses a risk to patients with a history of endocarditis, syphilis, Epstein-Barr virus infection, cytomegalovirus infection, or chronic hepatitis B. High-dose corticosteroid use can also result in exaggerated tissue damage.

Equipment and preparation

ALERT Informed consent is required.

Cryogun with nitrous oxide tank and 20- and 25-mm dermal tips ✧ liquid nitrogen with cotton-tipped applicators ✧ liquid nitrogen pressurized sprayer ✧ tissue freezing kit ✧ water-soluble lubricant (such as K-Y gel or Cryojel) ✧ cotton-tipped applicators ✧ timer or watch with a second hand ✧ vaginal speculum ✧ vaginal side-wall retractors or a condom or glove to place over the speculum (to avoid freezing the vaginal walls)

Premedicate the patient with a nonsteroidal anti-inflammatory drug, such as ibuprofen 800 mg, 1 hour before the procedure to decrease associated cramping and discomfort; most patients receive treatment in the office setting and don't need an anesthetic.

Essential steps

• Three basic scenarios exist, only the first of which is an indication for cryotherapy:
– the lesion is covered by the 20- or 25-mm probe

– the lesion extends beyond the probe and the ice ball can only extend to the lesion periphery but not uniformly beyond 4 mm of the extent of the lesion

– the lesion extends onto the vaginal fornices.

• Explain the procedure to the patient, and address concerns she might have.

• Assist the patient into the lithotomy position.

• Select a cryoprobe tip that will cover the lesion plus 5 mm beyond the lesion's borders.

• Select a flat or slightly conical tip to minimize inward migration of the squamocolumnar junction inside the os. Moisten the cryoprobe with warm water or saline solution and a thin layer of water-soluble lubricant to maintain good contact between the probe tip and the cervix.

• Turn on the gas and check the pressure. Insufficient pressure increases the time it takes the tissue to freeze.

• Apply the cryoprobe and begin freezing; start timing the freeze, and tell the patient you've started the procedure. When adherence occurs (after 5 seconds), apply gentle outward traction to center the probe in the cervix. Your goal is to prevent the vaginal walls from being affected without tearing the cryoprobe free.

• For benign cervicitis, freeze for one 3-minute period. For dysplastic CIN, freeze long enough to form an ice ball that extends at least 5 mm beyond the lesion. After the tissue thaws completely (5 to 10 minutes), repeat the entire process (called the freeze-thaw-refreeze cycle). Keep in mind that the timing isn't as important as formation of an adequate ice ball (also called cryolesion).

• Between freeze cycles, place the tip in warm water to increase efficacy.

• Tell the patient that pelvic and abdominal cramping is a normal, transient side effect. Expect tissues to flush during the thaw cycle.

Complications

Cramping and flushing commonly occur during the procedure. The squamocolumnar junction may be deeper in the os after the procedure, making subsequent examinations more difficult. Cervical stenosis may occur if a long tip is used. Rarely, infertility, bleeding, menstrual irregularities for up to 3 months, and infection occur.

Special considerations

• To produce an adequate cryolesion, make sure that the temperature at the periphery of the lesion and at 5-mm depth in the cervix reaches at least $-4°$ F ($-20°$ C) and is maintained for at least 1 minute. Adequate cryonecrosis at a depth of 5 mm requires a freeze-thaw-refreeze cycle of 5 minutes for each part of the cycle.

• For larger lesions, consider using a 25-mm probe, which may produce better results than a 20-mm probe. (See *Selecting the proper cryoprobe,* page 330.)

• Be aware that many cryosurgical units have a defrost function that causes the cryoprobe to detach less than 15 seconds after freezing stops; the gas must remain on to activate this defrost function.

• Keep in mind the following factors that require increased freeze time: increased size of the ice ball needed, low tank pressure, increased vascularity, extra keratin covering on the cervix (remove or moisten the keratin to decrease freeze time), and poor physical contact between the cryoprobe and lesion. The type of system used also affects freeze time.

SELECTING THE PROPER CRYOPROBE

Successfully freezing a lesion depends on selecting the appropriate cryoprobe tip. The shape of the tip determines the width and depth of the freeze area. Applying pressure to the cryoprobe allows the probe to freeze at a greater depth.

The first two illustrations here show the use of appropriately shaped cryoprobes. The final illustration shows an inappropriate cryoprobe. In this example, the probe doesn't cover the depth of the lesion.

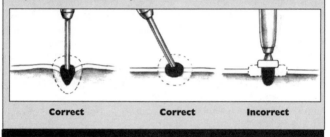

| Correct | Correct | Incorrect |

Patient teaching

• Tell the patient that cryosurgery will treat her cervical abnormality in the least invasive effective manner, preventing progression or worsening of the abnormality.

• Explain that a heavy watery discharge for at least 3 weeks — occasionally up to 8 weeks — can be normal; the discharge may be blood-tinged for a few days but should change to darker red to brown and lessen over time. Suggest that she wear a sanitary pad and change it at least every 4 hours. Also suggest that she douche with 1 tbs of vinegar in 1 cup of water or use a povidone-iodine vaginal suppository if odor becomes a problem.

• Tell her that she can resume normal activities but must refrain from sexual intercourse and from putting anything in the vagina, including tampons, for 2 weeks.

• Have her return to the office in 4 weeks for a postoperative examination, and tell her to follow up with a Pap test in 4 months; send her a reminder notice at that time.

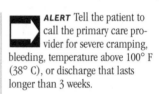 **ALERT** Tell the patient to call the primary care provider for severe cramping, bleeding, temperature above 100° F (38° C), or discharge that lasts longer than 3 weeks.

Cyst injection and removal

CPT code: 25111 excision of ganglion cyst, wrist, primary; 25112 recurrent; 26160 excision of lesion of tendon sheath or capsule (for example, cyst), hand or finger; 56420 I&D of Bartholin's gland abscess; 56740 excision of Bartholin's gland or cyst; 20600 arthrocentesis, aspiration, or injection of a small joint, bursa, or ganglion cyst (leg, fingers, toes); 20605 intermediate joint, bursa, or ganglion cyst (temporo-mandibular, acromioclavicular, wrist, elbow, ankle, olecranon bursa)

A ganglion cyst is a tumor that develops on or in a tendon sheath. Most commonly, the cause is chronic or recurrent inflammation from frequent strains or contusions at the site. Joints contain a thick, gel-like material. When this gel leaks from the joint into the weakened tendon sheath, it forms a cyst. Indications for removing the cyst are relieving discomfort and increasing joint mobility.

A Bartholin's cyst forms after inflammation of Bartholin's glands, resulting in an obstruction, edema, and pain. Causes include inspissated mucus, a congenitally narrow gland, and infection with *Neisseria gonorrhea*, *Staphylococcus*, *Streptococcus*, *Escherichia coli*, or *Trichomonas*. Signs and symptoms include labial swelling and pain, inguinal lymphadenopathy, dyspareunia, and a palpable mass.

Equipment and preparation

 ALERT Informed consent is required for injection and removal.

For injection: Antiseptic skin cleaner such as povidone-iodine ✧ sterile drape ✧ sterile latex gloves (unless patient is allergic to latex) ✧ 3- and 10-ml syringes ✧ 18G 1½" needle ✧ 22G or 25G 1½" needle ✧ 1% lidocaine (single-dose vials preferred because they contain no preservatives, decreasing the risk of allergic reaction) ✧ culture tube ✧ corticosteroid, short-acting (such as hydrocortisone 20 mg), intermediate (such as methylprednisolone 4 mg), or long-acting (such as dexamethasone 0.6 mg) ✧ sterile 4" × 4" gauze pads ✧ tape

For removal: Antiseptic skin cleaner, such as povidone-iodine ✧ sterile drape ✧ sterile latex gloves (unless patient is allergic to latex) ✧ 10- and 20-ml syringes ✧ 18G 1½" needle ✧ 25G 1½" needle ✧ 1% lidocaine, 5 to 10 ml (single-dose vials preferred because they contain no preservatives, decreasing the risk of allergic reaction) ✧ 250 ml normal sterile saline solution ✧ #11 scalpel ✧ sterile 4" × 4" gauze pads ✧ iodoform gauze ¼" or ½" wide ✧ sterile scissors ✧ sterile curved hemostats ✧ sterile forceps with teeth ✧ vaginal culture swab ✧ perineal pads

Essential steps

For injection

• Explain the procedure to the patient. Check the patient's history for allergies, especially to iodine and latex.

• Position the patient comfortably with the cyst clearly exposed.

• Clean the site and surrounding area with povidone-iodine solution.

• Apply the sterile drape, and put on sterile gloves.

• Use a small-gauge needle with the 3-ml syringe to draw up 2.5 ml of 1% lidocaine and 0.5 ml of corticosteroid. Agitate gently.

• Using the 10-ml syringe with the 18G needle, insert the needle into the cyst and aspirate. If the aspirate appears cloudy, send the specimen for culture and sensitivity and continue the procedure; if the return is bloody, remove the needle, apply a dressing, and end the procedure.

• Insert the needle of the syringe that contains lidocaine and corticosteroid, and aspirate for blood. If no blood appears, inject the medications.

• Remove the needle and apply a pressure dressing.

For removal of a Bartholin's cyst

• Explain the procedure to the patient.

• Check the patient's history for allergies, especially to iodine and latex.

• Instruct the patient to empty her bladder.

• Assist the patient to the lithotomy position, and drape the perineum appropriately.
• Clean the perineum with povidone-iodine solution.
• Set up a sterile field with open gauze, scalpel, needle, and syringes, and put on sterile gloves.
• Using the 10-ml syringe and 25G needle, draw up 5 to 10 ml of lidocaine.
• Insert the needle along the top of the cyst and aspirate. There should be no return. Inject as you withdraw the needle to obtain a field anesthesia effect.
• Use the scalpel to make an incision along the top of the cyst, ensuring that the incision is deep and long enough to permit easy drainage.
• Insert a gloved finger into the vaginal opening, positioning your finger medial to the abscess and applying gentle pressure to express all material possible.
• Use curved hemostats to aid inspection and to break any septa leading to fluid-filled cavities.
• Use the 20-ml syringe and 18G needle to irrigate the area with sterile saline solution.
• Fill in the cavity with iodoform gauze, leaving more than ¼″ (0.64 cm) extending from the cavity.
• Use a 4″ × 4″ gauze pad followed by a perineal pad to cover the site.

Complications

Infection, sepsis, recurrence, corticosteroid flare, atrophy of subcutaneous tissue

Special considerations

• Use only gentle pressure when expressing material from the cyst.
• Be sure to leave at least ¼″ of the iodoform gauze protruding from the cavity following cyst removal, to allow for removal of the gauze later.

Patient teaching

• For injection, tell the patient to leave the dressing on for 12 hours. Explain that redness, swelling, and warmth are normal. Tell her to rest and elevate the joint for 24 hours. If the cyst recurs, suggest cyst removal. Recommend a nonnarcotic analgesic, such as acetaminophen or ibuprofen, for pain, and tell the patient to follow up in 1 week.
• For removal, tell the patient that safe sex and careful perineal cleaning can help prevent recurrence. Tell her to remove half of the 4″ × 4″ gauze pads in 24 hours and the remaining pads after another 24 hours. Instruct her to change the gauze and perineal pads every 6 hours and as needed. Recommend a sitz bath with warm water four times a day for 1 week. Tell her to follow up in 1 week.

ALERT Tell the patient to call the primary care provider for signs of infection (rapidly increasing redness, swelling, pain, and warmth; cloudy yellow, green, or brown drainage; opening of wound; foul odor; red streak from wound area; or fever).

Defibrillation

CPT code: 92950 cardiopulmonary resuscitation (CPR)

Defibrillation delivers a controlled, untimed transcutaneous electric charge to the myocardium, depolarizing the heart muscle and often allowing the sinoatrial node to resume its inherent rhythm. Indications for defibrillation include ventricular fibrillation and pulseless ventricular tachycardia. Because no effective heart contractions occur during either of these arrhythmias, timing of the shock isn't important.

Defibrillation is always an emergency procedure. Its effectiveness depends on how quickly the rescuer starts the procedure and how well the underlying cause responds to the procedure.

Equipment

Defibrillator with anterior-posterior or transverse paddles (manual or external automatic defibrillator) or sterile internal myocardial paddles (if heart muscle is visible) ✧ conductive medium pads or gel ✧ electrocardiogram (ECG) monitor with recorder ✧ I.V. line and solution ✧ oxygen administration and suction equipment ✧ oral or nasal airway or intubation equipment ✧ hand-held resuscitation bag with 100% oxygen adapter and face mask ✧ transvenous or transthoracic pacemaker system ✧ emergency drugs, such as epinephrine, atropine, lidocaine, vasopressors

Essential steps

• Check that the patient is unresponsive.
• Open the airway, and assess for absence of spontaneous breathing.
• Provide two full ventilations.
• Assess for absence of carotid pulse (adult and child) or brachial pulse (infant).
• Call for help and initiate CPR until a monitor and defibrillator are available.
• Expose the chest wall.
• Apply the ECG monitor leads to the chest wall (avoiding paddle placement sites) or use "quick-look" paddles to determine cardiac rhythm. Quick-look paddles allow for single-lead interpretation of cardiac rhythm.
• For ventricular fibrillation or pulseless ventricular tachycardia, prepare to defibrillate.

• Apply conductive pads to chest wall, using transverse or anterior-posterior placement. If conductive pads aren't available, apply conductive gel to the paddles and place in the transverse or anterior-posterior position.
• Turn on the defibrillator.
• Select the appropriate energy level for defibrillation.
• Make sure the paddles are correctly placed.
• Warn everyone to step back from the patient. Then quickly scan the area to make sure that everyone and all unnecessary equipment are clear of the patient and bed.
• Charge the defibrillator for manual defibrillation or allow the external automatic defibrillator to determine its charge.
• Make sure the rhythm is still ventricular fibrillation or pulseless ventricular tachycardia.
• Activate the discharge buttons on the paddles of the manual defibrillator and keep the paddles on the chest wall until the paddles discharge.
• Assess the rhythm on the monitor and check the patient for a pulse.
• If defibrillation doesn't succeed, repeat three countershocks at increasing energy levels in rapid succession, after making sure everyone and all nonessential equipment are clear of the patient and bed.
• If the three rapid countershocks don't succeed, reinitiate CPR, provide manual ventilation, administer emergency drugs, and continue to defibrillate according to advanced cardiac life support (ACLS) protocol while transporting the patient to medical services.
• If defibrillation succeeds, assess the patient's vital signs, peripheral pulses, level of consciousness, and respiratory effort; administer emergency cardiac medications, oxygen or ventilation, and I.V. fluids; and continue cardiac monitoring while transporting the patient to medical services.

• Obtain a postdefibrillation ECG rhythm strip or 12-lead ECG.
• Document the patient's rhythm before defibrillation, time of each defibrillation, energy levels used, results of each defibrillation, and all other resuscitation measures used.

Complications

Death, chest wall injury or burns

Special considerations

• Make sure you're familiar with the defibrillator before using it.
• As needed, treat hypoxia, hypothermia, and acidosis — potential problems associated with ineffective defibrillation.
• Select correct energy levels sequentially from 200 to 360 joules per ACLS protocol for external defibrillation in adults. Use 2 joules/kg for children.
• Select 50 joules of energy for internal defibrillation.
• Announce "Charging defibrillator, stand clear" when charging the defibrillator.
• Maintain about 25 lb of pressure on each paddle during defibrillation.
• Don't defibrillate over a pacemaker or implanted cardioverter-defibrillator generator because doing so may interfere with the device's functioning.

Diaphragm fitting

CPT code: 57170 diaphragm or cervical cap fitting with instructions

The diaphragm is a barrier method of contraception that mechanically blocks sperm from entering the cervix. Its effectiveness ranges from 80% to 93% for new users and increases to 97% for long-term users. It's indicated for patients who prefer or require reversible contraception without medication. Contraindications include a history of toxic shock syndrome, vaginal stenosis, pelvic abnormalities, uterine prolapse, large cystocele or rectocele, allergy to spermicidal jellies or rubber, or being less than 6 weeks postpartum.

Equipment

Diaphragm fitting rings ✧ diaphragm ✧ lubricant (such as K-Y gel) ✧ diaphragm introducer (optional)

Essential steps

• After explaining the procedure to the patient, assist her into the lithotomy position.
• Insert your index and middle fingers as if performing a pelvic examination.
• Measure from the symphysis bone to the posterior of the cervix by touching the posterior fornix with your middle finger and raising your hand until the index finger touches the pubic arch.
• Use your thumb to hold your hand in place directly under the pubic bone.
• While maintaining your thumb position, withdraw your hand from the patient.
• Place one end of the diaphragm rim or fitting ring on the tip of the middle finger with the opposite side lying just in front of the thumb. This will give you the approximate diameter of the diaphragm. Diaphragms are manufactured in sizes of 60 to 90 mm, with the average being 75 to 80 mm.
• Lubricate the rim or dome of the fitting ring or diaphragm to lessen the discomfort of insertion.
• Fold the diaphragm in half with one hand by pressing the opposite

sides together. Hold the vulva open with the other hand.

• Slide the folded diaphragm into the vagina and toward the posterior fornix. It should fit from below the symphysis and cover the cervix. The proximal rim should fit behind the pubic arch with minimal pressure.

• Have the patient wiggle her hips to see if she feels the diaphragm in place. She shouldn't feel it.

• To remove the diaphragm, insert your index finger under the symphysis pubis and hook the diaphragm under the proximal rim. Gently pull the diaphragm down and out.

• Teach the patient how to insert and remove the diaphragm. Then leave the patient with the diaphragm in place so that she can practice inserting and removing it in private, leaving it in when she's done.

• Examine her to see if she inserted the diaphragm correctly.

Complications

Pregnancy from not using spermicidal jelly or from improperly placing the diaphragm (the result of poor technique or such body changes as a weight gain or loss of more than 15 pounds [6.8 kg] or surgery); recurrent urinary tract infections; discomfort or ulceration from an improper fit; teratogenic effects from the spermicide nonoxynol-9 (if the patient becomes pregnant)

Special considerations

• Although you shouldn't use spermicidal jelly for the demonstration, explain to the patient that she'll use it whenever she uses the diaphragm.

• You can obtain diaphragm fitting rings free from such companies as Ortho Pharmaceutical in sizes that increase in 5-mm increments.

• Several types of diaphragms exist. Most common in the United States,

the arching spring has a firm rim, needs no introducer, and is helpful to patients who have less pelvic support, cystocele, rectocele, or retroverted uterus. It tends to be easier to insert. The coil spring has a flexible rim and needs no introducer but requires good internal support and the cervix in the midplane or anterior position. The flat spring has flat-plane flexibility and may need an introducer. It's recommended for smaller women, those with a narrow pelvic shelf, and women who have never been pregnant.

Patient teaching

• Emphasize to the patient the importance of using the diaphragm with spermicidal jelly every time she has intercourse. Explain that she should apply about a teaspoon of spermicidal jelly (such as nonoxynol-9) to the concave surface and a thin layer around the rim.

• Teach her to insert one rim behind the pubic bone and the opposite rim behind the cervix and to confirm placement by feeling the cervix behind the dome.

• For subsequent coitus, she should leave the diaphragm in place and insert more spermicidal jelly into the vagina; she shouldn't douche.

• Tell her to leave the diaphragm in place at least 6 hours after the last session of intercourse but less than 24 hours.

• She should wash the diaphragm with mild soap and dry it after each use, soak it in a 10% bleach solution every other month, and inspect it at least once a month for holes and wear of the latex.

Dislocation reduction

CPT code: 21480 closed treatment of temporomandibular dislocation;

23650-55 of shoulder dislocation, with manipulation; 24600-5 of elbow dislocation; 26700-5 of metacarpophalangeal dislocation, single, with manipulation; 26770-75 of interphalangeal joint dislocation, single, with manipulation

Reduction and follow-up care for uncomplicated finger or toe dislocations can take place in the primary care setting. A patient with a shoulder, patella, or radial head dislocation needs a referral to an orthopedist after reduction in the primary care setting. A patient with a dislocation of a large joint or concurrent fracture requires a systemic analgesic or conscious sedation before reduction; such a procedure should be attempted only if neurologic or vascular compromise endangers the limb. Emergency departments can provide cardiac monitoring, oxygen, and resuscitation carts, allowing the use of I.V. analgesia (such as fentanyl) during reduction.

Equipment and preparation

Cleaning solution such as alcohol or povidone-iodine solution ◇ 3 ml lidocaine without epinephrine ◇ 5-ml syringe with 25G needle

Essential steps

• Obtain radiographic confirmation to rule out fractures and to determine the direction of dislocation.
• If necessary, use an assistant to help stabilize the patient. For a pediatric patient, the parents usually provide the best assistance and can help calm the child.
• As needed, use an oral narcotic or muscle relaxant or both, but have naloxone (Narcan) available and monitor the patient's vital signs and

airway patency during and after the procedure.

Finger or toe reduction

• Use a digital nerve block. Clean the digit with povidone-iodine or alcohol. Infiltrate up to 3 ml of lidocaine (without epinephrine), using a 25G needle for field anesthesia. (See "Anesthesia: Topical and local," page 323.)
• Grasp and stabilize the proximal segment in one hand.
• With your other hand, grasp and apply firm and steady longitudinal traction to the distal segment in the direction of angulation.
• Slowly move the distal segment in the opposite direction of the angulation while continuing to apply steady traction and pressure to the dorsal side.
• Continue moving the distal segment toward the neutral position until reduction occurs.
• Check joint stability.
• Apply an aluminum finger splint with tape to maintain the joint in position of function; you can tape a stable joint to the adjacent finger.
• As needed, obtain an X-ray to confirm positioning of the joint.

Shoulder reduction
First method

• With the patient in a supine position, grasp and support his upper arm above the elbow with both hands and support the forearm under your own arm against your body. Make sure the arm is adducted, externally rotated, and flexed.
• Apply firm, steady distracting axial traction to the arm, pulling it distally. ("Distracting" means to pull away from the skeletal attachment.)
• While maintaining traction, slowly ease the arm into the shoulder until reduction occurs. You may also need to provide some internal or external rotation or slight pressure directed

anteriorly from beneath the upper arm.

• As needed, ask an assistant to apply countertraction to stabilize the patient. Do this by wrapping a bed sheet around the patient's upper torso and having the assistant apply countertraction from the side opposite the affected shoulder.

• Obtain anteroposterior and axillary lateral X-rays to confirm reduction.

• Apply a sling and swath to prevent shoulder external rotation and abduction.

Second method (Stimson technique)

• Use this method for patients with recurrent dislocations. Place the patient in a prone position on the examination table with the involved extremity hanging off the table toward the floor.

• Apply steady traction to the distal extremity, either manually or with a 10- to 15-lb (4.5- to 6.8-kg) weight attached to the patient's wrist. Reduction should occur within a few minutes. You may need to provide some rotation or flexion of the extremity.

Patella reduction

• Place the patient in a supine position. Apply steady manual pressure to the lateral aspect of the patella with one hand while slowly extending the knee with the other hand until reduction occurs.

• Rule out patella fracture or rupture of the patellar or quadriceps tendon.

• Apply a knee immobilizer to prevent knee flexion.

Radial head subluxation in children (nursemaid's elbow)

• Rule out elbow, shoulder, and clavicle fracture or dislocation.

• Seat the child in the parent's lap. Explain to the parent that the child may experience brief pain with the procedure but then should experience immediate relief of symptoms once reduction occurs.

• Grasp the patient's wrist and distal forearm in one hand and support the elbow with the opposite hand, with the thumb over the radial head.

• Supinate the forearm, rotating the hand palm up.

• Flex the elbow until you feel a snap over the radial head, indicating that the orbicular ligament has reduced.

• The child shouldn't require a sling or immobilization.

Complications

Malposition or failure to maintain reduction, vascular compromise, neurologic compromise, opioid overdose

Special considerations

 COLLABORATION Attempt reduction of a large joint or a joint with a concurrent fracture only if acute vascular or neurologic compromise threatens the limb. Otherwise, refer the patient to an orthopedist or send him to the emergency department for reduction. Dislocations of the elbow, hip, knee (femorotibial), and ankle also require emergency referral unless acute neurovascular compromise exists. Most dislocations should be referred to an orthopedist after reduction.

Patient teaching

• Tell the patient to call or return at once if redislocation, loss of normal sensation of the limb (numbness and tingling), or increased pain occurs.

• Explain that the joint will probably swell for 24 to 48 hours after the injury and that keeping the joint elevated and applying ice for 20 minutes intermittently should minimize pain and swelling.

• Tell the patient with a patella or shoulder dislocation—especially a patient under age 30—that the risk of recurrence is high; explain the need for possible surgical treatment.

Doppler ultrasonography

CPT code: 93922 noninvasive physiologic studies of upper- or lower-extremity arteries, single-level, bilateral (includes ankle/brachial indices, Doppler waveform analysis, volume plethysmography, and transcutaneous oxygen tension measurement)

Doppler ultrasonography consists of an audio unit, volume control, and a transducer that detects the movement of red blood cells. It's used to determine arterial blood flow when blood perfusion may be compromised (for instance, in a cool, edematous, pale, cyanotic, or apparently pulseless extremity) and to determine placement for an arterial insertion.

Equipment

Doppler ✧ ultrasound transmission gel (not water-soluble lubricant) ✧ marking pen ✧ soft cloth and antiseptic solution or soapy water

Essential steps

• Position the patient comfortably with the affected area accessible.
• Mark the selected artery with the marking pen.
• Apply a small amount of coupling or transmission gel to the ultrasound probe.
• Position the probe on the skin directly over the selected artery.
• Set the volume control to the lowest setting. If your model doesn't have

a speaker, plug in the earphones and slowly raise the volume.
• To obtain the best signal, tilt the probe at a 45-degree angle from the artery, making sure to apply gel between the skin and the probe. Slowly move the probe in a circular motion to locate the center of the artery and the Doppler signal—a hissing noise at the heartbeat. Don't move the probe rapidly because this will distort the signal.
• After you've assessed the pulse, clean the probe with a soft cloth soaked in antiseptic solution or soapy water. Don't immerse the probe or bump it against a hard surface.

Complications

None common

Special considerations

• Don't place the Doppler probe over an open or draining lesion.
• Be sure to remove all conductive gel from the patient's skin.
• Be aware that failure to position the transducer properly can interfere with results.

Patient teaching

• Tell the patient that the worst discomfort is gel application.
• Explain the results and what options he has.
• If you detected good blood flow, teach the patient appropriate measures to prevent thrombosis (smoking cessation, elevation of the affected area, exercise, weight reduction).

Elliptical excision

CPT code: 11400-406 excision benign lesions on trunk, arms, or legs; 11420-426 on scalp, neck, hands, feet, or genitalia; 11600-

CHOOSING SUTURE MATERIALS

Sutures can be absorbable or nonabsorbable. Absorbable sutures are strands of suture material that eventually dissolve. Nonabsorbable sutures must be removed because the body can't dissolve them. This chart outlines various types of suture material and their indications for use.

Type of suture	Indications for use
Absorbable	
Plain gut	Rarely used due to its high tissue reactivity
Chromic catgut	Oral mucosa, vermilion border
Polyglycolic acid	Superficial closure of skin and mucosa
Nonabsorbable	
Silk	Tying off blood vessels
Nylon	Use and size of suture vary with location of wound: • 6-0 for eyelids and face • 5-0 for forehead, neck, and other delicate skin • 4-0 for neck, scalp, extremities, and back • 3-0 for running suture of scalp

606 excision malignant lesions on trunk, arms, or legs; 11620-626 on scalp, neck, hands, feet, or genitalia; (add 22 or 09922 for unusual or complex excision); 10080 I&D of pilonidal cyst, simple

In elliptical (also called fusiform) excision, the clinician can remove a skin lesion too large for a cutaneous punch and then suture the area closed, leaving behind a linear scar (larger lesions require a different form of excision and require skin flaps or grafts for closure). The location of the incision usually depends on the location of natural skin tension lines, which correspond with wrinkle lines. If such lines aren't readily apparent, gently pinching the skin in several directions should bring them out (this technique may not work with children and adolescents).

The goal of such surgery is to remove the lesion and leave as small a cosmetic defect as possible by following skin tension lines and, for lesions on the face, facial expressions. When deciding where to make the excision, the clinician must consider the depth of the skin; the impact of the excision on adjacent structures; the length, width, and orientation of the resulting scar; and the scar's effect on function. Placement of a shoulder incision, for instance, depends more on creating a scar that won't pull apart than on appearance. Ideally, the procedure will transform the oval-shaped wound left by the excision into a thin-line closure. Depending on the lesion's depth, the sutures may be absorbable or nonabsorbable or both. (See *Choosing suture materials.*)

Tools for marking the lesion before excision include a Devon skin marker, although the marker doesn't leave a very dark marking and tends to dry out when the cap is left off. Many clinicians prefer using an indelible marker, such as a Sharpie, although such markers can leave a tattoo if the ink isn't completely removed before closure.

USING THREE-POINT TRACTION

Making an elliptical excision requires that you maintain firm traction to the skin surface in more than one direction. The illustration below shows how to apply three-point traction to maintain multidirectional traction when making an elliptical excision. The arrows indicate the direction in which traction is being applied.

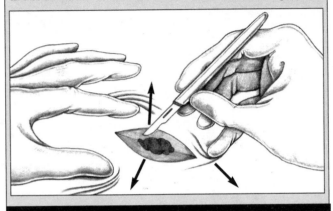

Equipment

Marker ✧ sterile gloves ✧ sterile drape ✧ masks ✧ protective eyewear ✧ antiseptic ✧ 2″ × 2″ or 4″ × 4″ gauze pads ✧ anesthetic ✧ #11 scalpel ✧ straight or curved iris scissors ✧ forceps or hook ✧ specimen container with 10% formalin ✧ electrocautery unit ✧ sutures ✧ suture needles

Essential steps

• Note the area in a circle at its clinical margins. Imagine a concentric circle around the first circle that includes the margin for normal skin. Use the marker to draw a final ellipse that's three times as long as it is wide.
• Wash and dry your hands, put on sterile gloves and a mask, and use eye protection.
• Administer the anesthetic, injecting it in a ring to obtain field anesthesia. Make sure that you anesthetize be-

yond the demarcated margins in anticipation of undermining.
• Use a gauze pad to apply antiseptic to the area, starting at the center and spiraling outward. Then drape the area to allow a clear view of the surgical site.
• Hold the scalpel like a pencil at a 90-degree angle, with the anterior belly of the blade in contact with the previously marked line. Apply three-point traction with the other hand, using firm, confident, vertical pressure at the corner of the ellipse. (See *Using three-point traction*.)
• Press down gently with the scalpel, and draw it through the skin in one firm, constant stroke, keeping the blade perpendicular to the skin surface (to avoid beveling the wound and margins). You don't have to cut through the skin's full thickness with a single stroke, but make sure you can see upper subcutaneous fat before trying to remove the specimen.
• Rarely, you may encounter a highly active blood vessel. If this happens,

UNDERMINING

Undermining, the technique of freeing the skin from underlying tissues, can decrease tension on the wound edge and is critical for obtaining acceptable cosmetic results after wound repair. Proper undermining minimizes scarring and keloid formation.

The level of undermining that should be done depends on the anatomic location of the wound and the natural plane of the wound. In general, undermine an area about the size of the widest part of the wound.

Blunt undermining
In blunt undermining, advance the scissors with the tips closed and then force them open. This causes blunt dissection of the underlying tissues.

Sharp undermining
In sharp undermining, a less-frequently used technique, use short, cutting strokes with a scalpel to separate the skin from underlying tissues.

Undermining tips
• Keep in mind that undermining increases the risk of bleeding. Make sure you can see the source of bleeding and can cauterize it safely.
• Treat the wound edge gently. Handle it with a single-pronged skin hook instead of forceps

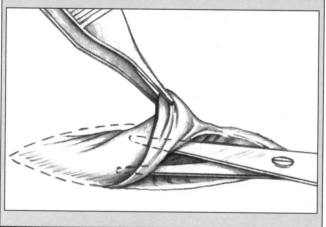

remove the blade and cauterize the affected site before continuing.
• After making the incisions, use a straight or curved iris scissors and forceps or hook and gently elevate one end of the fusiform ellipse.
• Insert the scissors through the subcutis and complete the incision through the subcutis along both sides of the specimen. Undermine the base completely and elevate the specimen. (See *Undermining*.)

• Place the specimen in a specimen container.
• Cauterize as needed to stop bleeding, but don't cauterize too much or the wound won't heal as quickly.
• Suture the wound closed (See "Suturing simple lacerations," page 359.)

Complications

Infection, scarring, pain

Special considerations

 COLLABORATION Refer the patient to a plastic surgeon for facial lesions greater than ¼" (0.6 cm); refer to a dermatologist for deep lesions.
• Keep in mind that wounds closed by approximation of the skin edges heal by primary intention.
• To speed healing and prevent crust formation, cover the wound with an occlusive or a semiocclusive dressing (particularly important for wounds created by a procedure).

Patient teaching

• Tell the patient to keep the sutures dry.
• Instruct him to remove the initial dressing in 24 hours and then clean it twice a day and cover it with ointment. The three-layer dressing consists of petroleum jelly or triple antibiotic ointment, a nonadherent dressing, and gauze followed by a tape covering. After the first day, tell him to replace the initial dressing with a smaller gauze bandage, being careful not to place the gauze itself directly over the wound (fibers in the gauze can get trapped in the wound edge, become matted, and delay healing).
• For suture removal, have him return in 3 to 6 days for a face wound, 7 to 10 days for an ear wound, and 5 to 10 days for a trunk or an extremity wound.
• Tell the patient to call the primary care provider for signs of infection (increasing redness, swelling, pain, and warmth; cloudy yellow, green, or brown drainage; opening of wound; foul odor; a red streak from wound area; or fever).

Fracture immobilization

CPT code: Casts: *29065 application, plaster, shoulder to hand (long arm); 29075 application, plaster, elbow to finger (short arm); 29085 application, plaster, hand and lower forearm (gauntlet); 29345 application, plaster, thigh to toes (long leg); 29355 application, plaster, thigh to ankle (cylinder); 29405 application, plaster, below knee to toes (short leg); 29425 application, plaster, walking or ambulatory type; 29440 adding walker to previously applied cast.* Splints: *29105 application of long-arm splint (shoulder to hand); 29125 application of short-arm splint (forearm to hand); 29130 application of finger splint; 29505 application of long-leg splint (thigh to ankle or toes); 29515 application of short-leg splint (calf to foot)*

Fractures must be properly immobilized to minimize discomfort, avoid any undue motion, ward off possible further injury, and allow time for proper healing of bones and ligaments.

Equipment

Disposable latex gloves (unless patient is allergic to latex) ✧ bucket of cool water ✧ tubular stockinette ✧ rolls of cast padding ✧ rolls of Fiberglas or plaster of Paris (from 1" to 6" rolls) ✧ sheet, towel, or gown to cover patient ✧ cast shoe for short-leg casts ✧ bandage scissors

Essential steps

• Measure a length of stockinette about 6" (15.2 cm) longer than the area you need to cast; this will allow for shortening of the stockinette as you pull it over the limb and for

some overlap at each end to turn down after you apply the cast material. Cut a thumb hole for an arm cast.
• Roll on the cast padding, overlapping by one-half the roll width with each turn. Start distally and roll proximally, leaving no gaps or wrinkles. Extend the padding about 2″ (5.1 cm) beyond the end of the planned cast. Apply extra padding over bony prominences and wounds and where the edge of the cast will be located.
• Maintain the limb in a neutral position unless otherwise indicated to correct the deformity. Preferred joint angles are 45 to 75 degrees of flexion for metacarpal, 10 degrees of flexion for distal interphalangeal, abduction for the thumb, 35 degrees of extension for the wrist, 90 degrees of flexion for the elbow, 10 to 15 degrees of flexion for the knee, 90 degrees of flexion for the ankle, and neutral for the subtalar.
• Wearing gloves, submerge a roll of casting material in water for a few seconds until saturated, briefly squeeze out excess water, and roll the first layer immediately. Start distally and roll proximally. Don't pull while wrapping; simply roll it on, overlapping the roll width by one-half with each turn. Gently mold with both hands around bony prominences, but don't squeeze hard enough to leave an impression in the cast.
• After applying the first layer, turn down the ends of the stockinette.
• Roll on the second layer of casting material, again overlapping by one-half with each turn. Take an extra turn or two over large joints, such as the knee and ankle, to provide extra reinforcement. If you reach the end of the cast before finishing the roll, continue back down the limb distally. Two or three layers are usually enough for upper-extremity Fiberglas casts; plaster casts require more layers. Lower-extremity casts also need

more layers, especially if the patient will bear any weight on the extremity. Pediatric casts need more reinforcement than adult casts.
• Keep the limb in the desired position until the cast hardens. Use bandage scissors to trim excess or rough edges before the material hardens completely. Fiberglas hardens within 5 minutes, allowing for weight bearing within 30 minutes. Plaster of Paris takes up to 24 hours to harden completely.

Complications

Neurologic or vascular compromise from excessively tight cast, skin irritation or breakdown from insufficient padding, fracture malunion or nonunion from poor cast positioning or molding, functional or ambulation impairment, or both, from joint malposition

Special considerations

• Keep in mind that Fiberglas is lighter and stronger, hardens more quickly, and is more radiolucent than plaster. Although plaster is cheaper and easier to mold than Fiberglas, it's also heavy, takes a long time to dry, and breaks down if it gets wet or worn down. Use plaster for temporary splints and in areas that require extensive molding to maintain the fracture position, especially in the hand. Applying Fiberglas without wetting it lengthens its drying time, giving you more time to mold or position a limb that's difficult to cast.
• When applying a short-arm cast, make sure the distal end doesn't extend past the metacarpophalangeal joint and add extra padding around the base of the thumb. Apply no more than two layers of cast material in the web space between the thumb and index finger, allowing room for the patient to pinch the thumb and

index finger together; having the patient pretend to hold a soda can will help him maintain the proper position. Keep the wrist extended at about 35 degrees to promote a grasping movement of the hand.

• When applying a thumb spica cast, apply a small tubular stockinette to the thumb and use less padding in the web space than you would for a short-arm cast.

• When applying a long-arm cast, add extra padding around the upper arm to prevent skin irritation. Provide a sling to prevent the cast edge from impinging on the underside of the upper arm.

• If applying a short-leg cast with the patient sitting on the examination table, take care to prevent ankle plantar flexion; you can use a special metal footrest designed for this purpose. Alternatively, place the patient in a prone position on the table with his knee flexed. Slightly angle the upper edge of the cast from the anterior, just below the tibial tubercle, to the posterior over the proximal calf to prevent the cast from impinging behind the knee when the patient flexes his knee. Make sure you can see all toes at the distal end of the cast. For a walking cast, reinforce the ankle and heel and add a plantar heel wedge to allow the foot to roll forward at heel strike. Apply a cast shoe to protect the toes and reduce wear on the cast.

Patient teaching

• Tell the patient to keep the cast dry; he can use a plastic bag to cover the cast when bathing adjacent areas and in wet weather.

• Tell him to elevate the injured limb as much as possible to limit swelling and to avoid extensive use or weight bearing unless instructed otherwise.

• Advise him not to push objects inside the cast to scratch (doing so may cause sores and infection) or to paint or varnish the cast (doing so will prevent air circulation around the skin), although he can have others sign the cast with a felt-tipped marker.

• Tell the patient to call the primary care provider for numbness, tingling, swelling, or pain (signs that the cast may be too tight, pinching nerves or constricting blood flow); irritation; skin breakdown at the cast's edges; painful or tight areas inside the cast.

Intra-articular and bursa corticosteroid injection

CPT code: 20550 injection sites include tendon sheath, ligaments, trigger points; 206000 arthrocentesis, aspiration, and/or injection of joint or bursa (for example, temporomandibular; acromioclavicular; wrist, elbow, or ankle; olecranon bursa); 20610 of major joint or bursa (for shoulder, hip, knee joint, subacromial bursa)

Often performed simultaneously with arthrocentesis, intra-articular corticosteroid injection can provide immediate relief from pain and swelling in the affected joint. Such injections typically provide only temporary relief, and the underlying cause still needs to be identified. Contraindications include suspected joint infection and recent fracture or known osteoporosis in the area. Corticosteroids used for injection include betamethasone, hydrocortisone, methylprednisolone, and triamcinolone. Because no corticosteroid has proved more effective, the choice lies with the clinician, based on cost and previous injection history.

Equipment

Povidone-iodine solution and alcohol sponges ✧ sterile latex gloves (unless

the patient is allergic to latex)
◇ drapes ◇ 1% or 2% lidocaine
solution without epinephrine, or fluoromethane spray, or both, for local
anesthesia ◇ sterile syringes (5- and
10-ml) ◇ 25G ⅝″ needle if performing local anesthesia with lidocaine ◇
18G and 20G 1½″ needles ◇ hemostat ◇ sterile 3″ × 3″ and 4″ × 4″
gauze pads ◇ corticosteroid

Essential steps

ALERT Informed consent is
required.

• Explain the procedure to the patient.
• Have all necessary equipment
ready.
• Place the patient in as comfortable
a position as possible to allow performance of the procedure.
• Carefully identify landmarks, and
mark the exact injection site by in-
denting the skin with the blunt end
of a ballpoint pen or a fingernail.
Such a marking won't readily wash
away.
• Clean the area with povidone-iodine solution and let it dry; repeat
this three times.
• Before injection, wipe the area with
the alcohol sponge to avoid getting
povidone-iodine in the joint.
• Using sterile technique, drape the
area and anesthetize it with topical
fluoromethane. If appropriate, use
the 25G ⅝″ needle to infiltrate the
subcutaneous skin with the lidocaine
solution (lidocaine may distort landmarks in smaller joints).
• Quickly insert the needle through
the skin to minimize patient discomfort. Avoid moving the needle from
side to side as it enters the joint. For
smaller joints, use a 22G needle with
a 3- to 5-ml syringe. For larger joints,
use an 18G needle.
• Aspirate as the needle advances
into the joint space or bursal sac un-

TWO-SYRINGE TECHNIQUE FOR INJECTING JOINTS

When you're performing joint injection with arthrocentesis, the two-
syringe technique can prove valuable.
After inserting a syringe into the joint
and aspirating joint fluid, attach a hemostat at the needle hub to stabilize
the needle while removing the syringe. Replace the syringe containing
the joint aspirate with a second syringe containing a corticosteroid and
inject the drug into the joint space.
When the injection is finished, remove the needle and apply pressure
and a sterile dressing.

til fluid flows freely to confirm the intra-articular or bursa location.
• Inject the corticosteroid into the
joint space.
• When performing joint injection
with arthrocentesis, use the two-
syringe technique. (See *Two-syringe
technique for injecting joints*.)
• To help distribute the corticosteroid
throughout the joint space, perform
passive range-of-motion exercises.
• Immobilize the joint, and provide
adequate analgesia for pain control.

Complications

The most serious complication is the
introduction of infection into the
area or the masking of an existing
infection; aseptic technique can help
reduce this risk. The patient should
not receive a corticosteroid injection
if infection is suspected.

Repeated injections may also result in necrosis of the joint space and
the juxta-articular bone, with subsequent joint destruction and instability. Other complications include tendon rupture, local soft-tissue atrophy,
hemarthrosis, and transient nerve
palsy.

High-dose or repeated corticosteroid injections may have long-term systemic effects. The patient may also experience corticosteroid arthropathy, a condition in which relief from symptoms results in the patient overusing the joint, causing further injury.

Special considerations

• You may inject large joints, such as the knee and shoulder, with the equivalent of 80 mg of methylprednisolone acetate with 1 to 2 ml of 1% lidocaine. Smaller joints require only 20 to 40 mg with 0.5 to 1.0 ml of 1% lidocaine.
• The patient shouldn't receive corticosteroid injections more than three times a year; more frequent injections may cause cartilage damage, systemic effects, and avascular necrosis.
• For corticosteroid injection, avoid direct contact with the skin or subcutaneous tissue to prevent skin atrophy. For intrabursal injection, inject the corticosteroid around—not into—the tendon or ligament. Because direct injection can lead to tendon or ligament rupture, reposition the needle if it meets resistance.

Patient teaching

• Explain to the patient that intra-articular injection is typically done in the office or emergency department and that he can go home after the procedure.
• Tell him to apply ice, compress the area with an elastic wrap, and elevate the joint to reduce swelling and pain. He should rest and immobilize the joint for several days after treatment. An immobilization device and crutches may encourage him to avoid overuse and weight-bearing activities

on the affected joint. Tell him to follow up within 1 week.

ALERT Tell the patient to call the primary care provider for signs of infection (increasing redness, swelling, pain, and warmth; unusual drainage; opening of wound; foul odor; a red streak from wound area; or fever) and warmth and increased pain and stiffness within the joint.

Papanicolaou test

CPT code: 88150 Pap smear interpretation — used by pathologist interpreting the specimen.

The Papanicolaou (Pap) test is most commonly used to detect cervical cancer. The cell sample can be placed on one or two glass slides, or Thinprep cells can be placed in a supplied bottle of fixative and then placed on slides by the laboratory.

Equipment

One or more slides or bottle ✧ spatula (wood if using slides, plastic if using Thinprep) ✧ cytobrush ✧ fixative for slide ✧ appropriate-sized speculum ✧ sterile latex gloves (unless patient is allergic to latex) ✧ drape

ALERT A cytobrush should always be used for a cervical or endocervical Pap, even on a pregnant patient.

Essential steps

ALERT Don't use any type of lubricant before a Pap test.
• Determine if the patient has any allergies, particularly to latex.
• Explain the procedure to the patient (if this is her first pelvic exami-

nation), and help her into the lithotomy position.

• Examine the vulva as well as Bartholin's and Skene's glands.

• Insert the speculum into the vagina, making sure you can see the entire cervix. If you can't, remove the speculum, insert your index finger into vagina and locate the cervix, and then reinsert the speculum.

• Insert the cytobrush into the endocervix, turning it 360 degrees. If you obtain a great deal of mucus, wipe it away without swabbing the endocervix.

• Take the spatula and lightly scrape around the ectocervix.

• Quickly place the cells on the slide, first with the spatula and then the cytobrush. To apply the cells, roll the brush across the surface of the slide or stroke both sides of the broom across the slide, placing the second stroke directly over the first.

• Apply fixative so that the cells don't dry out.

• If you're using Thinprep, use the same collection method, except use a plastic spatula. Once you've obtained the specimen, dip the spatula into the fixative, swish it around inside the bottle, and scrape off the cells. Then take the brush and move it in a circle in the bottle, wiping around the inside of the bottle 10 times.

• After finishing, remove the speculum from the vagina.

Complications

Discomfort, bleeding, flashbacks of trauma or abuse

Special considerations

• Look for lesions on the cervix and in the vaginal area, and include this area on the Pap smear, making a note of it on the Pap slip that's sent to the laboratory. Also note on the slip if any bleeding occurred, and note "contact bleeding" in the patient's chart. Don't use the term "friable," which can legally be misconstrued to mean a cancerous lesion, requiring colposcopy and biopsy.

• If the patient appears anxious or upset during the pelvic examination, stop at once, make eye contact, and ask if she wants you to stop. If she does, stop the examination, but discuss the importance of having a pelvic examination and Pap test at the next visit or with another provider. Once the patient has dressed, discuss your observations (for example, hands balled into fists, pallor, tears, and changes in breathing pattern) and ask if she wants to discuss anything. Think about your response in advance; you don't want to respond with hesitancy or silence if the patient discloses any trauma or abuse.

Removal of foreign body from the ear

CPT code: 69200 removal of foreign body from external auditory canal without general anesthesia; 30300 removal of foreign body, intranasal as office procedure. ICD-9: 931

Cerumen, or earwax, is the substance most commonly found in the external ear canal. Although not a foreign body, copious or hardened earwax may cause pressure or pain and conductive hearing loss in the affected ear and must be removed. Other small objects — including parts of toys, beans, nuts, coins, cotton applicator tips, and insects — may also lodge in the external ear. Children are at greater risk for foreign bodies in the ear than are adults.

Equipment

Otoscope ✧ ear curette, loop, or hook (plastic or wire) ✧ ear irrigation system (syringe with soft tubing, bulb syringe, or jet irrigation system [not always Food and Drug Administration approved]) ✧ basin of lukewarm water ✧ basin to catch irrigation fluid ✧ protective cover for patient ✧ viscous lidocaine, topical anesthetics, or mineral oil for ear instillation if foreign object is live insect ✧ carbamide peroxide or mineral oil for softening impacted wax (if needed). Optional: otic antibiotic or corticosteroid

Essential steps

• Before beginning, obtain a history of the complaint and related signs and symptoms. Ask the patient if he might have a perforated tympanic membrane.
• Inspect the external ear for signs of infection or injury.
• Using the otoscope, inspect the external ear canal for edema, erythema, and the presence and type of foreign body; determine the appropriate extraction method.
• Wash your hands, and prepare the equipment.
• Grasping the pinna of the ear, straighten the external ear canal by pulling the ear up and back (in an adult) or down and back (in a child).
• Gently insert the ear curette or loop into the external canal to grasp the object and gradually withdraw it.
• Instill viscous lidocaine, mineral oil, or topical anesthetic into the ear canal before extracting a live insect; the medication immobilizes the insect and reduces discomfort during extraction.
• If these are ineffective, instead try flushing out the object. However, if the object may swell (such as an organic foreign body), don't instill fluid into ear canal.
• Before flushing the ear canal, provide a protective covering for the patient and a drainage basin he can hold below his ear.
• Firmly flush the external ear canal with lukewarm water, using the syringe with soft tubing, bulb syringe, or jet irrigation system (use the jet system cautiously because of the risk of tympanic membrane injury).
• Don't force fluid directly at the tympanic membrane or you may injure it; instead, try to direct the flow past the object to flush the canal.
• Inspect the external ear canal for patency after extraction; repeat the procedure as needed until the canal is clear.
• Dry the external ear canal to reduce the risk of otitis externa.
• Instill a topical antibiotic or corticosteroid to control external edema, erythema, and infection.

Complications

Tympanic membrane rupture, laceration of the external ear canal, middle ear effusion with ear irrigation if tympanic membrane is perforated, otitis externa

Special considerations

• Don't push the foreign body toward the tympanic membrane during extraction because doing so could cause injury.
• Stop trying to extract the object if the patient experiences pain, severe vertigo, or nausea.
• Refer the patient to a primary care physician or otolaryngologist if the extraction effort wasn't successful or if the patient has a perforated tympanic membrane, myringotomy tubes, or chronic otitis media.
• If the patient has impacted earwax, consider instilling carbamide perox-

ide or mineral oil three times a day for 3 to 5 days to soften it.

Patient teaching

Tell the patient not to clean the external ear with a cotton-tipped applicator and not to place any small object into the ear canal.

Removal of foreign body from the eye

CPT code: 65205 removal of foreign body, external eye, conjunctival, superficial; 65210 removal of foreign body, external eye, conjunctival, embedded; 65220 removal of foreign body, external eye, conjunctival, corneal without slit lamp; 99070 eye tray: supplies and material provided by physician over and above what is usually included in office visit. ICD-9: 930.9

A patient who complains of eye pain, burning, and the feeling that he has something in his eye may have a foreign body in his eye, typically dust, dirt, or a metal, plastic, or wood particle. If the patient also displays photophobia and a tearing eye, he may have a corneal abrasion. People who take part in such activities as digging, drilling, hammering, welding, and woodworking without appropriate eye protection are at increased risk.

The clinician should evaluate a patient who complains of eye pain for one or more foreign bodies in the eye (some types of injuries can scatter fragments across the cornea). The foreign body typically lodges underneath the upper eyelid or in the superior temporal cul-de-sac where the upper lid attaches to the eyeball; foreign bodies can also lodge in the inferior cul-de-sac below the lower lid.

If the patient has a metallic object in the eye — especially from a high-velocity injury — an X-ray should be taken or a computed tomography scan of the orbit should be performed to make sure no object penetrated the eye itself. He shouldn't undergo magnetic resonance imaging if he has a metal object in his eye, although it may be indicated for a nonmetallic foreign body.

Equipment

Short-acting ophthalmic anesthetic solution (0.5% proparacaine) ✧ vision-screening device ✧ cotton-tipped applicators or eyelid retractor ✧ ophthalmoscope ✧ sterile fluorescein stain strips ✧ Wood's light or ophthalmoscope with a blue light ✧ tap water or sterile normal saline solution (for flushing the eye) ✧ ophthalmic antibiotic solution or ointment (usually broad-spectrum) ✧ eye patches or eye shield and adhesive tape (if indicated) ✧ binocular loupe or slit lamp (if available) ✧ small-gauge needle (may be attached to a syringe for stability)

ALERT *Don't* use fluorescein solution in place of fluorescein sodium stain strips. Use of fluorescein solution increases the risk of infection.

Essential steps

• Obtain a history of the injury and use of contact lenses and protective eyewear.
• Inspect the eye and lid for erythema, drainage, and hemorrhage; if you suspect intraocular perforation or open globe injuries, refer the patient to a primary care physician or ophthalmologist at once.
• Perform vision screening.
• Examine the pupillary reflex, extraocular movements, anterior and posterior chambers, and fundi.

• Wash your hands, and follow standard precautions.
• Open the affected eye, and instill 1 or 2 drops of short-acting ophthalmic anesthetic.
• While the patient looks down, evert the upper lid by placing the cotton-tipped applicator on the external upper lid, grasping the lashes, and turning the lid inside out over the applicator to expose the inner surface of the upper lid; you can also use the retractors to expose the conjunctiva.
• Examine the entire cornea, including the cul-de-sac, with an ophthalmoscope, slit lamp, or binocular loupe to locate and determine the depth of a foreign object.
• Use an oblique stream of tap water or sterile normal saline solution to flush the eye.
• Reexamine the entire conjunctiva to reassess the location and depth of the foreign body.
• Have the patient lie in a supine position with his eyes fixed so that the foreign body is at the highest position.
• Tell the patient not to move during removal; restrain his head if necessary.
• Use a saline-moistened cotton-tipped applicator to gently attempt to remove the foreign body without causing imbedding or scratching of the conjunctiva.
• If you can't remove the object with the applicator, gently attempt to dislodge the object with a small-gauge needle attached to a syringe for stability; under magnification, approach the object from the side rather than from the front to avoid scratching of the cornea.
• Gently irrigate the eye with saline solution to clean the area.
• Stain the conjunctiva with a fluorescein stain strip to assess for corneal abrasion.
• Apply ophthalmic antibiotic ointment.

• Cover the affected eye with an eye patch to promote patient comfort and protect the eye. Have the patient close both eyes and tightly tape two eye patches over the affected eye.
• Administer a tetanus booster, if indicated.
• Schedule a return office visit within 24 hours for reevaluation and restaining of the cornea.
• Document the type, number, and location of foreign bodies as well as removal procedures.

Complications

Corneal ulcer or abrasion, intraocular foreign body, uveitis, conjunctivitis (viral or bacterial)

Special considerations

• Use an ophthalmic magnet to remove metallic foreign bodies.
• Use a syringe or small-burr drill to remove rust rings.
• If you suspect intraocular perforation, cover the eye with a patch and protective shielding, have the patient rest the eye and elevate his head, and immediately refer him to an ophthalmologist.
• Refer the patient to an ophthalmologist if he has a metallic injury with rust rings that can't be removed, a corneal ulceration that won't heal, signs of uveitis, or vision loss.
• Signs of eye perforation include softness of the orbit on gentle palpation, any change in pupillary size or reaction, abnormality of the anterior chamber, and leakage of fluid from the chamber.
• Don't apply a topical corticosteroid or pain medications because they may mask changes or interfere with healing.
• Use an eye shield to protect the eye without putting pressure on the orbit.

• Encourage the patient to wear protective eyewear for occupational and recreational activities.
• Use a burr drill only if you're skilled in the procedure.
• If the patient complains of increased pain during the procedure, stop at once.

Skin lesion or skin tag removal

CPT code: 11300-303 shaving of epidermal or dermal lesion, single lesion on trunk, arms, or legs; 11305-308 on scalp, neck, hands, feet, or genitalia; 11400-406 excision of benign lesions on trunk, arms, or legs; 11420-426 on scalp, neck, hands, feet, or genitalia; 11600-606 excision of malignant lesions on trunk, arms, or legs; 11620-626 on scalp, neck, hands, feet, or genitalia (add 22 or 09922 for unusual or complex excision). CPT code: 11200 removal of skin tags, multiple fibrocutaneous tags, any area, < 15 lesions; 11201 each additional 10 lesions

A shave, scissor, or punch biopsy can be either incisional (removing only part of a lesion) or excisional (removing the entire lesion). In general, a clinician should remove the entire lesion, provided doing so allows for proper healing and an esthetically acceptable outcome.

The pathologist should receive an adequate specimen for diagnosis, for instance, a specimen that includes the dermis for a dermal lesion. Sometimes the pathologist also needs a portion of adjacent normal skin if the patient has a more complex skin disease, such as panniculitis; a wedge section can provide the larger and deeper specimen needed. The clinician should also provide as much detail about the site as possible.

A clinician who can't identify or doesn't plan to treat a lesion should not biopsy it; instead, the patient should be referred to someone who may be able to recognize the lesion, possibly saving the patient the discomfort and cost of biopsy. In addition, if a patient has a lesion that looks like skin cancer, he should be referred to a dermatologist, even though skin cancer isn't hard to recognize. The dermatologist has the background to choose the most appropriate treatment (including excision, radiation therapy, and chemotherapy) for a particular lesion.

Types of biopsy

The shave biopsy allows the clinician to take a specimen of a skin lesion that doesn't seem to extend deep into the dermis. It's a quick, easy way to remove superficial lesions and is ideal for raised lesions in the epidermis or superficial dermis, although if necessary, the procedure can extend down to the subcutis. The procedure is faster than a punch biopsy, generally requires only topical aluminum chloride to control bleeding, has a good cosmetic outcome, and can provide a relatively large specimen. However, it can leave a depressed scar if the biopsy goes too deep, result in pigment disturbance and, possibly, miss a deeper component of skin cancer. Most clinicians remove lesions with a sterilized razor blade; some prefer a #15 Bard-Parker blade. The inexpensive, sharp, flexible blade allows the clinician to curve the blade to match the surface of the lesion by applying pressure with the index finger and thumb. The clinician can then advance the blade across the base of the lesion with a steady sawing motion.

A variant of the shave biopsy, the scissor biopsy allows removal of small superficial growths, such as skin tags and filiform warts. It usually doesn't require local anesthesia. The clinician uses forceps with teeth to gently grasp and apply traction to the lesion, cuts the lesion at the base with iris scissors, and applies aluminum chloride and pressure to control bleeding.

For a punch biopsy, a specialized instrument is used to remove a cylindrical, full-thickness skin specimen. It's performed to obtain material for pathologic evaluation and to remove small cutaneous lesions quickly and effectively. Punches are available in sizes ranging from 1.5 to 10 mm and can be permanent or disposable; disposable punch biopsy instruments are preferable because they're sterile, inexpensive, and don't dull from repeated use. Because the instrument can only go as deep as the length of the cylinder, a biopsy that must include deeper fat or fascia may require two complete punches. The resulting wound may require suturing.

Punch biopsies generally produce a good cosmetic result, provide a deep specimen, and heal rapidly when sutured. However, they require sterile technique, specimen size is limited by the width and depth of the punch, and the wound may require extra time for suturing.

Equipment and preparation

70% isopropyl alcohol, povidone-iodine, or hexetidine ✧ local anesthesia ✧ 25G to 30G ½″ to 1″ needles and 3- to 5-ml syringe (for injecting the anesthetic) ✧ razor blade or #15 Bard-Parker blade ✧ aluminum chloride or electrocautery (to control bleeding) ✧ cotton-tipped applicators for shave biopsy ✧ punch, skin hook, or needle ✧ sharp scissors ✧ suture equipment ✧ sterile adhesive strips such as Steri-Strips ✧ three-layer pressure dressing with antibiotic ointment ✧ adhesive dressing overlay (for punch biopsy)

Essential steps

• After marking the biopsy site, clean the skin with antiseptic solution.
• Inject the local anesthetic if the lesion isn't elevated above the skin surface (the anesthetic usually raises the skin).
• For a punch biopsy, position the punch vertically over the area. Using your nondominant hand, apply perpendicular tissue traction. This results in an oval rather than a circular defect (a circular defect may result in a redundant cone of skin called a "dog-ear" on closure).
• Push the punch against the skin with firm, steady pressure, and simultaneously twist it clockwise. Continue this until you feel some give, indicating the descent of the punch into the fat layer.
• Withdraw the punch with the column of tissue. Remove the specimen gently (to avoid histologic artifacts).
• Use a skin hook or local anesthesia needle to elevate the plug of tissue, and transect the base with a pair of sharp scissors.
• To obtain the best cosmetic result and fastest healing, suture the biopsy site using simple interrupted or vertical mattress sutures. Typically, a 2-mm punch requires one suture, a 4- to 6-mm punch requires two sutures, and a 7- to 10-mm punch requires three to four sutures. Use 4-0 monofilament nylon sutures for wounds on the extremities and trunk and 5-0 and 6-0 monofilament nylon sutures with cutting P3 needles for biopsies taken from the face and anterior neck. (See "Suturing simple lacerations," page 359.) If necessary, reinforce the sutures on a wound under tension with sterile adhesive strips.

PERFORMING A SHAVE BIOPSY

This illustration of a shave biopsy shows how to position the scalpel so it's almost parallel to the skin surface.

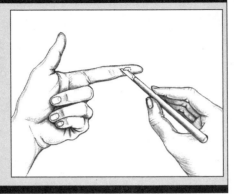

• Place a three-layer pressure dressing that contains triple antibiotic ointment (Polysporin) on the wound, followed by a nonadherent pad, gauze, and an adhesive dressing overlay.
• To perform a shave biopsy, fix the lesion and the surrounding tissue with your nondominant hand while passing the razor blade or scalpel under the lesion. Control the depth of the biopsy with the appropriate angle of entry. (See *Performing a shave biopsy*.)
• To control bleeding, apply 20% to 40% aluminum chloride directly to the wound with a cotton-tipped applicator or use electrocautery.

Complications

Infection, scarring, pain

Special considerations

 COLLABORATION Refer or consult with a dermatologist for deeper lesions, suspected neoplasms, and facial or penile lesions.
• Deeper shave biopsies can result in permanent depression at the biopsy site.

• If the patient has an atypical-appearing melanocytic lesion, *don't remove it with the shave procedure.* Instead, obtain a good specimen for pathology by performing a deep punch biopsy.
• Don't keep removing the punch from the biopsy site to check your progress or the specimen may have histologic artifacts.

Patient teaching

• Teach the patient how to care for the wound. He should gently clean the biopsy site daily with tap water and soap (with no rubbing or scrubbing) and then apply a little antibiotic ointment, preferably Polysporin rather than an ointment that contains neomycin, which carries a higher risk of allergic reaction. Tell him to continue wound care until the area completely heals.
• Tell him that the wound will appear uniformly pink or red when epithelialization is complete, and explain that keeping the wound covered and occluded promotes rapid healing and decreases the risk of scarring.
• If the punch biopsy site is in an area of tension, advise the patient to minimize activity to prevent bleeding and wound dehiscence.

ALERT Tell the patient to call the primary care provider for signs of infection (increasing redness, swelling, pain, and warmth; cloudy yellow, green, or brown drainage; opening of the wound; foul odor; a red streak leading from the site; or fever after 24 hours).

Skin scraping

CPT code: 87210 potassium hydroxide (KOH) testing of skin scraping

A skin scrape involves the gentle removal of a skin specimen that's then placed on a microscope slide for evaluation. This procedure is often used to confirm a diagnosis of a superficial fungal infection or arthropod infestation.

Equipment

#15 Bard-Parker surgical blade (if unavailable, use the edge of a glass microscope slide) ✧ alcohol sponge ✧ microscope slide and coverglass ✧ 5% to 20% KOH solution

Essential steps

• Position the patient comfortably with the area to be scraped accessible.
• Clean the area with an alcohol sponge.
• Lightly run the blade perpendicular to the skin; when the blade has collected enough of the superficial layer of the skin, wipe it across the slide. Make sure you use a gentle technique; the patient shouldn't experience pain or bleed.
• Place the coverglass on the slide.
• If you suspect a dermatophyte infection, apply KOH to the edge of the coverglass, allowing capillary action to draw the solution under.

• Gently heat the slide with a match until bubbles begin to expand.
• Blot excess KOH solution with lens paper.
• If you see hyphae (septated, tube-like structures), dermatophytes are present; pseudohyphae (tubelike structures without septa) and budding yeast forms indicate candidiasis.

Complications

None common

Special considerations

If KOH results are negative, collect a culture specimen and send it to the microbiology laboratory for growth and species identification.

Patient teaching

Just before scraping, tell the patient that you're about to scrape the skin but that the scraping won't cause pain. Explain that the scraping will help ensure proper diagnosis and treatment.

Soft-tissue aspiration

CPT code: 20600 arthrocentesis, aspiration, and/or injection: small joint, bursa, or ganglionic cyst (for example, fingers or toes); 20605 intermediate joint, bursa, or ganglionic cyst (for example, temporomandibular; acromioclavicular; wrist, elbow, or ankle; olecranon bursa); 20610 major joint or bursa (for example, shoulder, hip, knee joint, subacromial bursa)

Soft-tissue aspiration involves removing fluid or exudate from an area of soft tissue for evaluation and palliative care. It is used for conditions such as paronychia, cysts, and abscesses; specific indications include pain or swelling, or both, in soft tissue and hematoma from trauma. Contraindications include severe coagulopathies, swelling on the face, cellulitis, broken skin at the site, and prosthetic joint.

Equipment

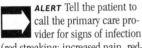 **ALERT** Informed consent is required.

Povidone-iodine solution and alcohol sponges ✧ sterile latex gloves (unless patient is allergic to latex) ✧ drape ✧ hemostat ✧ 10-ml syringe with 18G to 20G 1″ needle ✧ red-topped tube ✧ elastic bandage ✧ sterile 3″ × 3″ or 4″ × 4″ gauze pads ✧ tape

Essential steps

• Assemble equipment before beginning.
• Place the patient in as comfortable a position as possible to allow performance of the procedure.
• Clean the area with povidone-iodine solution and follow with alcohol.
• Attach an 18G or a 20G 1″ needle to a 10-ml syringe.
• Insert the needle, bevel down, into the leading edge of the swelling. Aspirate as you advance the needle.
• If the syringe becomes full and needs to be changed, use the two-syringe technique. Attach the hemostat to the needle hub to avoid needle rotation, remove the first syringe, replace it with an empty syringe, and continue aspirating.
• Place the aspirated fluid into a red-topped collection tube, and send it to the laboratory for analysis, if indicated.
• Apply a pressure dressing and compression device, such as an elastic bandage.

Complications

None common

Patient teaching

• Tell the patient to keep the pressure dressing intact for 24 hours and then remove it.
• Suggest applying heat for the first 24 hours for some relief from discomfort.

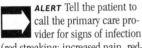 **ALERT** Tell the patient to call the primary care provider for signs of infection (red streaking; increased pain, redness, or warmth at the site; purulent drainage; or fever and chills).

Splinting and taping

CPT code: 29260-80 strapping: elbow, wrist, hand, or finger; 29530-50 ankle, knee, or toes; 99070 splinting

Splinting and taping can stabilize and immobilize acute injuries and provide symptomatic relief of chronic conditions, increasing patient comfort and preventing further injury. Acute injuries — such as sprains, strains, and fractures — typically require immediate joint stabilization; at the scene of the trauma, any rigid object can function as a splint. A temporary measure, splinting is initially preferred over circumferential casting for acute injuries because increased swelling within a circumferential cast can lead to vascular compromise, compartment syndrome, and distal swelling.

Inversion injuries, the most common cause of acute ankle injuries, typically occur in young adults who take part in recreational activities and sports. Fractures are more common in older adults. Chronic conditions such as overuse and repetitive-

GRADING ANKLE SPRAINS

Grading a sprain injury of the ankle allows uniform assessment and treatment for a wide variety of situations. This chart outlines grades currently used for ankle sprain injuries, the tissue damage involved, signs and symptoms of the injury, and treatment.

Tissue damage	Signs and symptoms	Treatment
Grade I Partial or complete tear of the anterior talofibular ligament	Local tenderness, minimal edema, but usually able to bear weight with no functional loss or joint instability	• Symptomatic treatment with elastic compression support to control edema • Intermittent removal of immobilization, with active range-of-motion (ROM) exercises, progressing as tolerated • Peroneal strengthening and exercise start at 2-3 weeks, depending on patient tolerance
Grade II Partial or complete tear of both the anterior talofibular and calcaneofibular ligaments	Painful weight bearing, minimal ligament function during examination, possible "popping" with injury, moderate to severe swelling, pain, ecchymosis, and mild joint instability	• Same as for Grade I, plus immobilization and non-weight bearing with an air splint or short-leg removable walking cast • Switch to hinged-joint immobilization at 2 weeks
Grade III Grade II injury plus a partial or complete tear of the posterior talofibular ligament	Ligamentous laxity, moderate to severe joint instability, complete interruption in alignment, inability to bear weight and often obvious deformity, diffuse joint swelling, pain initially but possibly no pain later	• Evaluation by an orthopedic surgeon • Short-leg walking cast for 3 weeks • Physical therapy including ROM exercises, peroneal strengthening, and proprioception training after 3 weeks • Possible cast for up to 6 weeks or surgical repair

motion injuries typically occur in the upper extremities and can usually be managed in a primary care setting or by an orthopedic specialist. Sprains vary based on the level of injury, disability, pain, and swelling. (See *Grading ankle sprains*.)

Chronic injuries typically affect the wrists and hands and usually result from tendosynovitis, as can occur with repetitive-motion injuries (carpal tunnel syndrome and tennis elbow). Splints increase the patient's comfort by keeping the joint in proper alignment.

When taking the patient's history, the clinician should obtain a description of the injury and the joint involved, how and when it occurred, the patient's level of activity right after the injury and at the time of evaluation, and a previous history of injury to the joint. Physical assessment should focus on the joint involved and its physical appearance, including swelling, obvious deformity, bleeding, and ecchymosis, possibly including a comparison with the other, uninjured extremity. The clinician should also assess the patient's neurovascular status and ask the patient if he can move the extremity.

Equipment

Tube stockinette in various diameters ✧ precast material or casting materials in various widths ✧ 4″ or 6″ elastic wraps ✧ 1″ to 2″ adhesive tape ✧ bucket of water ✧ soft padding material ✧ clean scissors ✧ sling for upper-extremity injuries ✧ aluminum splints for finger injuries ✧ wrist and finger splints for wrist or finger injuries ✧ knee immobilizer for knee injuries

Essential steps

• Have X-rays performed as appropriate to rule out fracture. Use the Ottawa ankle rules to determine if X-rays are needed; these rules can eliminate the need for up to 30% of X-rays with no missed clinically significant fractures. If the patient is under age 55, able to walk four steps at the time of injury and of evaluation, and has no tenderness over the posterior edge of the distal 2½″ (6.4 cm) or tip of either malleolus, an X-ray isn't required.
• After the X-ray has been read and the extent of the injury is known, prepare the patient for immobilization. Place him in as comfortable a position as possible that allows splinting or taping.
• Measure the splinting material against the patient and then add about 1½″ (3.8 cm) to the length of the splint to ensure a proper fit. Then fold the material into 10 to 15 overlapping layers.
• Apply a soft cotton bandage such as Webril to the extremity to protect the skin before applying the cast. Then moisten the plaster or casting materi-

al with cool water, apply it to the injured extremity, and mold the plaster to the extremity while maintaining the extremity in the proper position. Secure the splint with an elastic bandage and let it dry.

Complications

A splint that's wrapped too tightly can lead to vascular compromise, ischemia, and compartment syndrome of the affected extremity; making sure that the elastic bandage is snug but not tight can help prevent this, as can using a linear splint rather than a circular splint.

Exothermic burns can occur when the plaster begins to harden; the plaster should be removed at once if the patient complains of pain from the heat of the drying plaster. Pressure ulcers can result from plaster rubbing against bony prominences; Webril applied directly to the skin beneath the splint can help reduce this complication.

Special considerations

• Although several types of finger splints exist, the aluminum finger splint is most commonly used for isolated proximal and distal interphalangeal joint injuries. Place it on the injured finger and secure it with tape; for subsequent injuries, incorporate the splint into a volar arm splint.
• Use a volar arm splint for distal radial, ulnar, and carpal fractures and Grades II and III wrist sprains. Have the patient extend his wrist slightly, with the metacarpophalangeal joint flexed 60 to 70 degrees and the fingers flexed 10 to 20 degrees. Maintain this position until the splint hardens, and secure it with an elastic bandage. The splint should extend from the tip of the fingers to about 1¼″ to 1½″ (3.2 to 3.8 cm) distal to the elbow joint.

• Use the thumb spica splint for scaphoid fractures or injury to the ulnar collateral ligament of the thumb. Apply it to the radial (thumb side) surface of the forearm wrist, and wrap it around the thumb to the distal tip. Have the patient keep his thumb straight and in line with the axis of the radius, as if he's holding a can of soda, and maintain this position until the splint hardens.

• Apply an ulnar gutter splint for fourth and fifth metacarpal fractures (boxer's fracture). Place the splint along the ulnar aspect of the hand, from the distal interphalangeal joint to about 1¼″ to 1½″ from the elbow. Secure it with a 2″ or 3″ elastic bandage, and hold the arm in position until the splint hardens.

• For a splint on a lower extremity, the patient should be in a prone position, with the knee and ankle both flexed 90 degrees. Help him maintain this position until the splint hardens, and secure the splint with a large elastic bandage, usually 4″ or 6″.

• Use a posterior leg splint for Grades II and III ankle sprains, distal fibula and tibia fractures, crush injuries, foot fractures (excluding the toes), immobilization after reduction of a dislocated ankle or foot, and rupture of ankle or foot tendons with severe pain on weight bearing. Use 5″ to 6″ (12.7 to 15.3 cm) of plaster to extend the splint from the metatarsal joint to about 1½″ below the popliteal fossae, and secure the splint with an elastic bandage. You can also use a stirrup ankle splint for such injuries. Place a 5″ plaster splint over the plantar aspect of the foot and up both the medial and the lateral sides of the foreleg to the level of the fibula head.

• Use "buddy taping" or a hard-sole shoe for toe injuries. To "buddy tape" the injured toe, use 1″ (2.5 cm) of silk tape to tape the toe to the neighboring toe; this stabilizes and immobilizes the fracture or sprain.

• For chronic injuries, consider taping to stabilize and support the joint, particularly for an athlete. Taping immobilizes the area and provides supports, allowing the athlete to continue activities with minimal interference. Make sure the tape isn't too tight, and keep in mind that most taping loosens after activity, placing the joint at risk for further injury. Several methods of taping exist; a skilled professional (such as a trainer or sports medicine clinician) should perform such taping.

 COLLABORATION As appropriate, refer the patient to an orthopedic specialist for a custom-made splint; such a splint may be more comfortable than standard-sized splints.

Patient teaching

• Teach the patient the RICE regimen — rest, ice, compression, and elevation.

• Tell him to apply ice every 2 to 3 hours for 20 to 30 minutes for the first 24 hours. Then he can switch to moist heat (without wetting the cast) for the next 24 to 48 hours.

• Tell him to wear the splint except when sleeping or showering until he's reevaluated and to avoid activities that cause pain.

• Have him watch for signs of neurovascular compromise, such as coolness, swelling, and pain in the area around the splint or tape or if the area appears pale or dark in color. If he notes any, he should rest at once with the extremity elevated above his heart. Emphasize that swelling can occur swiftly with activity but will take much longer to subside. If swelling doesn't improve within 30 minutes, he should contact the primary care provider.

• Tell him to take acetaminophen or a nonsteroidal anti-inflammatory drug, or both, for pain, as directed.

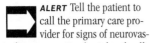 **ALERT** Tell the patient to call the primary care provider for signs of neurovascular compromise (peripheral pallor or blue-purple color, pain, coldness, swelling, or numbness and tingling) that don't resolve. The patient should remove the splint or tape and contact his primary care provider.

Suturing simple lacerations

CPT code: 12001-7 simple repair, superficial wounds on scalp, neck, axillae, external genitalia, trunk, and/or extremities; 12011-18 simple repair, superficial wounds on face, ears, eyelids, nose, lips, and/or mucous membranes; 12020 superficial dehiscence

Wounds closed with sutures may require the use of both absorbable and nonabsorbable sutures, such as polypropylene (Prolene) and nylon. Usually placed deeper within a wound, absorbable sutures absorb into the body over time; nonabsorbable sutures are used at the surface of the wound and require removal.

Suturing typically starts with a dermal layer of interrupted absorbable sutures (such sutures are especially important in high-tension areas, where the risk of pulling apart is greatest). The clinician should place the initial deep suture in the middle of the wound and then bisect each half in a sequential manner with other buried sutures.

Nonabsorbable sutures are used on the epidermal layer; these sutures allow for improved approximation and eversion of the wound edges, resulting in optimal cosmetic results. The clinician typically removes these sutures in 1 to 2 weeks, depending on their location.

A simple interrupted suture for the epidermal layer completely closes the wound. This type of suture offers the advantages of properly everting skin edges so that the wound lies flat when it spreads, lining up unequal wound edges, and allowing for regional variations in tension. It takes longer to close a wound with this suture than with a running suture such as a mattress suture.

Wounds closed by approximation of the skin edges heal by primary intention. Wounds heal faster under an occlusive or semiocclusive dressing, which prevents crust formation, which is especially important for wounds after a procedure.

Equipment

20- to 30-ml syringe with a 20G plastic cannula and irrigant ◇ smooth or multitooth forceps ◇ needle holder ◇ scissors ◇ scalpel, if needed ◇ appropriate sutures ◇ needles (round and tapered for mucosa, fascia, and muscle) ◇ injectable anesthesia (lidocaine or diphenhydramine, as appropriate) ◇ three-layer pressure dressing

Essential steps

• Position the patient in as comfortable a position as possible and allowing full visualization of the wound.
• Wash hands and apply gloves.
• Clean the wound with povidone-iodine solution in a circular pattern from the wound edges outward.
• Infiltrate a local anesthetic by inserting the needle along each side of the wound and injecting slowly as you withdraw the needle, to ensure uniform distribution.
• Examine the wound for foreign bodies or injury to underlying structures, such as a tendon or joint capsule.

• Use the syringe and cannula to irrigate the wound with chemical antiseptics or sterile saline irrigant.

• Trim and undermine wound edges as needed, to provide effective approximation.

• Using your dominant hand, grasp the suture needle securely with the needle holder. Use a toothed forceps in your other hand to stabilize the wound edge in a slightly everted position.

• Insert the needle at a right angle through the skin about 0.5 to 1.0 cm from the wound edge. Grasp the needle from the exterior with the needle holder. Before inserting the needle again, be sure the tissue layers are well approximated with minimal tension.

• Repeat the process and then tie the suture, being careful not to pull the suture edges too taut.

• Use scissors to trim jagged edges from the wound.

• As appropriate, place a vertical mattress suture in the middle of the wound and bisect each half sequentially with vertical mattress sutures. (See *Common suture techniques.*)

• After skin edges are approximated, fill in the remaining gaps with simple interrupted stitches.

• Types of closures that can be used include simple interrupted (good for dermal match); simple buried interrupted (good to relieve tension and close dead space); running superficial (for quick repair); running superficial locking (used in episiotomy repairs); vertical mattress (good for oral mucosa and thick skin); and horizontal mattress (good in fascia and to approximate thin fragile skin).

• If you have redundant cones of skin, called "dog-ears," remove them to optimize the cosmetic result. Excise the residual skin by making a small ellipse that extends the defect or by making an incision that lifts the dog-ear with the skin hook and drapes excess tissue over the side of the wound.

• To help equalize tension on wound edges, make a "hockey stick" incision, an angled incision that extends one end of the wound in the shape of a hockey stick. This incision creates a curvilinear line that allows for the approximation of skin edges without placing undue tension on any specific point along the line.

• After suturing the wound, compress the wound gently and look for residual bleeding. Use direct pressure for 5 minutes to minimize swelling and bleeding from the wound edge.

• Cover the site with a three-layer pressure dressing for 24 hours.

• Splint if necessary.

Drugs

• Administer antibiotics, such as cephalexin, if the area is infected.

• Administer tetanus prophylaxis if the patient hasn't been or doesn't know if he's been immunized within the past 5 years.

Complications

Dehiscence, infection, pain, scarring

Special considerations

 COLLABORATION Refer the patient to a plastic surgeon for debridement or if the wound has a large amount of dead space (expect drain placement). Refer the patient to a physician for complex lacerations or for artery, tendon, ligament, bone, or nerve involvement.

• Scalp sutures should be removed in 5 to 8 days; face sutures, in 3 to 5 days; abdomen and chest sutures, in 5 to 8 days; upper-extremity sutures, in 7 to 10 days; lower-extremity su-

COMMON SUTURE TECHNIQUES

The most commonly used suture techniques include the plain continuous, plain interrupted, and mattress sutures. The type of suture technique used depends on the site, shape, size, and depth of the wound.

In addition, the space left between sutures varies according to the location of the wound or the amount of tension expected to be applied to the wound. For instance, the space between sutures in most wounds is about 0.25 cm. Sutures would be placed even closer for facial wounds or in areas where high tension is anticipated, such as the elbow or knee.

These illustrations show four common suture techniques and the advantages of each.

Plain continuous
Plain continuous sutures provide even tension across the incision and are used for quick repair.

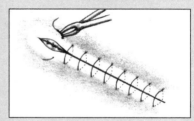

Plain interrupted
Plain interrupted sutures allow precise approximation of wound edges.

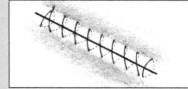

Horizontal mattress
Horizontal mattress sutures reduce dead space within the wound and reinforce subcutaneous tissue. These sutures decrease tension on the suture line and are commonly used to suture lax skin. Scarring is more likely with this technique.

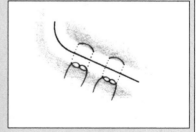

Vertical mattress
Vertical mattress sutures also reduce dead space within the wound and reinforce subcutaneous tissue. They're used in thick skin, such as in the palms or the soles, and in lax skin, but they're difficult to approximate and take more time to place.

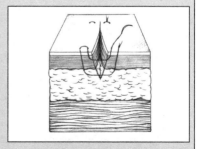

tures, in 7 to 14 days; and back sutures, in 10 to 14 days.
• To avoiding infection, the wound should be closed within 6 hours of injury.

Patient teaching

• Tell the patient to keep the sutures dry.
• Instruct him to remove the initial dressing in 24 hours and then clean it twice a day and cover it with ointment. The initial dressing is a three-layer dressing consisting of petroleum jelly or triple antibiotic ointment, a nonadherent dressing, and gauze followed by a tape covering. Next, tell him to replace the large dressing with a smaller gauze bandage when drainage no longer appears on the large dressing. Tell him to be careful not to place the gauze itself directly over the wound. Fibers in the gauze can get trapped in the wound edge, become matted, and delay healing.
• For suture removal, have him return in 3 to 6 days for face sutures, in 7 to 10 days for ear sutures, and in 5 to 10 days for trunk or extremity sutures.
• Tell the patient to call the primary care provider for signs of infection (increasing redness, swelling, pain, and warmth; cloudy yellow, green, or brown drainage; opening of wound; foul odor; a red streak from wound area; or fever).

Wart removal: Cryosurgery

CPT code: 17000 destruction any method (including laser, with/without surgical curettement/local anesthesia) of all benign/premalignant lesions any location, excluding cutaneous vascular proliferative lesions; 17003 multiple lesions; 17110 destruction of <14 flat warts, molluscum contagiosum, or milia; 17260 destruction of <0.5-cm malignant lesion from trunk, arms, or legs; 17261-66 indicates increasing lesion diameters; 17270 destruction of <0.5-cm malignant lesion from scalp, neck, hands, feet, genitalia; 17271-76 indicates increasing lesion diameters

Cryosurgery efficiently removes common skin lesions with minimal scar formation, pain, and pigment changes (in light-skinned patients). Cryosurgery uses freezing temperatures to destroy cells. Temperatures of 14° F (−10° C) to −4° F (−20 C°) destroy tissue; a temperature of −58° F (−50 C°) destroys malignant cells. In the procedure, a blister forms at the dermal-epidermal junction, and the skin superficial to the blister is left essentially bloodless and without sensation. The time needed for freezing varies with the type of skin lesion. (See *Freeze time guidelines.*) In particular, cryosurgery provides an excellent way to treat verruca vulgaris (common warts) and verruca plantaris (plantar warts). The clinician should use caution when treating warts in a child or an elderly patient who has had an exaggerated response and high levels of cryoglobulin (abnormal proteins that dissolve at body temperature but precipitate when cooled).

The procedure is contraindicated in patients with a sensitivity or adverse reaction to cryosurgery, in patients who won't accept the possibility of skin pigment changes, in areas that have compromised circulation or a great deal of hair (cryosurgery destroys hair follicles), and for lesions that require pathologic evaluation. It's relatively contraindicated for patients with collagen disorders, ulcerative colitis, glomerulonephritis, or

FREEZE TIME GUIDELINES

Cryosurgery involves use of the appropriate freeze time for the particular type of lesion to be removed. This table shows the times needed to freeze various types of skin lesions.

Keep in mind that if the freeze time noted yields insufficient coverage, allow the area to thaw after being frozen the first time, and then refreeze. Subsequent re-freezing obtains deeper penetration of the cold.

Type of lesion	Freeze time (in seconds)
Actinic keratosis	90
Condyloma acuminata	45
Molluscum contagiosum	25 to 30
Papular nevi	30 to 45
Seborrheic keratosis	30
Skin tags and polyps	30 to 45
Sebaceous hyperplasia	30 to 45
Lentigines (freckles)	10 to 15
Verruca plantaris (plantar warts; after debridement)	30 to 40

high cryoglobulin levels. It also poses a risk for patients with a history of endocarditis, syphilis, Epstein-Barr virus infection, cytomegalovirus infection, or chronic hepatitis B and for those taking high-dose corticosteroids.

Equipment

ALERT Informed consent is required.
Sterile drapes ✧ sterile latex gloves (unless patient is allergic to latex) ✧ tissue freezing kit or nitrous oxide cryosurgery unit ✧ 4″ × 4″ gauze pads soaked with water ✧ antiseptic skin cleaner, such as povidone-iodine ✧ cotton-tipped applicators ✧ water-soluble lubricant, such as K-Y gel ✧ topical antibiotic, such as triple antibiotic ointment ✧ dry 4″ × 4″ gauze pads ✧ tape

Essential steps

• Explain the procedure to the patient and assess for allergies, particularly to iodine and latex.
• Position the patient comfortably with the lesion easily accessible.
• Clean the area with antiseptic skin cleaner.
• Apply water-soaked gauze pads to the lesion for 5 to 10 minutes.
• Drape the lesion, and put on gloves.
• Use a cotton-topped applicator to apply lubricant.
• Freeze the lesion for 30 to 90 seconds at a time.
• Apply a topical antibiotic.
• Cover the area with gauze and tape.

Complications

Pigment changes, increased susceptibility to photodamage, ischemia, and
infection (rare)

Special considerations

• Choose the appropriate cryosurgical tip for the shape and depth of the
lesion. (See *Selecting the proper cryoprobe,* page 330.)
• Inform the patient with a wart that
wart removal requires two thaw times
of at least 45 seconds and that a blister will form. After the blister forms,
he should remove the top layer of the
skin from the blister with soap and
water, apply a thin coat of triple antibiotic ointment, and then cover the
area with an adhesive bandage.
• Use caution when treating the pal-
mar surface of the hand because cutaneous sensory nerves run superfi-
cially in the hands. If a nerve is affected, the patient usually recovers
within 6 weeks. When freezing an
area adjacent to a nerve, apply traction and advise the patient that sensory loss may occur.

 COLLABORATION Refer the
patient to a dermatologist for
mucosal and periorbital
cryosurgery because they require
shorter freezing times and may produce excessive swelling that may be
esthetically and functionally disabling.

Patient teaching

• Tell the patient to keep the skin
clean and dry. Explain the role of
skin in defending the body against
infection. Emphasize hygiene, sparing application of antibiotic ointment
to the site, and the importance of
keeping the site covered.
• Tell him which normal changes to
expect, including immediate redness,
swelling, and blisters in 16 to 36
hours that decrease within 72 hours.
Explain that crusting occurs within
72 hours and resolves within 1 week.
• Tell him that in that area, the skin
may become lighter or the hair less
plentiful but that only minimal scarring should occur. Advise him to wear
sunscreen on that area in particular.
• If sensory nerves were affected, reassure the patient that recovery typically occurs within 2 months.
• Tell him to follow up in 1 week to
check for resolution of the blister and
in 3 to 4 weeks for evaluation and,
possibly, retreatment.

 ALERT Tell the patient to
call the primary care provider for signs of infection
(increasing redness, swelling, pain,
and warmth; cloudy yellow, green, or
brown drainage; opening of wound;
foul odor; a red streak from the site;
or fever after 24 hours).

CHAPTER

Precautions

Preventing the spread of contagious disease

Standard precautions

The Guidelines for Isolation Precautions in Hospitals were developed by an advisory committee within the Centers for Disease Control and Prevention (CDC) known as the Hospital Infection Control Practices Advisory Committee (HICPAC). These guidelines contain two levels of precautions: *standard* precautions and *transmission-based* precautions.

Standard precautions are designed to decrease the risk of microorganism transmission from both recognized and unrecognized sources of infection. They should be followed at all times with every patient.

Standard precautions combine the major features of *universal* precautions, which were developed in response to the increasing incidence of human immunodeficiency virus, hepatitis B virus, and other blood-borne diseases, and *body substance isolation,* which was developed to decrease the risk of transmitting pathogens from moist body surfaces. Because standard precautions reduce the risk of transmission of blood-borne and other pathogens, many patients with diseases or conditions that previously required category- or disease-specific isolation precautions now only require standard precautions.

HICPAC and the CDC define the specific substances covered by standard precautions:
• blood
• all body secretions and excretions
• nonintact skin
• mucous membranes.

To implement standard infection control precautions, follow these steps.
• Wash your hands immediately if they become contaminated with blood or body fluids; also wash your hands before and after patient care and after removing gloves.
• Use a plain (nonantimicrobial) soap for routine hand washing.
• Wear gloves if you will or could come in contact with blood, specimens, tissue, body fluid, secretions or excretions, or contaminated surfaces or objects.
• Change your gloves between tasks and procedures on the same patient if you anticipate touching anything that might have a high concentration of microorganisms, and change them between patient contacts, to avoid cross-contamination. Gloves are available that contain substitutes for individuals with allergies to latex and polyvinyl chloride.
• Wear a gown, eye protection (goggles or glasses), and a mask during procedures likely to generate droplets of blood or body fluids, secretions, or excretions, such as surgery, endoscopic procedures, or dialysis.
• Carefully handle used patient care equipment that has been soiled with blood, body fluids, secretions, or excretions to avoid exposure to skin and mucous membranes, clothing contaminations, and transfer of microorganisms to other patients and environments.
• Ensure that procedures for routine care, cleaning, and disinfection of environmental surfaces and equipment are followed.
• Handle contaminated linens in a manner that prevents contamination and transfer of microorganisms. Keep them away from your body. Place in properly labeled containers. Ensure that linens are transported and processed according to facility policy.
• Handle used needles or other sharp implements carefully. Don't bend, break, reinsert them into their original sheaths, or unnecessarily handle them. Discard them intact immediately after use into an impervious dis-

posal box. These measures reduce the risk of accidental injury or infection.

• Use mouthpieces, resuscitation bags, or other ventilation devices in place of mouth-to-mouth resuscitation whenever possible.

• Place patients who can't maintain appropriate hygiene or who contaminate the environment in a private room. Notify infection control personnel.

• If you have an exudative lesion, avoid direct patient contact until the condition has resolved and you're cleared by the employee health provider.

• Because precautions can't be specified for every clinical situation, you must use your judgment in individual cases.

• If occupational exposure to blood is likely, you should receive the hepatitis B virus vaccine series.

Transmission-based precautions

Transmission-based precautions are divided into three types: airborne precautions, droplet precautions, and contact precautions.

Transmission-based precautions are followed in addition to standard precautions whenever a patient is known or suspected to be infected with highly contagious and epidemiologically important pathogens that are transmitted by air or droplets or by contact with dry skin or other contaminated surfaces. Some examples include measles (air), influenza (droplet), or GI, respiratory, skin, or wound infections (contact). In fact, transmission-based precautions replace all older categories of category- or disease-specific isolation, such as acid-fast bacillus isolation, neu-

tropenic isolation, contact isolation, blood and body fluid precautions, drainage and secretion precautions, and enteric precautions. One or more types of transmission-based precautions may be combined and followed when a patient has a disease that has multiple routes of transmission.

Airborne transmission-based precautions

To implement *airborne* transmission-based precautions in addition to standard precautions, follow these steps:

• Place the patient in a private room that has monitored negative air pressure in relation to surrounding areas (6 to 12 air exchanges per hour) and appropriate outdoor air discharge or high-efficiency filtration of room air. Order the room door closed, obtain an isolation cart with precaution instruction signs to place outside the room, and keep the patient in the room. If a private room isn't available, place the patient in a room with a patient who has an active infection with the same microorganism. Consult with infection control personnel if a private room isn't available.

• Wear respiratory protection (masks or face shields) when entering the room of a patient with a known or suspected respiratory infection. Persons immune to measles and varicella don't need to wear respiratory protection when entering the room of a patient with these illnesses.

• Limit patient transport and patient movement out of the room. If the patient must leave the room, have him wear a surgical mask.

Droplet transmission-based precautions

To implement *droplet* transmission-based precautions in addition to standard precautions, follow these steps:
• Place the patient in a private room or, if one isn't available, use a room with another patient who has an active infection with the same microorganism. If this isn't possible, consult infection control personnel. Special ventilation isn't necessary because droplets don't remain suspended in air.
• Wear a mask when working within 3′ (1 m) of the patient.
• Instruct visitors to stay 3′ from the infected patient.
• Limit movement of the patient from the room. If the patient must leave the room, have him wear a surgical mask.
• Additional precautions such as special respirators are necessary for preventing transmission of tuberculosis.

Contact transmission-based precautions

To implement *contact* transmission-based precautions in addition to standard precautions, follow these steps:
• Place the patient in a private room or, if one isn't available, use a room with another patient who has an active infection with the same microorganism. If this isn't possible, consult infection control personnel.
• Wear gloves whenever you enter the room. Always change gloves after contact with infected material. Remove gloves before leaving the patient's room, and wash your hands immediately with an antimicrobial soap or waterless antiseptic agent. Don't touch any contaminated surfaces after washing your hands.

• Wear a gown when entering the patient's room if you think your clothing will have extensive contact with the patient, environmental surfaces, or items in the patient's room or if the patient has diarrhea or is incontinent. Remove the gown before leaving the patient's room.
• Limit movement of the patient from the room.

Recommended barriers to infection

The list below presents the minimum requirements for using gloves, gowns, masks, and eye protection to avoid contacting and spreading pathogens. It assumes that you wash your hands thoroughly in all cases. Refer to your facility's guidelines and use your own judgment when assessing the need for barrier protection in specific situations.

Key

 Gloves

 Gown

 Mask

 Eyewear

Bleeding or pressure application to control it

 if soiling likely

 if splattering likely

 if splattering likely

Cardiopulmonary resuscitation

 if splattering likely

 if splattering likely

 if splattering likely

Central venous line insertion and venisection

Central venous pressure measurement

Chest drainage system change

if splattering likely

if splattering likely

if splattering likely

Chest tube insertion or removal

 if soiling likely

if splattering likely

if splattering likely

Colonoscopy, flexible sigmoidoscope

Coughing, frequent and forceful by patient; direct contact with secretions

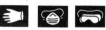

Dialysis, peritoneal (skin care at catheter site)

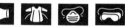

Dressing change for burns

Dressing removal or change for wounds with little or no drainage

Dressing removal or change for wounds with large amount of drainage

 if soiling likely

Fecal impaction, removal of

Gastric lavage

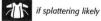 *if soiling likely*

Incision and drainage of abscess

if splattering likely

Intravenous or intraarterial line (insertion, removal, tubing change at catheter hub)

Intubation or extubation

 if splattering likely

 if splattering likely

 if splattering likely

Invasive procedures (lumbar puncture, bone marrow aspiration, paracentesis, liver biopsy) outside sterile field

Irrigation, indwelling urinary catheter

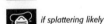

Irrigation, vaginal

 if soiling likely

Irrigation, wound

Joint or nerve injection

Lesion biopsy or removal

Linen, changing visibly soiled

 if soiling likely

Nasogastric tube, insertion or irrigation

 if soiling likely

 if splattering likely

 if splattering likely

Ostomy care, irrigation, and teaching

 if soiling likely

Pelvic exam and Papanicolaou test

Pressure ulcer care

Specimen collection (blood, stool, urine, sputum, wound)

Suctioning, nasotracheal or endotracheal

if soiling likely

if splattering likely

if splattering likely

Suctioning, oral or nasal

Tracheostomy suctioning and cannula cleaning

 if soiling likely

 if splattering likely

 if splattering likely

Wound packing

 if soiling likely

Checklist of reportable diseases

Certain contagious diseases must be reported to local and state public health officials and, ultimately, to the CDC. Typically, these diseases fit one of two categories — those reported individually on definitive or suspected diagnosis and those reported by the number of cases per week. The most commonly reported diseases include hepatitis, measles, viral meningitis, salmonellosis, shigellosis, syphilis, and gonorrhea.

In most states, the patient's primary care provider must report communicable diseases to health officials. In hospitals, the infection control practitioner or epidemiologist reports them. Therefore, you should know the reporting requirements and procedure. Fast, accurate reporting helps to identify and control infection sources, prevent epidemics, and guide public health policy.

The following list notes reportable diseases and conditions. Because disease reporting laws vary among states, the list isn't conclusive.
• Acquired immunodeficiency syndrome (AIDS)
• Amebiasis
• Animal bites
• Anthrax (cutaneous or pulmonary)
• Aseptic meningitis
• Botulism (food-borne, infant)
• Brucellosis
• Cholera
• Diphtheria (cutaneous or pharyngeal)
• Encephalitis (postinfectious or primary)
• Gastroenteritis (institutional outbreaks)
• Gonorrhea
• Group A beta-hemolytic streptococcal infections (including scarlet fever)
• Guillain-Barré syndrome
• Hepatitis A (include suspected source)
• Hepatitis B (include suspected source)
• Hepatitis C, formerly called non-A, non-B (include suspected source)
• Hepatitis, unspecified (include suspected source)
• Influenza
• Legionellosis (legionnaires' disease)
• Leprosy
• Leptospirosis
• Malaria
• Measles (rubeola)
• Meningitis (specify etiology)
• Meningococcal disease
• Mumps
• Pertussis
• Plague (bubonic or pneumonic)
• Poliomyelitis (spinal paralytic)
• Psittacosis

- Rabies
- Reye's syndrome
- Rheumatic fever
- Rocky Mountain spotted fever
- Rubella (congenital syndrome)
- Rubella (German measles)
- Salmonellosis (excluding typhoid fever)
- Shigellosis
- Smallpox
- Staphylococcal infections (neonatal)
- Syphilis (congenital less than 1 year)
- Syphilis (primary or secondary)
- Tetanus
- Toxic shock syndrome
- Trichinosis
- Tuberculosis
- Tularemia
- Typhoid fever
- Typhus (flea- and tick-borne)
- Varicella (chickenpox)
- Yellow fever

Drug hazards

Preventing and treating
adverse effects

Adverse or toxic drug reactions

Identifying and treating toxic drug reactions

The key to treating toxic drug reactions successfully is quickly and accurately identifying the drug, then immediately beginning appropriate treatment. (See *Managing toxic drug reactions,* pages 375 to 378.)

Identifying the most dangerous drugs

The following drugs cause roughly 90% of all reported reactions.

Anticoagulants

• heparin
• warfarin

Antimicrobials

• Cephalosporins
• Penicillins
• Sulfonamides

Bronchodilators

• Sympathomimetics
• theophylline

Cardiac drugs

• Antihypertensives
• Digoxin
• Diuretics
• Quinidine

Central nervous system drugs

• Analgesics
• Anticonvulsants
• Neuroleptics

• Sedative-hypnotics

Diagnostic agents

• X-ray contrast media

Hormones

• Corticosteroids
• Estrogens
• Insulin

Recognizing reactions in elderly patients

Elderly patients are especially susceptible to adverse reactions, such as urticaria, impotence, incontinence, GI upset, and rashes. Less common adverse reactions, such as anxiety, confusion, and forgetfulness, may be mistaken for typical elderly behaviors. The reactions described below are serious—you need to know how to recognize and deal with them.

Altered mental status

Agitation or confusion may follow the use of anticholinergics, diuretics, antihypertensives, and antidepressants. Paradoxically, depression may result from antidepressant drugs.

Anorexia

This is a warning sign of toxicity, especially from digitalis glycosides such as digoxin. Digitalis glycosides have a narrow therapeutic window.

Blood disorders

If the patient takes an anticoagulant, watch for signs of easy bruising or bleeding, such as excessive bleeding after tooth-brushing. Such signs may signal thrombocytopenia or blood dyscrasias. Other drugs that may
(Text continues on page 379.)

MANAGING TOXIC DRUG REACTIONS

Toxic reactions and clinical effects	Interventions	Selected causative drugs
Anemia, aplastic • Bleeding from mucous membranes, ecchymoses, petechiae • Fatigue, pallor, progressive weakness, shortness of breath, tachycardia progressing to heart failure • Fever, oral and rectal ulcers, sore throat without characteristic inflammation	• Stop drug, if possible. • Order vigorous supportive care, including transfusions, neutropenic isolation, antibiotics, and oxygen. • Colony-stimulating factors may be given. • In severe cases, a bone marrow transplant may be needed.	• altretamine • aspirin (long-term) • carbamazepine • chloramphenicol • co-trimoxazole • ganciclovir • Gold salts • hydrochlorothiazide • mephenytoin • methimazole • penicillamine • Phenothiazines • phenylbutazone • propylthiouracil • triamterene • zidovudine
Anemia, hemolytic • Chills, fever, back and abdominal pain (hemolytic crisis) • Jaundice, malaise, splenomegaly • Signs of shock	• Stop drug. • Order supportive care, including transfusions and oxygen. • Consider obtaining a blood sample for Coombs' tests.	• carbidopa-levodopa • levodopa • mefenamic acid • methyldopa • Penicillins • phenazopyridine • primaquine • quinidine • quinine • Sulfonamides
Bone marrow toxicity (agranulocytosis) • Enlarged lymph nodes, spleen, and tonsils • Septicemia, shock • Progressive fatigue and weakness, then sudden overwhelming infection with chills, fever, headache, and tachycardia • Pneumonia • Ulcers in the colon, mouth, and pharynx	• Stop drug. • Begin antibiotic therapy while awaiting blood culture and sensitivity results. • Order supportive therapy, including neutropenic isolation, warm saline gargles, and oral hygiene.	• Angiotensin-converting enzyme inhibitors • aminoglutethimide • carbamazepine • chloramphenicol • clomipramine • co-trimoxazole • flucytosine • Gold salts • penicillamine • Phenothiazines • phenylbutazone • phenytoin • procainamide • propylthiouracil • Sulfonylureas
Bone marrow toxicity (thrombocytopenia) • Fatigue, weakness, lethargy, malaise • Hemorrhage, loss of consciousness, shortness of breath, tachycardia	• Stop drug or reduce dosage. • Order corticosteroids and platelet transfusions. • Consider ordering platelet-stimulating factors.	• anistreplase • ciprofloxacin • cisplatin • colfosceril

(continued)

MANAGING TOXIC DRUG REACTIONS (continued)

Toxic reactions and clinical effects	Interventions	Selected causative drugs
Bone marrow toxicity (thrombocytopenia) (continued) • Sudden onset of ecchymoses or petechiae; large blood-filled bullae in the mouth		• etretinate • floxuridine • flucytosine • ganciclovir • Gold salts • heparin • interferons alfa-2a and alpha-2b • lymphocyte immune globulin • methotrexate • penicillamine • procarbazine • quinidine • quinine • Tetracyclines • valproic acid
Cardiomyopathy • Acute hypertensive reaction • Atrial and ventricular arrhythmias • Chest pain • Heart failure • Chronic cardiomyopathy • Pericarditis-myocarditis syndrome	• Discontinue drug, if possible. • Closely monitor patients receiving concurrent radiation therapy. • Institute cardiac monitoring at earliest sign of problems. • If patient is receiving doxorubicin, limit cumulative dose to less than 500 mg/m².	• cyclophosphamide • cytarabine • daunorubicin • doxorubicin • idarubicin • mitoxantrone
Dermatologic toxicity • May vary from phototoxicity to acneiform eruptions, alopecia, exfoliative dermatitis, lupus erythematosus-like reactions, toxic epidermal necrolysis	• Stop drug. • Order topical antihistamines and analgesics.	• Androgens • Barbiturates • Corticosteroids • Cephalosporins • Gold salts • hydralazine • Interferons • Iodides • Penicillins • pentamidine • phenolphthalein • Phenothiazines • phenylbutazone • procainamide • psoralens • Quinolones • Sulfonamides • Sulfonylureas • Tetracyclines • Thiazides

MANAGING TOXIC DRUG REACTIONS (continued)

Toxic reactions and clinical effects	Interventions	Selected causative drugs
Hepatotoxicity • Abdominal pain, hepatomegaly • Abnormal levels of alanine aminotransferase, aspartate aminotransferase, serum bilirubin, and lactate dehydrogenase • Bleeding, low-grade fever, mental changes, weight loss • Dry skin, pruritus, rash • Jaundice	• Reduce dosage or stop drug. • Order monitoring of vital signs, blood levels, weight, intake and output, and fluids and electrolytes. • Promote rest. • Perform hemodialysis, if needed. • Order symptomatic care: vitamins A, B complex, D, and K; potassium for alkalosis; salt-poor albumin for fluid and electrolyte balance; neomycin for GI flora; stomach aspiration for blood; reduced dietary protein; and lactulose for blood ammonia.	• amiodarone • asparaginase • carbamazepine • chlorpromazine • chlorpropamide • cytarabine • dantrolene • erythromycin estolate • ifosfamide • isoniazide • ketoconazole • leuprolide • methotrexate • methyldopa • mitoxantrone • niacin • phenobarbital • plicamycin • Quinolones • sulindac
Nephrotoxicity • Altered creatinine clearance (decreased or increased) • Blurred vision, dehydration (depending on part of kidney affected), edema, mild headache, pallor • Casts, albumin, or red or white blood cells in urine • Dizziness, fatigue, irritability, slowed mental processes • Electrolyte imbalance • Elevated blood urea nitrogen level • Oliguria	• Reduce dosage or stop drug. • Perform hemodialysis, if needed. • Order monitoring of vital signs, weight changes, and urine volume. • Give symptomatic care: fluid restriction and loop diuretics to reduce fluid retention, I.V. solutions to correct electrolyte imbalance.	• Aminoglycosides • Cephalosporins • cisplatin • Contrast media • Corticosteroids • cyclosporine • gallium • Gold salts (parenteral) • Nitrosoureas • Nonsteroidal anti-inflammatory drugs • penicillin • pentamidine isethionate • plicamycin • Vasopressors or vasoconstrictors
Neurotoxicity • Akathisia • Bilateral or unilateral palsies • Muscle twitching, tremor • Paresthesia • Seizures • Strokelike syndrome • Unsteady gait • Weakness	• Notify physician as soon as changes appear. • Reduce dosage or stop drug. • Monitor carefully for any changes in the patient's condition. • Order symptomatic care: Remain with the patient, reassure him, and protect him during seizures. Provide a quiet environment, draw shades, and speak in soft tones. Maintain the airway, and ventilate the patient as needed.	• Aminoglycosides • cisplatin • cytarabine • isoniazid • nitroprusside • polymyxin B injection • Vinca alkaloids

(continued)

MANAGING TOXIC DRUG REACTIONS (continued)

Toxic reactions and clinical effects	Interventions	Selected causative drugs
Ocular toxicity • Acute glaucoma • Blurred, colored, or flickering vision • Cataracts • Corneal deposits • Diplopia • Miosis • Mydriasis • Optic neuritis • Scotomata • Vision loss	• Notify physician as soon as changes appear. • Stop drug if possible. (Some oculotoxic drugs used to treat serious conditions may be given again at a reduced dosage after the eyes are rested and have returned to near normal.) • Monitor carefully for changes in symptoms. • Treat effects symptomatically.	• amiodarone • Antibiotics such as chloramphenicol • Anticholinergic agents • chloroquine • clomiphene • Corticosteroids • cyclophosphamide • cytarabine • Digitalis glycosides • ethambutol • hydroxychloroquine • lithium carbonate • methotrexate • Phenothiazines • quinidine • quinine • rifampin • tamoxifen • Vinca alkaloids
Ototoxicity • Ataxia • Hearing loss • Tinnitus • Vertigo	• Notify physician as soon as changes appear. • Stop drug or reduce dosage. • Monitor carefully for symptomatic changes.	• Aminoglycosides • Antibiotics, such as colistimethate sodium, erythromycin, gentamicin, kanamycin, and streptomycin • chloroquine • cisplatin • Loop diuretics • minocycline • quinidine • quinine • Salicylates • vancomycin
Pseudomembranous colitis • Abdominal pain • Colonic perforation • Fever • Hypotension • Severe dehydration • Shock • Sudden, copious diarrhea (watery or bloody)	• Discontinue drug and order another antibiotic, such as vancomycin or metronidazole. • Maintain fluid and electrolyte balance. • Check serum electrolyte levels daily. If pseudomembranous colitis is mild, order an ion exchange resin. • Monitor vital signs and hydration status.. • Immediately report signs of shock to physician. • Observe for signs of hypokalemia, especially malaise and weak, rapid, irregular pulse.	• Antibiotics

cause these reactions include antineoplastics such as methotrexate, antibiotics such as nitrofurantoin, and anticonvulsants, such as valproic acid and phenytoin. Tell your patient to report easy bruising immediately.

Dehydration

If the patient is taking diuretics, be alert for dehydration and electrolyte imbalance. Monitor blood levels of the drug, and give potassium supplements. Many drugs such as anticholinergics cause a dry mouth. Suggest sucking on sugarless candy for relief.

Orthostatic hypotension

Marked by light-headedness or faintness and unsteady footing, orthostatic hypotension can occur with the use of sedatives, antidepressants, antihypertensives, and antipsychotics. To prevent falls, warn the patient not to sit up or get out of bed too quickly, and to call for help with walking if he feels dizzy or faint.

Tardive dyskinesia

Characterized by abnormal tongue movements, lip pursing, grimacing, blinking, and gyrating motions of the face and extremities, this disorder may be triggered by psychotropic drugs, such as haloperidol or chlorpromazine.

Preventing drug overdose in renal failure

Impaired renal function can modify a drug's bioavailability, distribution, pharmacologic action, and elimination. Many drug dosages must be adjusted to avoid accidental overdose.

(See *Adjusting drug dosages in renal failure,* pages 380 to 385.)

Drug overdoses
General guidelines

If your patient has signs of acute drug toxicity, institute advanced life support measures as indicated. Administer the prescribed antidote, if available, and institute measures to block absorption and speed elimination of the drug. Consult with a regional poison control center for additional information about treatment of specific toxins. The steps below outline how to manage an acute overdose of ingested systemic drugs.

Starting advanced life support

• Establish and maintain an airway. This is usually done by inserting an oropharyngeal or endotracheal airway.
• If the patient isn't breathing, start ventilation with a bag-valve mask until a mechanical ventilator is available. Administer oxygen as indicated by pulse oximetry or arterial blood gas levels.
• Maintain circulation. Start an I.V. infusion, and obtain laboratory specimens to assess for toxic drug levels, electrolytes, and glucose levels as indicated.
For hypotension: Administer fluids and vasopressors such as dopamine (Intropin).
For hypertension: Prepare to administer antihypertensive agents (usually beta blockers if catecholamines were ingested). Prepare to treat arrhythmias as indicated for the specific toxin.
• Protect the patient from injury, and monitor for seizures. Observe the pa-
(Text continues on page 385.)

ADJUSTING DRUG DOSAGES IN RENAL FAILURE

To prevent an accidental drug overdose in a patient with renal failure, adjust dosages according to the severity of renal impairment, as shown in the chart below. (*Note:* "GFR" refers to glomerular filtration rate.)

Drug	Mild renal impairment (GFR > 50 ml/minute)		Moderate renal impairment (GFR 10 to 50 ml/minute)		Severe renal impairment (GFR < 10 ml/minute)	
	% of normal dose	Interval	% of normal dose	Interval	% of normal dose	Interval
acetaminophen	100%	q 4 hr	100%	q 6 hr	100%	q 8 hr
acetazolamide	100%	q 6 hr	100%	q 12 hr	Avoid	Avoid
acetohexamide	100%	q 12 hr	Avoid	Avoid	Avoid	Avoid
acyclovir	100%	q 8 hr	100%	q 24 hr	100%	q 48 hr
allopurinol	100%	q 8 hr	75%	q 8 hr	50%	q 8 hr
amantadine	100%	q 12 to 24 hr	100%	q 48 to 72 hr	100%	q 7 days
amikacin	60% to 90%	q 12 hr	30% to 70%	q 12 to 24 hr	20% to 30%	q 24 hr
amoxicillin	100%	q 6 hr	100%	q 6 to 12 hr	100%	q 12 to 16 hr
amphotericin B	100%	q 24 hr	100%	q 24 hr	100%	q 24 to 36 hr
ampicillin	100%	q 6 hr	100%	q 6 to 12 hr	100%	q 12 to 16 hr
aspirin	100%	q 4 hr	100%	q 4 to 6 hr	Avoid	Avoid
atenolol	100%	q 24 hr	100%	q 48 hr	100%	q 96 hr
azathioprine	100%	q 24 hr	100%	q 24 hr	100%	q 36 hr
betaxolol	100%	q 24 hr	100%	q 24 hr	50%	q 24 hr
bleomycin	100%	Varies	100%	Varies	50%	Varies
bretylium	100%	Continuous infusion	25% to 50%	Continuous infusion	Avoid	Avoid
captopril	100%	t.i.d.	100%	t.i.d.	50%	t.i.d.
carbamazepine	100%	q 6 to 8 hr	100%	q 6 to 8 hr	75%	q 6 to 8 hr
carbenicillin	100%	q 8 to 12 hr	100%	q 12 to 24 hr	100%	q 24 to 48 hr

ADJUSTING DRUG DOSAGES IN RENAL FAILURE
(continued)

Drug	Mild renal impairment (GFR > 50 ml/minute)		Moderate renal impairment (GFR 10 to 50 ml/minute)		Severe renal impairment (GFR < 10 ml/minute)	
	% of normal dose	Interval	% of normal dose	Interval	% of normal dose	Interval
cefaclor	100%	q 6 hr	50% to 100%	q 6 hr	33%	q 6 hr
cefadroxil	100%	q 8 hr	100%	q 12 to 24 hr	100%	q 24 to 48 hr
efamandole	100%	q 6 hr	100%	q 6 to 8 hr	100%	q 8 hr
cefonicid	50%	q 24 hr	25%	q 24 hr	25%	q 3 to 5 days
cefotaxime	100%	q 6 to 8 hr	100%	q 8 to 12 hr	100%	q 24 hr
cefoxitin	100%	q 8 hr	100%	q 8 to 12 hr	100%	q 24 to 48 hr
cephalexin	100%	q 6 hr	100%	q 6 to 8 hr	100%	q 12 hr
cephalothin	100%	q 6 hr	75%	q 6 hr	50%	q 6 hr
cephapirin	100%	q 6 hr	100%	q 6 to 8 hr	100%	q 12 hr
cephradine	100%	q 6 hr	50% to 100%	q 6 hr	50%	q 6 to 12 hr
chloral hydrate	100%	At bed-time	Avoid	Avoid	Avoid	Avoid
chlorpropamide	100%	q 24 hr	Avoid	Avoid	Avoid	Avoid
chlorthalidone	100%	q 24 hr	100%	q 24 hr	100%	q 48 hr
cimetidine	100%	q 6 hr	100%	q 8 hr	100%	q 12 hr
ciprofloxacin	100%	q 12 hr	100%	q 12 to 24 hr	100%	q 24 hr
cisplatin	100%	Varies	75%	Varies	50%	Varies
clofibrate	100%	q 6 to 12 hr	100%	q 12 to 18 hr	100%	q 24 to 48 hr
clonidine	100%	b.i.d.	100%	b.i.d.	50% to 75%	b.i.d.
colchicine	100%	Varies	100%	Varies	50%	Varies

(continued)

ADJUSTING DRUG DOSAGES IN RENAL FAILURE
(continued)

Drug	Mild renal impairment (GFR > 50 ml/minute)		Moderate renal impairment (GFR 10 to 50 ml/minute)		Severe renal impairment (GFR < 10 ml/minute)	
	% of normal dose	Interval	% of normal dose	Interval	% of normal dose	Interval
cyclophosphamide	100%	q 12 hr	100%	q 12 hr	100%	q 18 to 24 hr
diflunisal	100%	q 12 hr	100%	q 12 hr	50%	q 12 hr
digitoxin	100%	q 24 hr	100%	q 24 hr	50% to 75%	q 24 hr
digoxin	100%	q 24 hr	100%	q 36 hr	100%	q 48 hr
diphenhydramine	100%	q 6 hr	100%	q 6 to 9 hr	100%	q 9 to 12 hr
disopyramide	100%	q 6 hr	100%	q 12 to 24 hr	100%	q 24 to 40 hr
doxycycline	100%	q 12 hr	100%	q 12 to 18 hr	100%	q 18 to 24 hr
ethacrynic acid	100%	q 6 hr	100%	q 6 hr	Avoid	Avoid
ethambutol	100%	q 24 hr	100%	q 24 to 36 hr	100%	q 48 hr
ethosuximide	100%	q 12 hr	100%	q 12 hr	75%	q 12 hr
flucytosine	100%	q 6 hr	100%	q 12 to 24 hr	100%	q 24 to 48 hr
ganciclovir	100%	q 12 hr	100%	q 24 hr	100%	q 24 hr
gemfibrozil	100%	b.i.d.	50%	b.i.d.	25%	b.i.d.
gentamicin	60% to 90%	q 8 to 12 hr	30% to 70%	q 12 hr	20% to 30%	q 24 hr
guanethidine	100%	q 24 hr	100%	q 24 hr	100%	q 24 to 36 hr
hydralazine	100%	q 8 hr	100%	q 8 hr	100%	q 8 to 16 hr or q 12 to 24 hr*
hydroxyurea	100%	Varies	100%	Varies	50%	Varies
isoniazid	100%	q 24 hr	100%	q 24 hr	66% to 75%	q 24 hr

*Depending on whether patient is a fast or slow acetylator

ADJUSTING DRUG DOSAGES IN RENAL FAILURE
(continued)

Drug	Mild renal impairment (GFR > 50 ml/minute)		Moderate renal impairment (GFR 10 to 50 ml/minute)		Severe renal impairment (GFR < 10 ml/minute)	
	% of normal dose	Interval	% of normal dose	Interval	% of normal dose	Interval
kanamycin	60% to 90%	q 8 to 12 hr	30% to 70%	q 12 hr	20% to 30%	q 24 hr
ketorolac	100%	p.r.n.	100%	p.r.n.	50%	p.r.n.
lincomycin	100%	q 6 hr	100%	q 12 hr	100%	q 24 hr
lisinopril	100%	q 24 hr	50%	q 24 hr	25%	q 24 hr
lithium carbonate	100%	t.i.d. to q.i.d.	50% to 75%	t.i.d. to q.i.d	25% to 50%	t.i.d. to q.i.d.
loracarbef	100%	q 12 to 24 hr	50%	q 12 to 24 hr	100%	q 3 to 5 days
lorazepam	100%	t.i.d. to q.i.d.	100%	t.i.d. to q.i.d.	50%	t.i.d. to q.i.d.
meperidine	100%	Varies	75%	Varies	50%	Varies
meprobamate	100%	q 6 hr	100%	q 9 to 12 hr	100%	q 12 to 18 hr
methadone	100%	q 6 to 8 hr	100%	q 6 to 8 hr	50% to 75%	q 6 to 8 hr
methotrexate	100%	Varies	50%	Varies	Avoid	Avoid
methyldopa	100%	q 6 hr	100%	q 8 to 18 hr	100%	q 12 to 24 hr
metoclopramide	100%	Varies	75%	Varies	50%	Varies
metronidazole	100%	q 8 hr	100%	q 8 to 12 hr	100%	q 12 to 24 hr
mexiletine	100%	q 12 hr	100%	q 12 hr	50% to 75%	q 12 hr
mezlocillin	100%	q 4 to 6 hr	100%	q 6 to 8 hr	100%	q 8 hr
mitomycin	100%	Varies	100%	Varies	75%	Varies
moricizine	100%	q 8 hr	100%	q 8 hr	50% to 75%	q 8 hr
nadolol	100%	q 24 hr	50%	q 24 hr	25%	q 24 hr
nalidixic acid	100%	q.i.d.	Avoid	Avoid	Avoid	Avoid

(continued)

ADJUSTING DRUG DOSAGES IN RENAL FAILURE
(continued)

Drug	Mild renal impairment (GFR > 50 ml/minute)		Moderate renal impairment (GFR 10 to 50 ml/minute)		Severe renal impairment (GFR < 10 ml/minute)	
	% of normal dose	Interval	% of normal dose	Interval	% of normal dose	Interval
neostigmine	100%	q 6 hr	100%	q 6 hr	100%	q 12 to 18 hr
netilmicin	60% to 90%	q 8 to 12 hr	30% to 70%	q 12 hr	20% to 30%	q 24 hr
nicotinic acid	100%	t.i.d.	50%	t.i.d.	25%	t.i.d.
nitrofurantoin	100%	q.i.d.	Avoid	Avoid	Avoid	Avoid
oxazepam	100%	q.i.d.	100%	q.i.d.	75%	q.i.d.
penicillin G	100%	q 6 to 8 hr	100%	q 8 to 12 hr	Avoid over 10 million units/day	q 12 to 16 hr
pentamidine isethionate (parenteral)	100%	q 24 hr	100%	q 24 to 36 hr	100%	q 48 hr
phenobarbital	100%	t.i.d.	100%	t.i.d.	100%	q 12 to 16 hr
phenylbutazone	100%	t.i.d. to q.i.d.	100%	t.i.d. to q.i.d.	Avoid	Avoid
piperacillin	100%	q 4 to 6 hr	100%	q 6 to 8 hr	100%	q 8 hr
plicamycin	100%	Varies	75%	Varies	50%	Varies
primidone	100%	q 8 hr	100%	q 8 to 12 hr	50%	q 12 to 24 hr
probenecid	100%	q.i.d.	Avoid	Avoid	Avoid	Avoid
procainamide	100%	q 4 hr	100%	q 6 to 12 hr	100%	q 8 to 24 hr
propoxyphene	100%	q 4 hr	100%	q 4 hr	25%	q 4 hr
reserpine	100%	q 24 hr	100%	q 24 hr	Avoid	Avoid
spironolactone	100%	q 6 to 12 hr	100%	q 12 to 24 hr	Avoid	Avoid
streptomycin	100%	q 24 hr	100%	q 24 to 72 hr	100%	q 72 to 96 hr

ADJUSTING DRUG DOSAGES IN RENAL FAILURE
(continued)

Drug	Mild renal impairment (GFR > 50 ml/minute)		Moderate renal impairment (GFR 10 to 50 ml/minute)		Severe renal impairment (GFR < 10 ml/minute)	
	% of normal dose	Interval	% of normal dose	Interval	% of normal dose	Interval
streptozocin	100%	Varies	75%	Varies	50%	Varies
sulfamethoxazole	100%	q 12 hr	100%	q 18 hr	100%	q 24 hr
sulfisoxazole	100%	q 6 hr	100%	q 8 to 12 hr	100%	q 12 to 24 hr
sulindac	100%	b.i.d.	100%	b.i.d.	50%	b.i.d.
terbutaline	100%	t.i.d.	50%	t.i.d.	Avoid	Avoid
thiazides	100%	Daily to b.i.d.	100%	Daily to b.i.d.	Avoid	Avoid
ticarcillin	100%	q 8 to 12 hr	100%	q 12 to 24 hr	100%	q 24 to 48 hr
tobramycin	60% to 90%	q 8 to 12 hr	30% to 70%	q 12 hr	20% to 30%	q 24 hr
triamterene	100%	q 12 hr	100%	q 12 hr	Avoid	Avoid
trimethoprim	100%	q 12 hr	100%	q 18 hr	100%	q 24 hr
vancomycin	100%	q 1 to 3 days	100%	q 3 to 10 days	100%	q 10 days
vidarabine	100%	Continuous infusion	100%	Continuous infusion	75%	Continuous infusion

tient, and provide supportive care. Prepare to administer lorazepam, diazepam, or phenytoin.

Administering the antidote

The antidote is administered as soon as possible. Administer the prescribed antidote according to the class of drugs the patient has taken. Specific antidotes are described on the following pages.

Blocking drug absorption

• Gastric emptying is effective up to 2 hours after drug ingestion. Two methods are used: syrup of ipecac for a conscious patient who isn't expected to deteriorate and gastric lavage for a comatose patient or one who doesn't respond to syrup of ipecac.

• Adsorption with activated charcoal is used in place of emesis or lavage if the drug is well adsorbed by activated charcoal or after emesis or lavage to adsorb co-ingestants if the primary toxin isn't well adsorbed by activated charcoal.

• A cathartic may be given to speed transit of the poison through the GI tract. Whole-bowel irrigation with a balanced polyethylene glycol and electrolyte solution may be ordered if a sustained-release product was ingested.

Speeding drug elimination

• Gastric dialysis uses timed doses of activated charcoal for 1 to 2 days. The charcoal binds to the drug, thus facilitating its removal in feces.
• Diuresis is effective for some drug overdoses. Forced diuresis uses furosemide and osmotic diuretics, alkaline diuresis uses I.V. sodium bicarbonate, and acid diuresis uses oral or I.V. ascorbic acid or ammonium chloride.
• Peritoneal dialysis and hemodialysis are occasionally used in severe overdose.

Antidotes in poisoning or overdose

If your patient has signs of acute drug toxicity, institute advanced life support measures as indicated. Administer the prescribed antidote, if available, and take steps to block absorption and speed elimination of the drug. Consult with a regional poison control center for information on how to treat ingestion of a specific toxin. (See *Managing poisoning or overdose,* pages 387 to 392.)

Acetaminophen overdose

In an acute acetaminophen overdose, plasma levels of 300 µg/ml 4 hours after ingestion or 50 µg/ml 12 hours after ingestion are associated with hepatotoxicity. Clinical findings in an overdose include cyanosis, anemia, jaundice, skin eruptions, fever, emesis, CNS stimulation, delirium, and methemoglobinemia progressing to CNS depression, coma, vascular collapse, seizures, and death. Aceta-

minophen poisoning develops in stages:
• *stage 1 (12 to 24 hours after ingestion):* nausea, vomiting, diaphoresis, anorexia
• *stage 2 (24 to 48 hours after ingestion):* clinically improved but elevated liver function test results
• *stage 3 (72 to 96 hours after ingestion):* peak hepatotoxicity
• *stage 4 (7 to 8 days after ingestion):* recovery.

To treat acetaminophen toxicity, immediately induce emesis with syrup of ipecac if the patient is conscious, or with gastric lavage if he's comatose or doesn't respond to syrup of ipecac. Administer activated charcoal via a nasogastric tube. Oral acetylcysteine, a specific antidote for acetaminophen poisoning, is most effective if started within 12 hours after ingestion but can help if started as late as 24 hours after ingestion. Administer an oral loading dose of acetylcysteine, 140 mg/kg of body weight, followed by oral maintenance doses of 70 mg/kg of body weight every 4 hours for an additional 17 doses. Doses vomited within 1 hour of administration must be repeated. Remove charcoal by lavage before administering acetylcysteine because it may interfere with this antidote's absorption.

Acetylcysteine minimizes hepatic injury by supplying sulfhydryl groups that bind with acetaminophen metabolites. Hemodialysis may be helpful in removing acetaminophen from the body. Monitor laboratory parameters and vital signs closely. Cimetidine has been used investigationally to block acetaminophen's metabolism to toxic intermediates. Provide symptomatic and supportive measures (respiratory support and correction of fluid and electrolyte imbalances). Determine plasma acetaminophen levels at least 4 hours after

(Text continues on page 392.)

MANAGING POISONING OR OVERDOSE

Antidote and indications	Dosage	Nursing considerations
acetylcysteine (Mucomyst, Mucosil, Parvolex) • Treatment of acetaminophen toxicity	• *Adults and children*: 140 mg/kg P.O. initially, followed by 70 mg/kg every 4 hours for 17 doses (total of 1,330 mg/kg).	• Use cautiously in elderly or debilitated patients and in patients with asthma or severe respiratory insufficiency. • Don't use with activated charcoal. • Don't combine with amphotericin B, ampicillin, chymotrypsin, erythromycin lactobionate, hydrogen peroxide, oxytetracycline, tetracycline, iodized oil, or trypsin. Administer separately.
activated charcoal (Actidose-Aqua, Charcoaid, Charcocaps, Liqui-Char) • Treatment of poisoning or overdose with most orally administered drugs, except caustic agents and hydrocarbons	• *Adults*: initially, 1 g/kg (30 to 100 g) P.O., or 5 to 10 times the amount of poison ingested as a suspension in 180 to 240 ml of water. • *Children ages 1 to 12*: 20 to 50 g P.O. as single dose. • *Children under age 1*: 1 g/kg P.O. as single dose.	• Don't give to semiconscious or unconscious patients. • If possible, administer within 30 minutes of poisoning. Administer larger dose if patient has food in his stomach. • Don't give with syrup of ipecac because charcoal inactivates ipecac. If a patient needs syrup of ipecac, give charcoal after he has finished vomiting. • Don't give in ice cream, milk, or sherbet because they reduce adsorption capacities of charcoal. • Powder form is most effective. Mix with tap water to form a thick syrup. You may add a small amount of fruit juice or flavoring to make the syrup more palatable. • You may need to repeat the dose if the patient vomits shortly after administration.
aminocaproic acid (Amicar) • Antidote for alteplase, anistreplase, streptokinase, or urokinase toxicity	• *Adults*: initially, 5 g P.O. or as slow I.V. infusion, followed by 1 to 1.25 g/hour until bleeding is controlled. Don't exceed 30 g daily.	• Use cautiously with oral contraceptives and estrogens because they may increase the risk of hypercoagulability. • For infusion, dilute solution with sterile water for injection, normal saline solution, dextrose 5% in water (D_5W), or Ringer's solution. • Monitor coagulation studies, heart rhythm, and blood pressure.
amyl nitrite • Antidote for cyanide poisoning	• *Adults*: 0.2 or 0.3 ml by inhalation for 30 to 60 seconds every 5 minutes until patient regains consciousness.	• Amyl nitrite is effective within 30 seconds, but its effects last only 3 to 5 minutes. • To administer, wrap ampule in cloth and crush. Hold near the patient's nose and mouth so that he can inhale vapor. • Monitor the patient for orthostatic hypotension. • The patient may experience headache after administration.

(continued)

MANAGING POISONING OR OVERDOSE *(continued)*

Antidote and indications	Dosage	Nursing considerations
atropine sulfate • Antidote for anticholinesterase toxicity	• *Adults:* initially, 1 to 2 mg by direct I.V. injection, then 2 mg every 5 to 60 minutes until symptoms subside. In severe cases, initial dose may be as much as 6 mg every 4 to 60 minutes, as needed. Administer over 1 to 2 minutes.	• Atropine sulfate is contraindicated for patients with glaucoma, myasthenia gravis, obstructive uropathy, or unstable cardiovascular status. • Monitor intake and output to assess for urine retention.
botulism antitoxin, trivalent equine • Treatment of botulism	• *Adults and children:* 2 vials I.V. Dilute antitoxin 1:10 in D_5W, $D_{10}W$, or normal saline solution before administration. Give first 10 ml of diluted solution over 5 minutes; after 15 minutes, you may increase rate.	• Obtain an accurate patient history of allergies, especially to horses, and of reactions to immunizations. • Test the patient for sensitivity (against a control of normal saline solution in opposing extremity) before administration. Read results after 5 to 30 minutes. A wheal indicates a positive reaction, requiring patient desensitization. • Keep epinephrine 1:1,000 available in case of allergic reaction.
deferoxamine mesylate (Desferal) • Adjunctive treatment of acute iron intoxication	• *Adults and children:* initially, 1 g I.V. or I.M., followed by 500 mg I.M. or I.V. every 4 hours for two doses; then 500 mg I.M. or I.V. every 4 to 12 hours. Don't infuse more than 15 mg/kg/hour. Don't administer more than 6 g in 24 hours.	• Don't administer the drug to patients with severe renal disease or anuria. Use cautiously in patients with impaired renal function. • Keep epinephrine 1:1,000 available in case of allergic reaction. • Use I.M. route if possible. Use I.V. route only when the patient is in shock. • To reconstitute for I.M. administration, add 2 ml of sterile water for injection to each ampule. Make sure the drug dissolves completely. To reconstitute for I.V. administration, dissolve as for I.M. use but in normal saline solution, D_5W, or lactated Ringer's solution. • Monitor intake and output carefully. Warn patient that his urine may turn red. • Reconstituted solution can be stored for up to 1, week at room temperature. Protect from light.

MANAGING POISONING OR OVERDOSE (continued)

Antidote and indications	Dosage	Nursing considerations
digoxin immune Fab (ovine) (Digibind) • Treatment of potentially life-threatening digoxin or digitoxin intoxication	• *Adults and children:* give I.V. over 30 minutes or as a bolus if cardiac arrest is imminent. Dosage varies according to amount of drug ingested; average dose is 10 vials (400 mg), but if toxicity resulted from acute digoxin ingestion and neither serum digoxin level nor estimated ingestion amount is known, increase dose to 20 vials (760 mg). • Package inserts or reference books contain charts and formulas to calculate dose based on number of tablets ingested or serum digoxin level.	• Use cautiously in patients allergic to ovine proteins because the drug is derived from digoxin-specific antibody fragments obtained from immunized sheep. Perform skin test before administering. • Use only in patients in shock or cardiac arrest with ventricular arrhythmias, such as ventricular tachycardia or fibrillation; with progressive bradycardia, such as severe sinus bradycardia; or with second- or third-degree atrioventricular block unresponsive to atropine. • Infuse through a 0.22-micron membrane filter, if possible. • Refrigerate powder for reconstitution. If possible, use reconstituted drug immediately, although you may refrigerate it for up to 4 hours. • Drug interferes with digitalis immunoassay measurements, resulting in misleading standard serum digoxin levels until the drug is cleared from the body (about 2 days). • Total serum digoxin levels may rise after administration of this drug, reflecting fat-bound (inactive) digoxin. • Monitor potassium levels closely.
edetate calcium disodium (Calcium Disodium Versenate, Calcium EDTA) • Treatment of lead poisoning in patients with blood levels > 50 μg/dl	*For blood levels of 51 to 100 μg/dl* • *Adults and children:* 1 g/m^2, I.M. or I.V. daily for 3 to 5 days. For I.V. infusion, dilute in D_5W or normal saline solution and give over 1 to 2 hours. *For blood levels >100 μg/dl* • *Adults and children:* 1.5 g/m^2, I.M. or I.V. daily for 3 to 5 days, usually with dimercaprol. For I.V. infusion, dilute in D_5W or normal saline solution and administer over 1 to 2 hours. If necessary, repeat course 2 to 3 weeks later.	• Don't give to patients with severe renal disease or anuria. • Avoid using I.V. route in patients with lead encephalopathy because intracranial pressure may increase; use I.M. route. • Avoid rapid infusion; I.M. route is preferred, especially for children. • If giving a high dose, give with dimercaprol to avoid toxicity. • Force fluids to facilitate lead excretion except in patients with lead encephalopathy. • Before giving, obtain baseline intake and output, urinalysis, blood urea nitrogen, and serum alkaline phosphatase, calcium, creatinine, and phosphorus levels. Then monitor these values on first, third, and fifth days of treatment. Monitor electrocardiogram periodically. • If procaine hydrochloride has been added to I.M. solution to minimize pain, watch for local reaction.

(continued)

MANAGING POISONING OR OVERDOSE *(continued)*

Antidote and indications	Dosage	Nursing considerations
methylene blue • Treatment of cyanide poisoning	• *Adults and children:* 1 to 2 mg/kg of 1% solution by direct I.V. injection over several minutes. May repeat dose in 1 hour.	• Don't give to patients with severe renal impairment or hypersensitivity to drug. • Use with caution in glucose-6-phosphate dehydrogenase deficiency; may cause hemolysis. • Avoid extravasation; S.C. injection may cause necrotic abscesses. • Warn the patient that methylene blue will discolor his urine and stools and stain his skin. Hypochlorite solution rubbed on skin will remove stains.
naloxone hydrochloride (Narcan) • Treatment of respiratory depression caused by opioid drugs • Treatment of postoperative narcotic depression • Treatment of asphyxia neonatorurn	*For respiratory depression caused by opioid drugs* • *Adults:* 0.4 to 2 mg I.V., S.C., or I.M. May repeat every 2 to 3 minutes, as needed. *For postoperative narcotic depression* • *Adults:* 0.1 to 0.2 mg I.V. every 2 to 3 minutes, as needed. • *Children:* 0.01 mg/kg I.V., I.M., or S.C. Repeat as necessary every 2 to 3 minutes. If patient doesn't improve with initial dose of 0.01 mg/kg, he may need up to 10 times this dose (0.1 mg/kg). *For asphyxia neonatorum* • *Neonates:* 0.01 mg/kg I.V. into umbilical vein. Repeat every 2 to 3 minutes for three doses, if necessary.	• Use cautiously in patients with cardiac irritability or narcotic addiction. • Monitor respiratory depth and rate. Be prepared to provide oxygen, ventilation, and other resuscitative measures. • If neonatal concentration (0.02 mg/ml) isn't available, dilute adult concentration (0.4 mg) by mixing 0.5 ml with 9.5 ml of sterile water or normal saline solution. • Respiratory rate increases within 2 minutes. Effects last 1 to 4 hours. • Duration of narcotic may exceed that of naloxone, causing the patient to relapse into respiratory depression. • You may administer drug by continuous I.V. infusion to control adverse effects of epidurally administered morphine. • You may see "overshoot" effect—the patient's respiratory rate after receiving drug exceeds his rate before respiratory depression occurred. • Naloxone is the safest drug to use when the cause of respiratory depression is uncertain. • This drug doesn't reverse respiratory depression caused by diazepam. • Although generally believed ineffective in treating respiratory depression caused by nonopioid drugs, naloxone may reverse coma induced by alcohol intoxication, according to recent reports.

MANAGING POISONING OR OVERDOSE *(continued)*

Antidote and indications	Dosage	Nursing considerations
pralidoxime chloride (Protopam Chloride) • Antidote for organophosphate poisoning and cholinergic drug overdose	• *Adults*: I.V. infusion of 1 to 2 g in 100 ml of normal saline solution over 15 to 30 minutes. If the patient has pulmonary edema, administer by slow I.V. push over 5 minutes. Repeat in 1 hour if weakness persists. If the patient needs additional doses, administer them cautiously. If I.V. administration isn't possible, give I.M. or S.C., or 1 to 3 g P.O. every 5 hours. • *Children*: 20 to 40 mg/kg I.V.	• Don't give to patients poisoned with carbaryl (Sevin), a carbamate insecticide, because it increases Sevin's toxicity. • Use with caution in patients with renal insufficiency, myasthenia gravis, asthma, or peptic ulcer. • Use in hospitalized patients only; have respiratory and other supportive equipment available. • Administer antidote as soon as possible after poisoning. Treatment is most effective if started within 24 hours of exposure. • Before administering, suction secretions and make sure airway is patent. • Dilute drug with sterile water without preservatives. Give atropine along with pralidoxime. • If the patient's skin was exposed, remove his clothing and wash his skin and hair with sodium bicarbonate, soap, water, and alcohol as soon as possible. He may need a second washing. When washing the patient, wear protective gloves and clothes to avoid exposure. • Observe the patient for 48 to 72 hours after he ingested poison. Delayed absorption may occur. Watch for signs of rapid weakening in the patient with myasthenia gravis being treated for overdose of cholinergic drugs. He may pass quickly from cholinergic crisis to myasthenic crisis and require more cholinergic drugs to treat the myasthenia. Keep edrophonium available.
protamine sulfate • Treatment of heparin overdose	• *Adults*: usually 1 mg for every 78 to 95 units of heparin, based on coagulation studies. Dilute to 1% (10 mg/ml) and give by slow I.V. injection over 1 to 3 minutes. Don't exceed 50 mg in 10 minutes.	• Use cautiously after cardiac surgery. • Administer slowly to reduce adverse reactions. Have equipment available to treat shock. • Monitor the patient continuously, and check vital signs frequently. • Watch for spontaneous bleeding (heparin "rebound"), especially in patients undergoing dialysis and in those who have had cardiac surgery. • Protamine sulfate may act as an anticoagulant in extremely high doses.

(continued)

MANAGING POISONING OR OVERDOSE (continued)

Antidote and indications	Dosage	Nursing considerations
syrup of ipecac (ipecac syrup) • Induction of vomiting in poisoning	• *Adults*: 15 ml P.O., followed by 200 to 300 ml of water. • *Children over age 1*: 15 ml P.O., followed by about 200 ml of water or milk. • *Children under age 1*: 5 to 10 ml P.O., followed by 100 to 200 ml of water or milk. Repeat dose once after 20 minutes, if necessary.	• Syrup of ipecac is contraindicated for semicomatose, unconscious, and severely inebriated patients and for those with seizures, shock, or absent gag reflex. • Don't give after ingestion of petroleum distillates or volatile oils because of the risk of aspiration pneumonitis. Don't give after ingestion of caustic substances such as lye because further injury can result. • Before giving, make sure you have ipecac syrup, not ipecac fluid extract (14 times more concentrated, and deadly). • If two doses don't induce vomiting, consider gastric lavage. • If the patient also needs activated charcoal, give charcoal after he has vomited, or charcoal will neutralize the emetic effect. • Suggest to parents of children over age 1 that they keep 1 oz (30 ml) of syrup of ipecac available.

overdose. If they indicate hepatotoxicity, perform liver function tests every 24 hours for at least 96 hours.

Analeptic overdose (amphetamines, cocaine)

Individual responses to overdose with analeptic drugs vary widely. Toxic doses also vary, depending on the drug and the route of ingestion.

Signs and symptoms of overdose include restlessness, tremor, hyperreflexia, tachypnea, confusion, aggressiveness, hallucinations, and panic; fatigue and depression usually follow the excitement stage. Other effects may include arrhythmias, shock, altered blood pressure, nausea, vomiting, diarrhea, and abdominal cramps; death is usually preceded by seizures and coma.

Treat overdose symptomatically and supportively: If oral ingestion is recent (within 4 hours), use gastric lavage or syrup of ipecac to empty the stomach and reduce further absorption. Follow with activated charcoal. Monitor vital signs and fluid and electrolyte balance. If the drug was smoked or injected, focus on enhancing drug elimination and providing supportive care. Administer sedatives as needed. Urine acidification may enhance excretion. A saline cathartic (magnesium citrate) may hasten GI evacuation of unabsorbed sustained-release drug.

Anticholinergic overdose

Clinical effects of an anticholinergic overdose include such peripheral effects as dilated, nonreactive pupils; blurred vision; flushed, hot, dry skin; dry mucous membranes; dysphagia; decreased or absent bowel sounds; urine retention; hyperthermia; tachycardia; hypertension; and increased respiratory rate.

Treatment is primarily symptomatic and supportive as needed. If the patient is alert, induce emesis (or use gastric lavage), and follow with a saline cathartic and activated charcoal to prevent further drug absorption. In severe cases, physostigmine may be administered to block central antimuscarinic effects. Give fluids as needed to treat shock. If urine retention occurs, catheterization may be necessary.

Anticoagulant overdose

Clinical effects of an oral anticoagulant overdose vary with severity. They may include internal or external bleeding or skin necrosis, but the most common sign is hematuria. Excessively prolonged prothrombin time or minor bleeding mandates withdrawal of therapy; withholding one or two doses may be adequate in some cases. Treatment to control bleeding may include oral or I.V. phytonadione (vitamin K_1) and, in severe hemorrhage, fresh frozen plasma or whole blood. Menadione (vitamin K_3) isn't as effective. Use of phytonadione may interfere with subsequent oral anticoagulant therapy.

Antihistamine overdose

Drowsiness is the usual clinical sign of antihistamine overdose. Seizures, coma, and respiratory depression may occur with severe overdose. Certain histamine antagonists such as diphenhydramine also block cholinergic receptors and produce modest anticholinergic symptoms, such as dry mouth, flushed skin, fixed and dilated pupils, and GI symptoms, especially in children. Phenothiazine-type antihistamines such as promethazine also block dopamine receptors. Movement disorders mimicking Parkinson's disease may be seen.

Treat overdose with gastric lavage followed by activated charcoal. Syrup of ipecac is generally not recommended because acute dystonic reactions may increase the risk of aspiration. In addition, phenothiazine-type antihistamines may have antiemetic effects. Treat hypotension with fluids or vasopressors, and treat seizures with phenytoin or diazepam. Watch for arrhythmias, and treat accordingly.

Barbiturate overdose

A barbiturate overdose causes unsteady gait, slurred speech, sustained nystagmus, somnolence, confusion, respiratory depression, pulmonary edema, areflexia, and coma. Typical shock syndrome with tachycardia and hypotension, jaundice, hypothermia followed by fever, and oliguria may occur.

Maintain and support ventilation and pulmonary function as necessary; support cardiac function and circulation with vasopressors and I.V. fluids as needed. If the patient is conscious and the gag reflex is intact, induce emesis (if ingestion was recent) by administering syrup of ipecac. If emesis is contraindicated, perform gastric lavage while a cuffed endotracheal tube is in place to prevent aspiration. Follow with administration of activated charcoal and saline cathartic. Measure intake and output, vital signs, and laboratory parameters; maintain body temperature. The patient should be rolled from side to side every 30 minutes to avoid pulmonary congestion.

Alkalinization of urine may be helpful in removing the drug from the body; hemodialysis may be useful in severe overdose.

Benzodiazepine overdose

An overdose of benzodiazepines produces somnolence, confusion, coma, hypoactive reflexes, dyspnea, labored breathing, hypotension, bradycardia, slurred speech, and unsteady gait or impaired coordination.

Support blood pressure and respiration until drug effects subside; monitor vital signs. Mechanical ventilatory assistance via an endotracheal tube may be required to maintain a patent airway and support adequate oxygenation. Flumazenil, a specific benzodiazepine antagonist, may be useful. Use I.V. fluids or vasopressors, such as dopamine and phenylephrine, to treat hypotension as needed. If the patient is conscious and his gag reflex is intact, induce emesis (if ingestion was recent) by administering syrup of ipecac.

If emesis is contraindicated, perform gastric lavage while a cuffed endotracheal tube is in place to prevent aspiration. After emesis or lavage, administer activated charcoal with a cathartic as a single dose. Dialysis is of limited value.

CNS depressant overdose

Signs of central nervous system (CNS) depressant overdose include prolonged coma, hypotension, hypothermia followed by fever, and inadequate ventilation even without significant respiratory depression. Absence of pupillary reflexes, dilated pupils, loss of deep tendon reflexes, tonic muscle spasms, and apnea may occur.

Treatment of overdose involves support of respiration and cardiovascular function; mechanical ventilation may be necessary. Maintain adequate urine output with adequate hydration while avoiding pulmonary edema. Empty gastric contents by inducing emesis. For lipid-soluble drugs such as glutethimide, charcoal and resin hemoperfusion are effective in removing the drug; hemodialysis and peritoneal dialysis are of minimal value. Because of the significant storage of glutethimide in fat tissue, blood levels commonly show large fluctuations with worsening of symptoms.

Digitalis glycoside overdose

Clinical effects of a digitalis glycoside overdose are primarily related to the GI, cardiovascular, and central nervous systems.

Severe overdose may cause hyperkalemia, which may develop rapidly and result in life-threatening cardiac effects. Cardiac signs of digoxin toxicity may occur with or without other toxicity signs and commonly precede other toxic effects. Because cardiotoxic effects also can occur in heart disease, determining whether these effects result from an underlying heart disease or digoxin toxicity may be difficult. Digoxin has caused almost every kind of arrhythmia; various combinations of arrhythmias may occur in the same patient. Patients with chronic digoxin toxicity commonly have ventricular arrhythmias, atrioventricular (AV) conduction disturbances, or both. Patients with digoxin-induced ventricular tachycardia have a high mortality because ventricular fibrillation or asystole may result.

If toxicity is suspected, the drug should be discontinued and serum drug level measurements obtained. Usually, the drug takes at least 6 hours to be distributed between plasma and tissue and reach equilibrium; plasma levels drawn earlier may show higher digoxin levels than those present after the drug is distributed into the tissues.

Other treatment measures include immediate emesis induction, gastric lavage, and administration of activated charcoal to reduce absorption of the remaining drug. Multiple doses of activated charcoal (such as 50 g every 6 hours) may help reduce further absorption, especially of any drug undergoing enterohepatic recirculation. Some clinicians advocate cholestyramine administration if digoxin was recently ingested; however, this may not be useful if the ingestion is life-threatening. Any interacting drugs probably should be discontinued.

Ventricular arrhythmias may be treated with I.V. potassium (replacement doses; but not in patients with significant AV block), I.V. phenytoin, I.V. lidocaine, or I.V. propranolol. Refractory ventricular tachyarrhythmias may be controlled with overdrive pacing. Procainamide may be used for ventricular arrhythmias that don't respond to the above treatments. In severe AV block, asystole, and hemodynamically significant sinus bradycardia, atropine restores a normal rate.

Administration of digoxin-specific antibody fragments (digoxin immune Fab [Digibind]) treats life-threatening digoxin toxicity. Each 40 mg of digoxin immune Fab binds about 0.6 mg of digoxin in the bloodstream. The complex is then excreted in the urine, rapidly decreasing serum levels and therefore cardiac drug concentrations.

Iron supplement overdose

Iron supplements represent a major source of poisoning, especially in small children. In fact, as little as 1 g of ferrous sulfate can kill an infant.

Symptoms of poisoning result from iron's acute corrosive effects on the GI mucosa as well as the adverse metabolic effects caused by iron overload.

Four stages of acute iron poisoning have been identified, and signs and symptoms may occur within the first 10 to 60 minutes of ingestion or may be delayed several hours.

The first findings reflect acute GI irritation and include epigastric pain, nausea, and vomiting. Diarrhea may present as green, followed by tarry, stools and then as melena. Hematemesis may be accompanied by drowsiness, lassitude, shock, and coma. Local erosion of the stomach and small intestine may further enhance the absorption of iron.

If death doesn't occur in the first phase, a second phase of apparent recovery may last 24 hours.

A third phase, which can occur 4 to 48 hours after ingestion, is marked by CNS abnormalities, metabolic acidosis, hepatic dysfunction, renal failure, and bleeding diathesis. This may progress to circulatory failure, coma, and death.

If the patient survives, the fourth phase consists of late complications of acute iron intoxication and may occur 2 to 6 weeks after overdose. Severe gastric scarring, pyloric stenosis, or intestinal obstruction may be present.

Patients who develop vomiting, diarrhea, leukocytosis, or hyperglycemia and have an abdominal X-ray positive for iron within 6 hours of ingestion are likely to be at risk for serious toxicity. Empty the stomach by inducing emesis with syrup of ipecac, and perform gastric lavage.

If patients have had multiple episodes of vomiting or the vomitus contains blood, avoid ipecac and perform lavage. Some clinicians add sodium bicarbonate to the lavage solution to convert ferrous iron to ferrous carbonate, which is poorly absorbed. Disodium phosphate has also been used; however, some children may develop life-threatening hyperphosphatemia or hypercalcemia. Other possible treatments include lavage with normal saline solution, administration of a saline cathartic, surgical removal of tablets, and chelation therapy with deferoxamine mesylate. Hemodialysis is of little value. Supportive treatment includes monitoring acid-base balance, maintaining a patent airway, and controlling shock and dehydration with appropriate I.V. therapy.

Nonsteroidal anti-inflammatory drug overdose

Clinical manifestations of overdose with nonsteroidal anti-inflammatory drugs include dizziness, drowsiness, paresthesia, vomiting, nausea, abdominal pain, headache, sweating, nystagmus, apnea, and cyanosis.

To treat an ibuprofen overdose, empty the stomach at once by inducing emesis with syrup of ipecac or gastric lavage. Administer activated charcoal by nasogastric tube. Provide symptomatic and supportive measures, including respiratory support and correction of fluid and electrolyte imbalances. Monitor laboratory tests and vital signs closely. Alkaline diuresis may enhance renal excretion. Dialysis is of minimal value because ibuprofen is strongly protein-bound.

Opiate overdose

Rapid I.V. administration of opiates may result in overdose because of the delay in maximum CNS effect (30 minutes). The most common signs of morphine overdose are respiratory depression with or without CNS depression and miosis (pinpoint pupils). Other acute toxic effects include hypotension, bradycardia, hypothermia, shock, apnea, cardiopulmonary arrest, circulatory collapse, pulmonary edema, and seizures.

To treat acute overdose: First, establish adequate respiratory exchange via a patent airway and ventilation as needed; then administer a narcotic antagonist (naloxone) to reverse respiratory depression. (Because the duration of action of morphine is longer than that of naloxone, repeated doses of naloxone are necessary.) Naloxone shouldn't be given unless clinically significant respiratory or cardiovascular depression is present. Monitor vital signs closely.

If the patient presents within 2 hours of an oral overdose, empty the stomach immediately by inducing emesis (with syrup of ipecac) or using gastric lavage. Use caution to avoid any risk of aspiration. Administer activated charcoal via a nasogastric tube for further removal of the drug in an oral overdose.

Provide symptomatic and supportive treatment (continued respiratory support and correction of fluid or electrolyte imbalance). Monitor laboratory parameters, vital signs, and neurologic status closely.

Phenothiazine overdose

CNS depression due to phenothiazine overdose is characterized by deep, unarousable sleep and possible coma, hypotension or hypertension, extrapyramidal symptoms, abnormal involuntary muscle movements, agitation, seizures, arrhythmias, electrocardiogram changes, hypothermia or hyperthermia, and autonomic nervous system dysfunction.

Treatment is symptomatic and supportive, including maintaining vital signs, a patent airway, stable body temperature, and fluid and electrolyte balance.

Don't induce vomiting; phenothiazines inhibit the cough reflex, so aspiration may occur. Use gastric lavage and then activated charcoal and saline cathartics. Dialysis doesn't help. Regulate body temperature as needed. Treat hypotension with I.V. fluids: Don't give epinephrine. Treat seizures with parenteral diazepam or barbiturates, arrhythmias with parenteral phenytoin, and extrapyramidal reactions with benztropine or parenteral diphenhydramine.

Salicylate overdose

Clinical effects of salicylate overdose include metabolic acidosis with respiratory alkalosis, hyperpnea, and tachypnea due to increased carbon dioxide production and direct stimulation of the respiratory center.

To treat aspirin overdose, empty the patient's stomach immediately by inducing emesis with syrup of ipecac if the patient is conscious, or by gastric lavage. Administer activated charcoal via a nasogastric tube. Provide symptomatic and supportive measures (respiratory support and correction of fluid and electrolyte imbalances). Closely monitor laboratory values and vital signs. Enhance renal excretion by administering sodium bicarbonate to alkalinize urine. Use a cooling blanket or sponging if the patient's rectal temperature is above 104° F (40° C). Hemodialysis is effective in removing aspirin but is

used only in severe poisoning or in those at risk for pulmonary edema.

Tricyclic antidepressant overdose

An overdose of tricyclic antidepressants is commonly life-threatening, particularly when combined with alcohol. The first 12 hours after ingestion are a stimulatory phase characterized by excessive anticholinergic activity (agitation, irritation, confusion, hallucinations, hyperthermia, parkinsonian symptoms, seizures, urine retention, dry mucous membranes, pupillary dilation, constipation, and ileus). This phase precedes CNS depressant effects, including hypothermia, decreased or absent reflexes, sedation, hypotension, cyanosis, and cardiac irregularities, including tachycardia, conduction disturbances, and quinidine-like effects on the electrocardiogram.

The severity of an overdose is best indicated by a widening of the QRS complex, which usually represents severe toxicity; obtaining serum measurements usually isn't helpful. Metabolic acidosis may follow hypotension, hypoventilation, and seizures.

Treatment is symptomatic and supportive, including maintaining a patent airway, stable body temperature, and fluid and electrolyte balance. Induce emesis if the patient is conscious; follow with gastric lavage and activated charcoal to prevent further absorption. Dialysis is of little use. Treat seizures with parenteral diazepam or phenytoin, arrhythmias with parenteral phenytoin or lidocaine, and acidosis with sodium bicarbonate. Don't give barbiturates; they may enhance CNS and respiratory depressant effects.

Interactions
Dangerous drug interactions

Drugs can interact to produce undesirable, even hazardous, effects. Such interactions can decrease therapeutic efficacy or cause toxicity. (See *Dangerous drug combinations,* pages 399 to 402.)

Drug-food interactions

acebutolol (Sectral): Food in general. *Slightly decreases drug absorption and peak concentrations.*

amiloride hydrochloride (Midamor): Potassium-rich diet. *May rapidly increase serum potassium levels.*

antihypertensive drugs: Licorice. *Decreases antihypertensive effect.*

bacampicillin hydrochloride (Spectrobid powder for oral suspension): Food in general. *Decreases drug absorption.*

buspirone hydrochloride (BuSpar): Food in general. *May decrease presystemic drug clearance.*

Grapefruit juice. *May increase serum levels.*

caffeine (Caffedrine, NoDoz, Quick Pep, Vivarin): Caffeine-containing beverages and food. *May cause sleeplessness, irritability, nervousness, and rapid heartbeat.*

calcium glubionate (Neo-Calglucon syrup): Bran, cereals (whole grain), dairy products, rhubarb, spinach. *Large quantities interfere with calcium absorption.*

captopril (Capoten): Food in general. *Reduces drug absorption by 30% to 40%.*

cefuroxime axetil (Ceftin tablets): Food in general. *Increases drug absorption.*

choline and magnesium salicylate (Trilisate): Food that lowers urinary pH. *Decreases urinary salicylate excretion, and increases plasma levels.*

Food that raises urinary pH. *Enhances renal salicylate clearance, and diminishes plasma salicylate concentration.*

demeclocycline hydrochloride (Declomycin): Dairy products, food in general. *Interferes with absorption of oral forms of demeclocycline.*

dextroamphetamine sulfate (Dexedrine elixir): Fruit juice. *Lowers blood drug levels and efficacy.*

dicumarol: Diet high in vitamin K. *Decreases prothrombin time.*

digoxin (Lanoxin tablets, Lanoxicaps): Food high in bran fiber. *May reduce bioavailability of oral digoxin.*

Food in general. *Slows drug absorption rate.*

dyclonine hydrochloride (Dyclone 0.5% and 1% topical solutions, USP): Food in general. *Topical anesthesia may impair swallowing, enhancing risk of aspiration; food shouldn't be ingested for 60 minutes.*

erythromycin base (ERYC, PCE dispertab tablets): Food in general. *Optimum blood levels are obtained on a fasting stomach; administration is preferable 30 minutes before or 2 hours after meals.*

estramustine phosphate sodium (Emcyt): Dairy products, calcium-rich foods. *Impair drug absorption.*

etodolac (Lodine): Food in general. *Reduces peak concentration by approximately 50%, and in-*

(Text continues on page 402.)

DANGEROUS DRUG COMBINATIONS

If possible, avoid administering the drug combinations shown below to prevent dangerous drug interactions.

Drug	Interacting drug	Possible effect
Aminoglycosides amikacin gentamicin kanamycin neomycin netilmicin streptomycin tobramycin	Parenteral cephalosporins • ceftazidime • ceftizoxime • cephalothin	Possible enhanced nephrotoxicity
	Loop diuretics • bumetanide • ethacrynic acid • furosemide	Possible enhanced ototoxicity
Amphetamines amphetamine benzphetamine dextroamphetamine methamphetamine	Urine alkalinizers • potassium citrate • sodium acetate • sodium bicarbonate • sodium citrate • sodium lactate • tromethamine	Decreased urinary excretion of amphetamine
Angiotensin-converting enzyme (ACE) inhibitors captopril enalapril lisinopril	indomethacin Nonsteroidal anti-inflammatory drugs (NSAIDs)	Decreased or abolished effectiveness of antihypertensive action of ACE inhibitors
Barbiturate anesthetics methohexital thiopental	Opiate analgesics	Enhanced central nervous system and respiratory depression
Barbiturates amobarbital aprobarbital butabarbital mephobarbital pentobarbital phenobarbital primidone secobarbital	valproic acid	Increased serum barbiturate levels
Beta-adrenergic blockers acebutolol atenolol betaxolol carteolol esmolol levobunolol metoprolol nadolol penbutolol pindolol propranolol timolol	verapamil	Enhanced pharmacologic effects of both beta-adrenergic blockers and verapamil

(continued)

DANGEROUS DRUG COMBINATIONS (continued)

Drug	Interacting drug	Possible effect
carbamazepine	erythromycin	Increased risk of carbamazepine toxicity
carmustine	cimetidine	Enhanced risk of bone marrow toxicity
ciprofloxacin	Antacids containing magnesium or aluminum hydroxide	Decreased plasma levels and effectiveness of ciprofloxacin
clonidine	Beta-adrenergic blockers	Enhanced rebound hypertension following rapid clonidine withdrawal
cyclosporine	Hydantoins	Reduced plasma levels of cyclosporine
Digitalis glycosides	Loop and thiazide diuretics	Increased risk of cardiac arrhythmias due to hypokalemia
	Thiazide-like diuretics	Increased therapeutic or toxic effects
digitoxin	quinidine	Decreased digitoxin clearance
digoxin	amiodarone	Decreased renal clearance of digoxin
	quinidine	Enhanced clearance of digoxin
	verapamil	Elevated serum digoxin levels
dopamine	phenytoin	Hypertension and bradycardia
epinephrine	Beta-adrenergic blockers	Increased systolic and diastolic pressures; marked decrease in heart rate
erythromycin	astemizole	Increased risk of arrhythmia
	carbamazepine	Decreased carbamazepine clearance
	theophylline	Decreased hepatic clearance of theophylline
ethanol	disulfiram furazolidone metronidazole	Acute alcohol intolerance reaction
furazolidone	Amine-containing foods Anorexiants	Inhibits MAO, possibly leading to hypertensive crisis

DANGEROUS DRUG COMBINATIONS (continued)

Drug	Interacting drug	Possible effect
heparin	Salicylates NSAIDs	Enhanced risk of bleeding
levodopa	furazolidone	Enhanced toxic effects of levodopa
lithium	Thiazide diuretics NSAIDs	Decreased lithium excretion
meperidine	MAO inhibitors	Cardiovascular instability and increased toxicity
methotrexate	probenecid	Decreased methotrexate elimination
	Salicylates	Increased risk of methotrexate toxicity
Monoamine oxidase (MAO) inhibitors	Amine-containing foods Anorexiants meperidine	Risk of hypertensive crisis
Nondepolarizing muscle relaxants	Aminoglycosides Inhalational anesthetics	Enhanced neuromuscular blockade
Nonsedating antihistamines astemizole terfenadine	erythromycin ketoconazole	Decrease metabolism of antihistamine; risk of cardiac arrhythmia
Potassium supplements	Potassium-sparing diuretics	Increased risk of hyperkalemia
quinidine	amiodarone	Increased risk of quinidine toxicity
Sympathomimetics	MAO inhibitors	Increased risk of hypertensive crisis
Tetracyclines	Antacids containing magnesium, aluminum, or bismuth salts Iron supplements	Decreased plasma levels and effectiveness of tetracyclines
theophylline	carbamazepine	Reduced theophylline levels
	cimetidine	Increased theophylline levels
	ciprofloxacin	Increased theophylline levels
	erythromycin	Increased theophylline levels
	phenobarbital	Reduced theophylline levels
	rifampin	Reduced theophylline levels

(continued)

DANGEROUS DRUG COMBINATIONS (continued)

Drug	Interacting drug	Possible effect
warfarin	testosterone	Possible enhanced bleeding caused by increased hypoprothrombinemia
	Barbiturates carbamazepine	Reduced effectiveness of warfarin
	amiodarone Certain cephalosporins chloral hydrate cholestyramine cimetidine clofibrate co-trimoxazole dextrothyroxine disulfiram	Increased risk of bleeding
	erythromycin glucagon metronidazole phenylbutazone quinidine quinine Salicylates sulfinpyrazone Thyroid drugs Tricyclic antidepressants	Increased risk of bleeding
	ethchlorvynol glutethimide griseofulvin	Decreased pharmacologic effect
	rifampin trazodone	Decreased risk of bleeding
	methimazole propylthiouracil	Increased or decreased risk of bleeding

creases time to peak concentration by 1.4 to 3.8 hours.

etretinate (Tegison capsules): Dairy products, high lipid diet. *Increases drug absorption.*

famotidine (Pepcid oral suspension): Food in general. *Slightly increases bioavailability.*

felodipine (Plendil): Grapefruit juice, doubly concentrated. *Increases bioavailability more than twofold.*

fenoprofen calcium (Nalfon pulvules and tablets): Dairy products, food in general. *Delays and diminishes peak blood levels.*

ferrous sulfate (Feosol, Slow-Fe): Dairy products, eggs. *Inhibits iron absorption.*

fluoroquinolone antibiotics, such as ciprofloxacin (Cipro), norfloxacin (Noroxin), ofloxacin (Floxin): Food in general (particularly dairy products). *May decrease absorption of oral fluoroquinolones.*

flurbiprofen (Ansaid): Food in general. *Alters rate of absorption but not extent of drug availability.*

fosinopril sodium (Monopril): Food in general. *May slow rate but not extent of drug absorption.*

glipizide (Glucotrol): Food in

general. *Delays absorption by about 40 minutes.*

hydralazine hydrochloride (Apresoline tablets): Food in general. *Increases plasma levels.*

hydrochlorothiazide (Esidrix, HydroDIURIL): Food in general. *Enhances GI drug absorption.*

ibuprofen (Advil, Children's Advil suspension, Motrin, Nuprin, PediaProfen suspension, Rufen): Food in general. *Reduces rate but not extent of absorption.*

isotretinoin (Accutane): Dairy products, food in general. *Increases absorption of oral isotretinoin.*

isradipine (DynaCirc): Food in general. *Significantly increases time to peak by about 1 hour with no effect on bioavailability.*

ketoprofen (Orudis capsules): Food in general. *Slows absorption rate, delays and reduces peak concentrations.*

levodopa-carbidopa (Sinemet tablets): High-protein diet. *May impair levodopa absorption.*

Food in general. *Increases the extent of availability and peak concentrations of sustained-release levodopa-carbidopa.*

levothyroxine sodium (Synthroid injection): Soybean formula (infant's). *May cause excessive fecal loss.*

lidocaine hydrochloride (Xylocaine): Food in general. *Topical anesthesia may impair swallowing, enhancing risk of aspiration; avoid food ingestion for 60 minutes.*

liotrix (Thyrolar): Soybean formula (infant's). *May cause excessive fecal loss.*

lovastatin (Mevacor): Grapefruit juice. *Increases serum levels.*

meclofenamate (Meclomen): Food in general. *Decreases rate and extent of drug absorption.*

methenamine mandelate (Mandelamine granules): Food that raises urinary pH. *Reduces essential antibacterial activity.*

methotrexate sodium (Rheumatrex): Food in general. *Delays absorption, and reduces peak concentration of oral methotrexate sodium.*

minocycline hydrochloride (Minocin): Dairy products. *Slightly decreases peak plasma concentration levels and delays them by 1 hour.*

misoprostol (Cytotec): Food in general. *Diminishes maximum plasma concentrations.*

monoamine oxidase (MAO) inhibitors, such as isocarboxazid (Marplan tablets), phenelzine (Nardil), or tranylcypromine (Parnate tablets); drugs that also inhibit MAO, such as amphetamines, furazolidone (Furoxone), isoniazid (Laniazid), or procarbazine (Matulane capsules): Anchovies, avocados, bananas, beans (broad, fava), beer (including alcohol-free and reduced-alcohol), caviar, cheese (especially aged, strong, unpasteurized), chocolate, sour cream, canned figs, pickled herring, liver, liqueurs, meat extracts, meat prepared with tenderizers, raisins, sauerkraut, sherry, soy sauce, red wine, yeast extract, yogurt. *Can cause hypertensive crisis.*

moricizine hydrochloride (Ethmozine): Food in general. *Administration 30 minutes after a meal delays rate but not extent of drug absorption.*

nifedipine (Procardia XL tablets): Food in general. *Slightly alters early rate of drug absorption.*

Grapefruit juice. *May increase bioavailability and drug levels.*

nitrofurantoin (Macrodantin capsules): Food in general. *Increases drug bioavailability.*

pancrelipase (Cotazym capsules): Food with a pH greater than

5.5. *Dissolves protective enteric coating.*

pentoxifylline (Trental): Food in general. *Delays drug absorption but doesn't affect total absorption.*

phenytoin (Dilantin): Charcoal-broiled meats. *May decrease blood drug levels.*

polyethylene glycol and electrolyte solution (GoLYTELY, NuLYTELY): Food in general. *For best results, no solid food should be consumed during 3- to 4-hour period before drinking solution.*

propafenone hydrochloride (Rythmol): Food in general. *Increased peak blood levels and bioavailability in a single-dose study.*

propranolol hydrochloride (Inderal): Food in general. *Increases bioavailability of oral propranolol.*

ramipril (Altace): Food in general. *Reduces rate but not extent of drug absorption.*

salsalate (Disalcid, Mono-Gesic, Salflex): Food that lowers urinary pH. *Decreases urinary excretion, and increases plasma levels.*

Food that raises urinary pH. *Increases renal clearance and urinary excretion of salicylic acid.*

selegiline hydrochloride (Eldepryl): Food with high concentration of tyramine. *May precipitate hypertensive crisis if daily dosage exceeds recommended maximum.*

sodium fluoride (Luride): Dairy products. *Forms calcium fluoride, which is poorly absorbed.*

sulindac (Clinoril tablets): Food in general. *Slightly delays peak plasma concentrations of biologically active sulfide metabolite.*

tetracycline hydrochloride (Achromycin V): Dairy products, food in general. *Interferes with absorption of oral tetracycline.*

theophylline (Quibron-T Dividose, Quibron-T/SR Dividose, Respbid, Slo-Bid, Theo-Dur, Theo-24, Theolair-SR, Theo-X, Uniphyl): Caffeine-containing beverages, chocolate, cola. *Large quantities increase adverse effects of theophylline.*

High-lipid diet. *Reduces plasma concentration levels, and delays time of peak plasma levels.*

Charcoal-broiled foods, especially meats; cruciferous (cabbage family) vegetables; and high-protein and low-carbohydrate diets. *Large quantities may increase hepatic metabolism of theophylline.*

tolmetin sodium (Tolectin): Dairy products. *Decrease total tolmetin bioavailability by 16%.*

Food in general. *Decreases total tolmetin bioavailability by 16% and reduces peak plasma concentrations by 50%.*

trazodone hydrochloride (Desyrel): Food in general. *May affect bioavailability, including amount of drug absorbed and peak plasma levels.*

triazolam (Halcion): Grapefruit juice. *May increase serum levels.*

verapamil hydrochloride (Calan SR, Isoptin SR): Food in general. *Decreases bioavailability but narrows peak-to-trough ratio.*

warfarin sodium (Coumadin, Panwarfin): Diet high in vitamin K. *Decreases prothrombin time.*

Charcoal-broiled meats. *May decrease blood drug levels.*

Drug-alcohol interactions

Drug-alcohol interactions are more than just potentiated CNS depression. Combined with NSAIDs, alcohol is highly irritating to the stomach; combined with some diuretics and cardiac medications, it may

EFFECTS OF MIXING DRUGS AND ALCOHOL

Drug	Effects
• Analgesics • Antianxiety drugs • Antidepressants • Antihistamines • Antipsychotics • Hypnotics	Deepened central nervous system (CNS) depression
• Monoamine oxidase inhibitors	Deepened CNS depression; possible hypertensive crisis with certain types of beer and wine containing tyramine (Chianti, Alicante)
• Oral antidiabetic agents	Disulfiram-like effects (facial flushing, headache), especially with chlorpropamide; inadequate food intake may trigger increased antidiabetic activity
• Cephalosporins • metronidazole • disulfiram	Facial flushing, headache

cause a steep drop in blood pressure. (See *Effects of mixing drugs and alcohol.*)

Compatibility of drugs with tube feedings

Some feeding formulas such as Ensure may break down chemically when combined with a drug such as Dimetapp Elixir. Increased formula viscosity—and a clogged tube—can occur from giving Klorvess, NeoCalglucon Syrup, Dimetane Elixir, Phenergan Syrup, or Sudafed Syrup with a feeding formula.

Drug preparations such as ferrous sulfate or potassium chloride liquids are incompatible with some formulas, causing clumping and other problems when mixed in a tube. Still other combinations may alter the bioavailability of some drugs, such as phenytoin.

To avoid incompatibility problems, follow these guidelines:
• Never add a drug to a feeding formula container.
• Always check the compatibility of an ordered drug and the feeding formula before administering.

• Infuse 30 ml of water before and after giving a single drug dose through the tube.
• Flush the feeding tube with 5 ml of water between drug doses if you're giving more than one drug.
• Dilute highly concentrated liquids with 60 ml of water before giving.
• Instill drugs in liquid form when possible. If you must crush a tablet, crush it into fine dust and dissolve it in warm water. (Never crush and liquefy enteric-coated tablets or timed-release capsules.)
• Time drug and formula administration intervals appropriately; you may need to withhold tube feeding and supply medication by mouth to an empty stomach or with food.

Recognizing and treating acute toxicity

Treatment of substance abuse is a long-term process beset with relapses. You need to understand the signs and symptoms of toxicity before you can take steps to help the patient recover from his addiction. (See *Managing acute toxicity,* pages 406 to 410.)

MANAGING ACUTE TOXICITY

Substance	Signs and symptoms	Interventions
alcohol (ethanol) • Beer and wine • Distilled spirits • Other preparations, such as cough syrup, aftershave, or mouthwash	• Ataxia • Seizures • Coma • Hypothermia • Alcohol breath odor • Respiratory depression • Bradycardia • Hypotension • Nausea and vomiting	• Induce vomiting or perform gastric lavage if ingestion occurred in the previous 4 hours. Give activated charcoal and a saline cathartic. • Start I.V. fluid replacement and administer dextrose 5% in water, thiamine, B-complex vitamins, and vitamin C to prevent dehydration and hypoglycemia and to correct nutritional deficiencies. • Pad bed rails and apply cloth restraints to protect the patient from injury. • Give an anticonvulsant such as diazepam to control seizures. • Watch the patient for signs and symptoms of withdrawal, such as hallucinations and alcohol withdrawal delirium. If these occur, consider giving chlordiazepoxide, chloral hydrate, or paraldehyde. (Be sure to administer paraldehyde with a glass syringe or glass cup to avoid a chemical reaction with plastic.) • Auscultate the patient's lungs frequently to detect crackles or rhonchi, possibly indicating aspiration pneumonia. If you note these breath sounds, consider antibiotics. • Monitor the patient's neurologic status and vital signs every 15 minutes until he's stable. Assist with dialysis if his vital functions are severely depressed.
Amphetamines • Amphetamine sulfate (Benzedrine): bennies, greenies, cartwheels • Dextroamphetamine sulfate (Dexedrine): dexies, hearts, oranges • Methamphetamine: speed, meth, crystal	• Dilated reactive pupils • Altered mental status (from confusion to paranoia) • Hallucinations • Tremors and seizure activity • Hyperactive deep tendon reflexes • Exhaustion • Coma • Dry mouth • Shallow respirations • Tachycardia • Hypertension • Hyperthermia • Diaphoresis	• If the drug was taken orally, induce vomiting or perform gastric lavage; give activated charcoal and a sodium or magnesium sulfate cathartic. • Lower the patient's urine pH to 5 by adding ammonium chloride or ascorbic acid to his I.V. solution. • Force diuresis by giving the patient mannitol. • Give a short-acting barbiturate such as pentobarbital to control stimulant-induced seizures. • Restrain the patient, especially if he's paranoid or hallucinating, so he won't injure himself or others. • Give haloperidol I.M. to treat agitation or assaultive behavior. • Give an alpha-adrenergic blocker such as phentolamine for hypertension. • Watch for cardiac arrhythmias. If these develop, consider propranolol or lidocaine to treat tachyarrhythmias or ventricular arrhythmias, respectively. • Treat hyperthermia with tepid sponge baths or a hypothermia blanket. • Provide a quiet environment to avoid overstimulation. • Be alert for signs and symptoms of withdrawal, such as abdominal tenderness, muscle aches, and long periods of sleep. • Observe suicide precautions, especially if the patient shows signs of withdrawal.

MANAGING ACUTE TOXICITY (continued)

Substance	Signs and symptoms	Interventions
Antipsychotics • Chlorpromazine (Thorazine) • Phenothiazines • Thioridazine (Mellaril)	• Constricted pupils • Photosensitivity • Extrapyramidal effects (dyskinesia, opisthotonos, muscle rigidity, ocular deviation) • Dry mouth • Decreased level of consciousness (LOC) • Decreased deep tendon reflexes • Seizures • Hypothermia or hyperthermia • Dysphagia • Respiratory depression • Hypotension • Tachycardia	• Expect to perform gastric lavage if the patient ingested the drug within the past 6 hours. (Don't induce vomiting because phenothiazines have an antiemetic effect.) Consider activated charcoal and a cathartic. • Give diphenhydramine to treat extrapyramidal effects. • Give physostigmine salicylate to reverse anticholinergic effects in severe cases. • Replace fluids I.V. to correct hypotension; monitor the patient's vital signs often. • Monitor his respiratory rate, and give supplemental oxygen to treat respiratory depression. • Give an anticonvulsant such as diazepam or a short-acting barbiturate such as pentobarbital sodium to control seizures. • Keep the patient's room dark to avoid exacerbating his photosensitivity.
Anxiolytic sedative-hypnotics • Benzodiazepines (Valium, Librium)	• Confusion • Drowsiness • Stupor • Decreased reflexes • Seizures • Coma • Shallow respirations • Hypotension	• Induce vomiting or perform gastric lavage; consider activated charcoal and a cathartic. • Give supplemental oxygen to correct hypoxia-induced seizures. • Replace fluids I.V. to correct hypotension; monitor the patient's vital signs often. • For benzodiazepine overdose, or to reverse the effect of benzodiazepine-induced sedation or respiratory depression, give flumazenil (Romazicon).
Barbiturate sedative-hypnotics • Amobarbital sodium (Amytal sodium): blue angels, blue devils, blue birds • Phenobarbital (Luminal): phennies, purple hearts, goofballs • Secobarbital sodium (Seconal): reds, red devils	• Poor pupil reaction to light • Nystagmus • Depressed LOC (from confusion to coma) • Flaccid muscles and absent reflexes • Hyperthermia or hypothermia • Cyanosis • Respiratory depression • Hypotension • Blisters or bullous lesions	• Induce vomiting or perform gastric lavage if the patient ingested the drug within 4 hours; consider activated charcoal and a saline cathartic. • Maintain his blood pressure with I.V. fluid challenges and vasopressors. • If the patient has taken a phenobarbital overdose, give sodium bicarbonate I.V. to alkalinize his urine and speed the drug's elimination. • Apply a hyperthermia or hypothermia blanket to help return the patient's temperature to normal. • Prepare your patient for hemodialysis or hemoperfusion if toxicity is severe. • Perform frequent neurologic assessments, and check your patient's pulse rate, temperature, skin color, and reflexes often. • Notify the physician if you see signs of respiratory distress or pulmonary edema. • Watch for signs and symptoms of withdrawal, such as hyperreflexia, tonic-clonic seizures, and hallucinations. Provide symptomatic relief of withdrawal symptoms. • Protect the patient from injuring himself.

(continued)

MANAGING ACUTE TOXICITY *(continued)*

Substance	Signs and symptoms	Interventions
cocaine • Cocaine hydrochloride: crack, freebase	• Dilated pupils • Confusion • Alternating euphoria and apprehension • Hyperexcitability • Visual, auditory, and olfactory hallucinations • Spasms and seizures • Coma • Tachypnea • Hyperpnea • Pallor or cyanosis • Respiratory arrest • Tachycardia • Hypertension or hypotension • Fever • Nausea and vomiting • Abdominal pain • Perforated nasal septum or mouth sores	• Calm the patient by talking to him in a quiet room. • If cocaine was ingested, induce vomiting or perform gastric lavage; give activated charcoal followed by a saline cathartic. • Give the patient a tepid sponge bath, and administer an antipyretic to reduce fever. • Monitor his blood pressure and heart rate. Expect to give propranolol for symptomatic tachycardia. • Administer an anticonvulsant such as diazepam to control seizures. • Scrape the inside of his nose to remove residual amounts of the drug. • Monitor his cardiac rate and rhythm — ventricular fibrillation and cardiac standstill can occur as a direct cardiotoxic result of cocaine ingestion. Defibrillate the patient, and initiate cardiopulmonary resuscitation, if indicated.
glutethimide • Doriden: Ciba, CB (street names for drug)	• Small, reactive pupils • Nystagmus • Drowsiness • Irritability • Impaired thought processes (memory, judgment, attention span) • Slurred speech • Twitching, spasms, and seizures • Hypothermia • CNS depression (from unresponsiveness to deep coma) • Apnea • Respiratory depression • Hypotension • Paralytic ileus • Poor bladder control	• If the drug was taken orally, induce vomiting or perform gastric lavage; give activated charcoal and a cathartic. • Maintain the patient's blood pressure with I.V. fluid challenges and vasopressors. • Assist with hemodialysis or hemoperfusion if the patient has hepatic or renal failure or is in a prolonged coma. • Administer an anticonvulsant such as diazepam for seizures. • Perform hourly neurologic assessments: Coma may recur because of the drug's slow release from fat deposits. • Be alert for signs of increased intracranial pressure, such as decreasing LOC and widening pulse pressure. Consider mannitol I.M. • Watch for signs and symptoms of withdrawal, such as hyperreflexia, tonic-clonic seizures, and hallucinations, and provide symptomatic relief of withdrawal symptoms. • Protect the patient from injuring himself.

MANAGING ACUTE TOXICITY (continued)

Substance	Signs and symptoms	Interventions
Hallucinogens • Lysergic acid diethylamide (LSD): hawk, acid, sunshine • Mescaline (peyote): mese, cactus, big chief	• Dilated pupils • Intensified perceptions • Agitation and anxiety • Synesthesia • Impaired judgment • Hyperactive movement • Flashback experiences • Hallucinations • Depersonalization • Moderately increased blood pressure • Increased heart rate • Fever	• Reorient the patient repeatedly to time, place, and person. • Restrain the patient to protect him from injuring himself and others. • Calm the patient by talking to him in a quiet room. • If the drug was taken orally, induce vomiting or perform gastric lavage; give activated charcoal and a cathartic. • Give diazepam I.V. to control seizures.
Narcotics • Codeine • Heroin: junk, smack, H, snow • Hydromorphone hydrochloride (Dilaudid): D, lords • Morphine: Mort, M, monkey, Emma	• Constricted pupils • Depressed LOC (but the patient is usually responsive to persistent verbal or tactile stimuli) • Seizures • Hypothermia • Slow, deep respirations • Hypotension • Bradycardia • Skin changes (pruritus, urticaria, flushed skin)	• Give naloxone until the drug's CNS depressant effects are reversed. • Replace fluids I.M. to increase circulatory volume. • Correct hypothermia by applying extra blankets; if the patient's body temperature doesn't increase, use a hyperthermia blanket. • Reorient the patient often. • Auscultate the lungs often for crackles, possibly indicating pulmonary edema. (Onset may be delayed.) • Administer oxygen via nasal cannula, mask, or mechanical ventilation to correct hypoxemia from hypoventilation. • Monitor cardiac rate and rhythm, being alert for atrial fibrillation. (This should resolve when hypoxemia is corrected.) • Be alert for signs of withdrawal, such as piloerection (goose flesh), diaphoresis, and hyperactive bowel sounds. • Institute safety measures to prevent patient injury.

(continued)

MANAGING ACUTE TOXICITY (continued)

Substance	Signs and symptoms	Interventions
phencyclidine (PCP) • Angel dust, peace pill, hog	• Blank stare • Nystagmus • Amnesia • Decreased awareness of surroundings • Recurrent coma • Violent behavior • Hyperactivity • Seizures • Gait ataxia • Muscle rigidity • Drooling • Hyperthermia • Hypertensive crisis • Cardiac arrest	• If the drug was taken orally, induce vomiting or perform gastric lavage; instill and remove activated charcoal repeatedly. • Acidify the patient's urine with ascorbic acid to increase drug excretion. • Expect to continue to acidify urine for 2 weeks because signs and symptoms may recur when fat cells release PCP stores. • Give diazepam and haloperidol to control agitation or psychotic behavior. • Institute safety measures to protect the patient from injury. • Administer diazepam to control seizures. • Institute seizure precautions. • Provide a quiet environment and dimmed light. • Give propranolol for hypertension and tachycardia, and give nitroprusside for severe hypertension. • Closely monitor urine output and serial renal function tests. Rhabdomyolysis, myoglobinuria, and renal failure may occur in severe intoxication. • If renal failure develops, prepare the patient for hemodialysis.

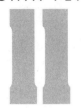

CHAPTER

Financial and legal issues

Handling the business of health care

Avoiding legal pitfalls

The nurse practitioner (NP) who wants to work in private practice can look forward to exciting opportunities as well as risks and challenges. This chapter addresses the legal risks you'll face in setting up a private practice. It also covers the challenges of providing and documenting quality of care and obtaining reimbursement for your services.

Now that private practice is a credible option for NPs, any NP who wants to open her own practice must anticipate potential legal problems and take measures to prevent them. Such awareness and risk avoidance is the legal equivalent of preventive medicine. Below you'll find an attorney's perspective on setting up a private practice, with cases to illustrate some of the legal pitfalls.

Who's the boss?

Karen Able, an obstetric-gynecologic nurse practitioner (NP), and Cheryl Best, a family NP, agree to open a practice together. Both are experienced NPs who've known each other for 5 years. Although they haven't worked together, each knows that the other is well respected in the community. They agree that they'll be equal partners in the practice, but they decide not to draw up a partnership agreement.

However, a friend of Best's suggests that she really should have a written agreement with Able. On her friend's advice, Best talks to an attorney, who tells her he charges $150 per hour plus a $450 fee for the partnership agreement — and that Able will need her own attorney. Able and Best decide to forgo the expenses of attorneys

at this stage. They choose a location for the practice, pick out furniture, buy equipment, and hire a receptionist. They're in business.

After about 3 months, Best notices that half of Able's patients lack insurance and that many patients don't pay at the time of service and owe the practice money. Also, the practice is facing mounting laboratory bills for Papanicolaou tests and other expensive gynecologic tests from Able's patients. In contrast, most of Best's patients have insurance, and Best has told those who don't that they — not the practice — have to provide payment for office visits and laboratory charges.

Best talks to Able about the situation. Able, who sees her patient roster growing, says she hasn't wanted to offend patients by demanding payment. Best tells her that if the situation continues, they'll go broke; neither has been able to draw much of a paycheck, and Best's husband has been pressuring her to use better business savvy to help the practice survive. Best suggests that Able have her patients pay outstanding bills before offering further service.

Making decisions together

When an NP starts a practice alone, she makes the administrative and business decisions. When two or more people work together, however, each has an opinion on how the business should operate. As the case above demonstrates, this can lead to problems. Money — how to collect it and how to spend it — is often at the root of such problems. In fact, magazines on medical practice management and the civil courts point to money disagreements as the reason for most partnership breakups.

A clear decision-making process can help avoid such disagreements. Each of the three basic ways of organizing a private practice has its own decision-making process. If the practice is a *sole proprietorship* run by just one NP, she, of course, makes the decisions. In a *partnership*, the partners must set up a specific decision-making process together and agree to abide by it. If the practice is a *corporation*, bylaws establish the chain of command within the corporation.

In their partnership, Able and Best never specified which partner would make what decisions and didn't have guidelines for resolving a deadlock. If they had drawn up an administrative chart that they both could agree to early in planning their business and had consulted attorneys as needed, they might have avoided this pitfall.

What makes someone an employee?

Peter Jones, NP, has worked for David Harding, MD, for 5 years. He notices that a nearby town is growing in size and lacks a health care provider. Jones, who is familiar with the current sources of reimbursement for NPs, writes a business plan and determines that he could support himself if he left Harding's employ and set up a private practice.

Jones asks Harding to supply, for a fee, medical backup support for his practice, and they draw up an agreement. Harding also offers to cover one session a week at the new practice for a percentage of the reimbursed charges. Is Harding an employee?

Employee or independent contractor?

What distinguishes an employee from an independent contractor? One difference is the responsibilities of the employer. An employer must withhold payroll taxes — income, Medicare, Social Security, and unemployment — for an employee. An employ-

er has to pay workers' compensation for an employee injured on the job. In some states, small businesses must offer health benefits to employees. An employer may be held responsible for employee malpractice and thus should carry professional liability insurance to cover employees.

A business that hires the services of an independent contractor doesn't carry such expensive responsibilities. Can Jones avoid those responsibilities with Harding? Legally, it depends. Under the circumstances described, Harding *is* an employee of Jones because Jones, not Harding, will:

• control when and where the job is done

• hire the medical assistant that Harding will work with

• supply the equipment necessary to do the job

• suffer financial losses if the work doesn't produce income for the practice.

Given the costs of maintaining an employee, Jones can save money if he uses Harding as an independent contractor. In this case, Harding would be considered an independent contractor if he provides consultation as needed, at an hourly rate, over the telephone. To make sure the Internal Revenue Service (IRS) views Harding as an independent contractor, Jones should ask Harding to:

• bill him periodically for work done using Harding's office stationery

• bill varying amounts (a standard weekly or monthly fee will look like a salary to the IRS)

• not work at Jones' place of business.

Jones can't avoid these requirements by simply writing a contract that states the arrangement is one of independent contractors rather than employer-employee. Some business owners have tried this tactic, but it doesn't impress the IRS. If the IRS determines that Jones is an employer and hasn't provided proper coverage for all his employees, it could fine him and create other business headaches. If Harding suffers an injury at Jones' place of business, Harding can ask for — and very possibly may receive — workers' compensation for his injuries and lost wages. (See *Employee or independent contractor?*)

What makes someone a patient?

Mary White, a family NP in private practice, receives a message to call Judy Burke, a nurse, at home. Burke and White used to work together, and White remembers her as a talented, competent nurse; Burke, in turn, has always respected White's judgment.

Burke wants to talk with White about her 6-year-old son, James, who has an earache. He has a history of earaches from infections; amoxicillin has cleared up these infections in the past. Burke reports that James is otherwise completely healthy. Burke works the evening shift, and her son attends first grade during the day. As a result, she can't take him to his pediatrician until the end of the month, which is 2 weeks away. She also wants to avoid the $20 copayment. White remembers meeting James once at a picnic but has never seen the child in her office. Burke asks White to prescribe amoxicillin for James as a favor. They both know that Burke's health maintenance organization insurance won't reimburse White for an office visit. Is James a patient of White?

Avoiding malpractice litigation

In most situations like this case, White could probably proceed with caution to treat the child over the telephone with no ill effects to the child or to her malpractice history. (See *Elements of malpractice.*) However, White would be held liable in court in the small percentage of cases in which:
• the mother made an incorrect diagnosis
• the infecting organism proved resistant to amoxicillin, the antibiotic used in the past
• the child had some other problem that White would have detected from taking a history and performing a physical examination at her office.

If White gives any advice to Burke or prescribes medication, White is taking on a professional relationship with James, and James is considered White's patient. White is then liable for any breach in the standard of care that causes injury to James. It doesn't

ELEMENTS OF MALPRACTICE

To prove malpractice, the patient or plaintiff must prove certain elements to a jury or judge.

Establishing duty: Creating a client or professional relationship

These relationships can arise in unexpected ways, including:
- over the telephone
- at a social gathering
- by supervising another's treatment
- by providing sample medication
- by giving advice or opinions to family or friends.

Breach of duty: The neglect or failure to fulfill in a proper manner the duties of an office, job, or position

A nurse practitioner (NP) can be accused of breach of duty for negligence or behavior that falls below the appropriate standard of care for NPs under similar circumstances. This is the most litigated issue. In general, you're considered not to have committed a breach of duty if expert witnesses recognize the treatment as reasonably prudent and acceptable under similar conditions and circumstances. Expert witnesses are currently practicing or recently retired (less than 5 years) professionals with similar backgrounds (for instance, an NP for NP standards and a physician for physician standards).

Breach of duty can also include sexual misconduct — behavior the patient reasonably interprets as being romantic, intended for sexual arousal, or sexual in nature. To avoid such charges, you should focus on what a patient may interpret from your actions, always have a witness present, and establish a strong anti–sexual-harassment policy or follow your practice's policy. You should also remember that even something as minor as meeting at a bar and flirting with a patient who goes to your medical practice — even if that patient hasn't

seen you professionally — may be interpreted as sexual misconduct.

Terminating a professional relationship with a patient, especially in the managed care arena, may be considered a breach of duty. You can combat this by scrupulously following a clear termination protocol. The protocol must include notification of the patient by telephone and letter as well as a specific procedure to transfer the patient to another primary care provider (PCP) without a gap in medical care. Some states' statutes hold a PCP responsible for 60 days after termination of a relationship or until a course of treatment is completed.

Prescribing inappropriate or excessive amounts of medications can lead to a breach-of-duty charge that is hard to defend against. Medications must be in the best interest of the patient, within standards of practice, and within established prescribing guidelines. To combat this type of risk, know drug schedules (check the *Physician's Desk Reference* if you're unsure) and be aware of patients who may cause problems (for instance, those who request specific drugs or insist on continuing the same drug; those who repeatedly lose prescriptions or medications; and those who come in with the same complaint they've had previously and request the same drug). Of course, prescribing drugs for oneself is also illegal.

Dispensing drug samples can also lead to a breach of duty. Each package you dispense must be labeled with the patient's name, the date dispensed, the PCP's name, and all relevant prescribing information. Manufacturers can provide some of this information in their package inserts, but the PCP is liable for the remaining information. Although scheduled drugs are more likely to bring about legal

(continued)

ELEMENTS OF MALPRACTICE *(continued)*

action, a practice's inventory must list all drugs — even non-narcotic drugs. This inventory must be kept for a minimum of 2 years past the date of purchase and must include the date of purchase, manufacturer, quantity, and drug disbursements. The practice must report all inventory discrepancies to the Drug Enforcement Agency.

Proximal causation: The causal link between the practitioner's failure to conform to treatment standards and harm to the patient

Deviation from established guidelines of practice, coupled with an adverse event, can provide proximal causation. An example would be ordering a drug to be given as eyedrops when it's only approved as eardrops. The NP who wrote the order will likely be held responsible if the patient suffers harm.

Damages: Actual injury to the patient

There are many type of damages. Special damages are those which actually were caused by the injury and include things like medical bills and loss of wages. General damages are directly attributed to a legal wrong but are abstract in nature, such as pain and suffering or a worsening lifestyle. Punitive damages, also called exemplary damages, are compensation in excess of actual damages that are a form of punishment to the wrongdoer and reparation to the injured.

---

matter that James is the patient of another provider, that White receives no compensation for treating James, or that she offers advice on the phone.

To protect herself, White must either politely refuse to give advice, inform Burke to call her son's pediatrician, or ask Burke to bring James to her office to go through the usual new-patient evaluation before prescribing an antibiotic or any other treatment for James. If Burke brings James to her office, White could then follow up with him as she would with her other patients.

The lesson here may seem obvious, but you may feel obliged to deliver care to friends and acquaintances who "just want a little advice" but aren't patients. It's easy to forget that an NP is professionally responsible for any health care advice given. To protect yourself against litigation, you must follow the normal evaluation process.

Telephone triage protocols

Giving appropriate advice

Every day, health care providers receive phone calls from patients seeking help and advice over the phone. If you're answering such calls, protocols or algorithms can give you specific guidelines that allow you to gather the information you need, offer appropriate advice to the caller, and protect yourself and the practice from liability. Specifically, the way a caller answers a question determines what you'll ask next. Then, based on the information you gather, you should be able to do two things: first, assess the caller's symptoms and classify them as emergent, urgent, or nonurgent and, second, determine the appropriate disposition or outcome — the recommended level of care, education, and follow-up the caller needs.

Ideally, using protocols increases consistency in the assessment and disposition of calls regardless of which provider takes the call. That is why a practice should have comprehensive, current, user-friendly, symptom-based, and readily available written guidelines. To increase the quality of care, the medical partners in a practice should periodically review calls to identify weaknesses in the protocols.

The type of protocol you're following affects what advice you can give. More conservative protocols typically result in more patients being advised to go to the primary care provider's office or to the emergency department. Less conservative protocols allow you and other providers to use more judgment, which may result in fewer office or emergency department visits; such protocols help contain costs but may result in greater legal vulnerability. You also need to consider whether a caller falls into a high-risk group (such as juveniles, pregnant women, and the elderly) when giving advice.

When advising patients, make sure that following a protocol doesn't require you to function outside your scope of practice and license. Your state's nursing practice act should provide guidance for independent decision making and assessment.

Giving appropriate advice also requires you to phrase both questions and suggestions carefully, avoiding diagnosing over the phone. For instance, you might say, "Is there anything else going on that I haven't asked about? From what you're describing, this is what concerns me, _____. Because of that, I recommend _____." You might also say, "From what you're describing, it sounds like there are some things I can offer you to make your child

more comfortable. I also want to tell you a few things to watch for. Please call back if they occur or if you have any other questions or concerns." Try to provide the level of care that offers the caller the most comfort and peace of mind given the diagnostic possibilities his symptoms suggest.

Three basics of triage

Telephone triage won't work effectively unless three things happen. First, providers must answer or return all calls as soon as possible. Someone must have the authority to decide what calls are emergent at the first point of contact. Otherwise, a delay in getting back to a caller may result in the aggravation of an injury and cause liability. Second, all providers must perform a thorough assessment to help avoid negative outcomes. That is why a medically trained professional is involved in the triage process instead of just anyone who can read questions and follow an algorithm. (See *Using a telephone triage log,* page 418.) Third, providers must document all calls in detail.

Documentation

Call documentation serves several functions. Thorough documentation can provide the caller's primary care provider (PCP) with information about the patient's complaint, possibly identifying a problem the PCP didn't know about. It can also provide other team members with information about the call if the caller should phone back for affirmation or more detailed assistance. Finally, it can serve as protection against legal liability, working as well as a system of taping calls if the documentation is thorough enough.

USING A TELEPHONE TRIAGE LOG

Date/Time: _5/5/00 9 PM_ Phone# Current: _555-5555_ Home: _555-5555_

Patient Name: _Heidi Knipp_ Caller: _John E. Knipp_ Relation: _Father_

Address: _555 Ember Circle, Ember CO 10999_

Patient DOB/Age: _5/5/97_ SS#: _555-55-5555_ Wt (< 18 y.o.): _45 lbs_

Allergies: _NKDA_

PMH: _denies_

Current med list, including herbals/supplements: _Multivitamin_

Chief complaint

Symptoms/Assessment: _fever 101.2°F (orally)_

(OLDCART acronym) Onset: _just now_ Location: _systemic_

Duration: _unknown_ Characteristics: _cranky_

Aggravated by: _unknown_ Relieved by: _nothing tried_

Treatments tried/Time seeking treatment (why now?): _wants antibiotics now_
because going out of town tomorrow

Protocol/Algorithm used: _Fever_

Recommended: _self-care measures_ Caller Accepted: (Yes)/No

Endpoint accepted by patient:

Call 911 Nearest ED ED

Specialist (e.g., Poison Control/Ophthalmologist):_____

PCP: _Joy S. Kair_ Call/See in: < 4 hr < 24 hr < 72 hr (PRN)

Self-care advice given on: _fever_

Per protocol/reference: _fever_

Potential complications of nontreatment:_____

Caller agreed to followup phone call: (Yes)/No

Callback scheduled for: (time/person) _5/6/00 before noon_

Notes: _Advised of rationale for no antibiotics at this time &_
signs/symptoms of concern.

PCP signature: _Joy S. Kair, FNP_

Such documentation works best if documentation forms aren't only thorough but also easy to use. This encourages all providers to document completely (unfortunately, many providers don't thoroughly document, leaving themselves and the practice open to liability). Forms for documentation can be designed to work by exclusion or inclusion of abnormal findings and need to be retained for up to 10 years, depending on your state's statute of limitations. The caller should also have the right not to have his PCP informed or be told at the beginning of the call that his PCP will get a record of the call.

Recording calls

One way to keep track of calls is to record them. Although expensive, it's a worthwhile way to help control risk, providing a record of what both the provider and the caller said. Even if only some calls are recorded but quality assurance is done on some of those calls, the provider can establish a standard of care and a record of following call-center policy. However, if no record exists, it becomes the caller's word against the provider's word. Call records can also help detect weaknesses in the system, allowing the call center to enhance training and algorithms.

Making protocols work

Telephone triage protocols ensure that all providers offer consistent and accurate health care information to callers. Ways to make protocols more effective include:
• promoting staff involvement in refining protocols
• using resource books that outline telephone advice protocols
• customizing commercial protocols for specific use
• making protocols physically convenient (for instance, having them in a three-ring binder alphabetized by signs and symptoms or in a computer program that searches for key words and includes space for documenting calls)
• having protocols available at every telephone station
• ensuring that all practitioners know where protocols are and how they're organized.
    The following Web sites may help:

• *Arent Fox Telemedicine and the Law* — This site has information about support technologies and telemedicine and includes federal and state legislation as well as links to related sites. Its address is *http://www.arentfox.com/telemedicine.html*.
• *The SpringNet Legal connection* — This site is designed to increase awareness of legal issues and includes information on delegation, documentation, and protection. It's at *http://www.springnet.com/legal.html*.

HEDIS and primary care

Quality of care

As the health care system continues to change, primary care providers (PCPs) face a new challenge — not just providing and documenting quality care but also effectively communicating that quality to consumers. One of the most important tools for providing standardized information about the performance of managed health care plans to the public is the Health Plan Employer Data and Information Set (HEDIS). Developed by the National Committee for Quality Assurance (NCQA), a non-profit organization that accredits managed health care plans, HEDIS lets the public compare managed health care plans. To rate plans, HEDIS uses standardized specifications for 71 clinical performance measures, procedure utilization, and patient satisfaction.
    How does this affect you? As a PCP, you must deal with managed health care plans. If a health plan isn't accredited by either NCQA (the primary accrediting agency for health plans) or the Joint Commission for Accreditation of Healthcare Organizations

(JCAHO), many companies — and Medicare and Medicaid — won't contract with that health plan. You also play a part in that accreditation; the NCQA gathers data from health plans nationwide, and those health plans gather data from medical practices, such as yours. Date sources include:
• patient satisfaction surveys
• medical record audits by health maintenance organization personnel sent to practice sites
• phone surveys of patients (some plans use nurse-auditors)
• Current Procedural Terminology (CPT) codes used by practices to bill for procedures and visits
• *International Classification of Diseases, 9th edition, Clinical Modification* (ICD-9-CM) diagnostic codes used by the NCQA to define target populations (These codes and CPT codes are included with each entry in chapter 8, Primary care procedures.)
• functional status surveys
• PCP entries in patient records.

Currently, the NCQA reports only aggregate data, reflecting the performance of entire health plans. However, consumers want more detailed information about specific medical practices, even individual practitioners. In time, they're likely to get such information, increasing the pressure on PCPs to provide and document quality care. The shift from voluntary to mandatory compliance (mandatory, if a health plan wants to remain accredited) for preventive care and health maintenance screening pressures PCPs to also focus on providing and documenting preventive care.

Specific performance measures

The NCQA has defined specific aspects of care to audit so that it can quantify data. These benchmarks are research-proven practices (for instance, performing annual dilated retinal examinations in diabetics diagnosed for more than 5 years) that increase the level of health in a given population. Knowing what these benchmarks are and what specific items the NCQA will audit lets you demonstrate the quality of care you provide. Specific sections of HEDIS under the PCP's control include:
• adult cancer screening
• post–myocardial infarction (MI) care with beta-adrenergic blockers
• cholesterol management
• depression pharmacotherapy
• chronic illness management
• diabetic retinal eye examination
• elderly health maintenance
• immunization
• mental illness follow-up
• perinatal care
• smoking cessation.

Below you'll find information on HEDIS performance measures and data sources that you can use to help you to best display your level of care.

Adult cancer screening

Performance measures for adult cancer screening focus on a mammogram in the past 2 years for women between ages 52 and 69 and a Papanicalaou (Pap) test in the past 3 years for those between ages 21 and 64. For various reasons, many patients neglect to act on these referrals. But follow-up contact by a PCP's office reinforces the need for the tests and boosts compliance rates. Health plans collect data on cancer screening from CPT codes on bills and medical record audits. Simply referring a patient for screening isn't enough; only completed mammographies and Pap tests are tallied.

Post–myocardial infarction care with beta-adrenergic blockers

The performance measure in post–myocardial infarction care with beta-adrenergic blockers applies to patients diagnosed with acute MI. Specifically, auditors look for the prescription of beta-adrenergic blockers within 7 days of discharge. Patients are excluded if they have an allergy or contraindication to beta blockers, were readmitted to a hospital within 7 days of discharge, or were transferred to a subacute care facility.

Cholesterol management

The cholesterol management audit selects patients who've had an acute cardiovascular event within the past year. The performance measure criteria is a low-density lipoprotein (LDL) screening within the past year. In 2000, auditors began checking for an LDL level below 130 mg/dl in patients who had an acute cardiovascular event in the past year.

Depression pharmacotherapy

Depression pharmacology selects records of patients treated with antidepressants. The three elements audited are three follow-up office visits during the 12-week period after a new episode, at least 12 weeks of antidepressant medication, and completion of a 6-month treatment course.

Chronic illness management

HEDIS measures for chronic illness management focus on six chronic conditions: MI or acute cardiovascular event, diabetes, schizophrenia, manic-depressive illness, paranoia, and depression. The performance measures address specific aspects of these illnesses.

Diabetic retinal eye examination

Auditors for the diabetic retinal eye examination use administrative data to locate entries with the ICD-9 code for diabetes and then eliminate patients under age 31. They then review patient charts and check for the eye examination CPT billing code within the past year.

Elderly health maintenance

The first performance measure for elderly health maintenance is influenza immunization within the past year in older adults (auditors exclude those who have a history of egg allergy or Guillain-Barré syndrome, are residents in hospice care, or are insured commercially or through Medicaid). The second criterion uses a patient survey form that measures functional status and allows the compilation of data on each patient over several years. Using a five-point scale, patients answer the following four questions:

• How would you rate your own health?
• In the past month, have emotional problems interfered with your daily activities?
• In the past month, has your physical health interfered with your daily activities?
• In the past month, has pain interfered with your daily activities?

Immunization

Health plans vary enormously on immunization rates. Although 65% of 2-year-olds overall have had their recommended vaccinations, the rates for specific plans range from 21% to 94%. The immunization performance measure checks the immunization status at ages 2 and 13. Specific criteria for 2-year-olds are four shots of diphtheria and tetanus toxoid and pertussis vaccine, three polio vaccines, one dose of measles-mumps-rubella vaccine (MMR), one varicella vaccine, a minimum of two haemophilus b conjugate vaccines, and two hepatitis B vaccines. By age 13, each child should have received a second dose of MMR, a third hepatitis B vaccine, and a tetanus-diphtheria booster.

PCPs should clearly document the reason for not vaccinating because auditors exclude from the data children who shouldn't be immunized. Contraindications include immunocompromised status, an anaphylactic reaction to neomycin (for MMR or varicella), an anaphylactic reaction to neomycin, streptomycin or polymyxin B (for inactivated polio vaccine [IPV]), an anaphylactic reaction to baker's yeast (for hepatitis B), or a history of anaphylactic reaction to the specific vaccine. Keep in mind that an anaphylactic reaction to eggs is no longer considered an absolute contraindication to MMR and influenza vaccination because the vaccinations use only a small amount of egg protein, making the risk of a reaction minimal. (See chapter 12, Health promotion, for more detail about immunizations.)

Mental illness follow-up

The mental illness follow-up performance measure audits records of patients who were hospitalized for manic depression, paranoia, or schizophrenia. The criterion is an outpatient visit to a mental health provider within 30 days of discharge. Patients under 6 years old, those transferred to a subacute care facility, and those readmitted within 30 days of discharge are excluded.

Perinatal care

Auditors look at two aspects of primary care during pregnancy: a visit in the first trimester and a postpartum checkup within 6 weeks of delivery. Specifically, they look for CPT codes or evidence of obstetric screening tests within the appropriate date ranges for patients who've given birth. Although the performance measures for perinatal care define a timeframe for the visits, they don't specify the type of practitioner; the patient may see a physician assistant, a nurse practitioner, a family doctor, a nurse-midwife, or an obstetrician.

Smoking cessation advice

NCQA audits on smoking randomly select patient surveys for adults who report they're current smokers or have recently quit. The auditor then asks these patients if they've received smoking cessation advice from a PCP.

Promoting preventive care

You and other PCPs aren't the only ones working hard to promote preventive care measures; managed health care companies and the government have taken steps, too. For instance, one managed health care company has nurse-auditors call patients who seem to lack specific preventive care measures (including immunization, mammography, Pap tests, dilated retinal examination, and perinatal care) to verify the information and to tell them about general guidelines for the specific preventive health measure. The government provides information and documentation forms through the U.S. Public Health Service to encourage frequent preventive health care checks.

However, the PCP is still the patient's main point of contact for preventive care. The following tips can help you promote and document preventive care measures.

• To remind you to conduct screenings, perform recommended tests, and take other appropriate measures, place simple forms in a set place in each patient's medical record. Make sure they're easy to document with the date and a note if needed. The U.S. Public Health Service has developed health maintenance flowcharts for the Put Prevention into Practice program that you can use. These and other resources are available to help you provide quality preventive care.

(See *Provider resources for preventive care.*)

• Use the medical groups' business card to record the patient's next appointment and remind him of the appointment.

• Develop a system to send out reminder postcards for such procedures as childhood immunizations, mammograms, Depo-Provera injections, and dilated retinal examinations. While the patient is in the office, jot down on a postcard the patient's name and the date of the next examination or procedure and place the card in a file (divided into months) for later mailing by office staff.

• Use office staff or a computer to phone patients to make appointments or to remind them of appointments. Such calls also increase compliance with referral appointments (such as for mammography) that many patients don't keep.

• Keep a copy of CPT codes available where you and others document to ensure proper payment and credit is given by auditors.

• Review documentation specifications for billing and for performance measures. Make sure immunization records include each immunization and the date (using a chart that lists the immunization schedule with boxes to fill in the date and batch number helps personnel remember to immunize the patient and to complete documentation). Forms that indicate the date and results of mammograms and Pap tests also help. Even though you don't have to include a copy of a mammogram report in the patient's chart, it's good practice to do so. Remember that a referral alone isn't enough; performance measures only indicate if mammograms and Pap tests have been completed.

• Make sure that at least one person — usually the office manager — is clearly designated to evaluate HEDIS compliance practices and re-

PROVIDER RESOURCES FOR PREVENTIVE CARE

The following organizations provide resources your practice can use to help you provide the best preventive care to your patients.

• The U.S. Public Health Service has a program called Put Prevention Into Practice that offers health maintenance flowcharts, patient reminder forms, and posters to display in the practice's office that emphasize prevention. Some are free, but a minimal fee is charged for some bulk orders. Contact: Agency on Health Care Policy and Research Publications, P.O. Box 8547, Silver Spring, MD 20907; 800-358-9295; *www.ahcpr.gov*

• The Joint Commission of American Hospital Organization (JCAHO) also uses outcomes-related data in accreditation. For providers in hospitals, long-term and home care settings, health care networks, and behavioral health care, JCAHO measures include clinical performance, health status, and patient satisfaction. Quality Check, a directory of JCAHO-accredited organizations and performance reports, is available on the Internet at *www.jcaho.org*. Contact: JCAHO, P.O. Box 75751, Chicago, IL 60675-5751; 630-792-5085

• The National Committee for Quality Assurance Publications provides information on the Health Plan Employer Data and Information Set and more. Its web address is *www.ncqa.org*. Contact: National Committee for Quality Assurance Publications, P.O. Box 533, Annapolis Junction, MD 20701-0533; 800-839-6487

sults. This person should routinely audit patient records, remind PCPs when charts don't reflect preventive screening and health maintenance, refine documentation forms or systems within the practice, and orient auditors to those forms or systems.

Understanding what steps PCPs can take to provide quality care—

and knowing that the public can compare the quality of care different health plans offer—encourages all PCPs to offer the highest quality care, not just the most cost-effective care. This allows us to improve the health of all our patients, one patient at a time.

NP scope of practice

Nurse practitioner (NP) care generally focuses on management of common acute disorders and injuries as well as stable chronic diseases. As part of this care, the NP orders, conducts, and interprets diagnostic and laboratory tests; prescribes treatments; and educates and counsels patients. Some NPs specialize in specific areas like women's health or pediatrics, which add explicit activities to their scope of practice. In addition, some NPs pursue additional training and perform advanced clinical procedures that can further expand their scope of practice, though not beyond that defined by each state's nurse practice act. For information on a specific state's scope of practice and prescriptive authority, see *NP scope of practice survey*.

Reimbursement for NP services

Medical practices need to provide and document quality care. However, they also need to receive reimbursement for that care. Most health care plans reimburse nurse practitioners (NPs) and doctors based on diagnostic and procedural codes. Therefore, an important part of receiving appropriate reimbursement is having an effective coding system in place that avoids

undercoding (and lost revenues) as well as overcoding (and the risks of fines, accusations of fraud, and denial of payment). Efficient coding captures all potential revenues and diagnoses appropriate for a service contract.

Each service, procedure, or supply should be identified with a code that describes the diagnosis, symptom, complaint, condition, problem, or follow-up care as defined by the Health Care Financing Administration (HCFA). You can use the *International Classification of Diseases, 9th edition, Clinical Modification* (ICD-9-CM) or ICD-9 codes and the most recent Current Procedural Terminology (CPT) manual to effectively code medical diagnoses and procedures. Make sure the ICD-9 codes are as specific as possible. Approximately 100 three-digit codes are valid; all others require further digits to obtain credit and payment for the care provided. For follow-up care and ancillary services, use V codes listed in these resources. If your practice provided only these services, the V code should precede the diagnostic code to indicate this.

To make sure the practice receives reimbursement, make sure documentation meets the coding criteria. Keep in mind that the most common reasons for denial of reimbursement include lack of a diagnosis (ICD-9) code, lack of a procedure (CPT) code, and failure of diagnosis and procedure codes to correspond. Make sure you also attach required progress notes to charts, or the practice could face fines, denial, or return of payment if charts are audited.

Although the practitioner chooses the codes, the billing department must also keep up with the latest coding developments. You can find such updates on the HCFA Web site *(www.hcfa.gov)* or in Medicare newsletters. The method of billing

NP SCOPE OF PRACTICE SURVEY

The map below provides a state-by-state summary of the degree of independence for all aspects of the nurse practitioner (NP) scope of practice, including diagnosing and treating (except prescribing). A state-by-state analysis of the degree of independence for the prescriptive authority aspect of the NP scope of practice.

Legal scope of practice for Advanced Practice Nurses

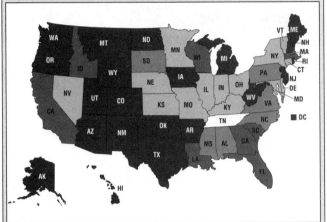

■ States with nurse practitioner* title protection and a board of nursing having sole authority in the scope of practice with no statutory or regulatory requirements for doctor collaboration, direction, or supervision: **Alaska, Arizona, Arkansas, Colorado, Hawaii, Iowa, Maine, Michigan, Montana, New Hampshire, New Jersey, New Mexico, North Dakota, Oklahoma, Oregon, Rhode Island, Texas, Utah, Washington, Washington, D.C., West Virginia, Wyoming**

■ States with nurse practitioner* title protection and a board of nursing having sole authority in the scope of practice, but the scope of practice has a requirement for doctor collaboration: **Connecticut, Delaware, Illinois, Indiana, Kansas, Kentucky, Ohio, Maryland, Minnesota, Missouri, Nebraska**, Nevada, New York, Vermont**

■ States with nurse practitioner* title protection and a board of nursing having sole authority in the scope of practice, but the scope of practice has a requirement for doctor supervision: **California, Florida, Georgia, Idaho, Louisiana, Massachusetts, South Carolina, Wisconsin**

■ States with nurse practitioner** title protection, but the scope of practice is authorized by the board of nursing and the board of medicine: **Alabama, Mississippi, North Carolina, Pennsylvania, South Dakota, Virginia**

□ States without nurse practitioner* title protection where APNs function under a broad nurse practice act: **Tennessee**

(continued)

---

* The information may apply to other APNs (clinical nurse specialists, nurse-midwives, and nurse-anesthetists).
** States with ARNP board. Washington, D.C., is included as a state in this table.
Adapted with permission from *The Nurse Practitioner* 24(1):18-19, January 2000.

NP SCOPE OF PRACTICE SURVEY *(continued)*

The map below provides a state-by-state analysis of the degree of independence for the prescriptive authority aspect of the NP scope of practice.

Prescriptive authority for Advanced Practice Nurses

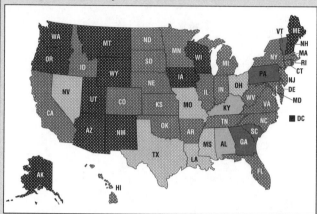

States where nurse practitioners* can prescribe (including controlled substances) independent of any required doctor involvement in prescriptive authority: **Alaska, Arizona, Iowa, Maine, Montana, New Hampshire, New Mexico, Oregon, Utah‡, Washington‡, Washington, D.C., Wisconsin, Wyoming**

States where nurse practitioners* can prescribe (including controlled substances) with some degree of doctor involvement or delegation of prescription writing: **Arkansas, California, Colorado, Connecticut, Delaware, Florida§, Georgia, Hawaii, Idaho, Illinois§, Indiana, Kansas‡, Maryland, Massachusetts, Michigan, Minnesota, Nebraska**, New Jersey, New York, North Carolina, North Dakota, Oklahoma, Pennsylvania, Rhode Island, South Carolina&, South Dakota, Tennessee§, Vermont, West Virginia**

States where nurse practitioners* can prescribe (excluding controlled substances) with some degree of doctor involvement or delegation of prescription writing: **Alabama, Kentucky, Louisiana, Missouri, Mississippi, Nevada, Ohio&, Texas, Virginia**

States where nurse practitioners* have no statutory or regulatory prescribing authority: none

States where nurse practitioners* also have the authority to dispense drug samples according to statute or rules and regulations: **Alaska, Arizona, Arkansas, California, Colorado, Connecticut, Delaware, Florida, Hawaii, Idaho, Illinois, Indiana, Iowa, Kansas, Louisiana, Maine, Maryland, Massachusetts, Michigan, Minnesota, Mississippi, Missouri, Montana, Nebraska, Nevada, New Hampshire, New Jersey, New Mexico, New York, North Carolina, North Dakota, Ohio&, Oklahoma, Oregon, South Dakota, Tennessee, Texas, Utah, Virginia, Washington, West Virginia, Wisconsin, Wyoming**

---

*The information may apply to other APNs (clinical nurse specialists, nurse midwives and nurse anesthetists). Washington, D.C., is included as a state in this table.

‡ Schedule IV and/or V medications only
& In narrowly specified situations
§ Pending approval of rules and regulations

and the type of electronic billing software your practice uses also influence reimbursement, turnaround time and, ultimately, productivity.

Types of reimbursement

There are many possible methods of reimbursement for nurse practitioner (NP) services. Each method has specific rules and requirements that must be followed precisely to generate payment.

Salary

If you work for an employer, you may receive an hourly wage or salary for your services. In this situation, the employer — not you — is responsible for billing various payment sources and receiving revenues from third-party payers, although your salary may include productivity incentives. However, several methods exist for re-imbursing NPs for their services, methods that require precise adherence to their rules for reimbursement to take place. Even if you're currently in a salaried position, it helps to understand these methods.

ALERT Make sure you're paid efficiently for your services by becoming familiar with the rules of the reimbursement plan for which you are providing services before you see patients. Even if you're on salary, you may be held to certain standards of revenue generation to justify your salary. Also, find out how the practice handles deductibles, copayments, and other out-of-pocket patient revenues; many practices use that information when calculating overall productivity levels. Pay attention to the mix of patients the practice assigns to you. If you only receive low-income and Medicaid patients and those with

unpaid debts, you'll generate less revenue, making you look less productive than you actually are. Lost clinic revenue from denied third-party payment could also result in a salary reduction or termination.

Regardless of how you're reimbursed, make sure you comply with state Board of Nursing (BON) regulations. Each state has a specific definition, scope of practice, qualifications, collaboration requirements, and prescriptive and diagnostic authority standards for NPs. These requirements are subject to change. To get updated requirements, contact your state BON. (You'll also find this information in each January issue of Springhouse's journal *The Nurse Practitioner*.)

Medicare

Although not all NPs provide services to Medicare patients, Medicare regulations — written by the Health Care Financing Administration (HCFA) — serve as a template for many aspects of health care delivery and reimbursement policies in the private sector and also with other age groups. You can go to the HCFA Web site at *www.hcfa.gov* for updates.

ALERT According to the HCFA Final Rule on reimbursement of NP services issued in late 1998, to bill Medicare directly for services, an NP must:
• have a master's degree in nursing
• be a registered professional nurse licensed as an NP in accordance with laws in the state where she provides services
• be certified as an NP by the American Nurses Credentialing Center or another nationally recognized certifying organization.

Two distinct reimbursement rates exist for NP services: *incident-to* reimbursement and *direct* reimbursement. Incident-to reimbursement pays for services performed by an NP under the supervision of a doctor and reimburses at a higher rate (however, incident-to reimbursement requires that the doctor be on-site during the billing incident). Rates of direct reimbursement for NP services depend on the *International Classification of Diseases, 9th edition,* code and Current Procedural Terminology code used for billing, adjusted down by a percentage from the payment base used for doctors. Different codes exist for the office (99201-99205 for new patients and 99211-99215 for established patients) and for nursing home visits (99301-99303 for new patients, 99311-99313 for routine visits, and 99314-99315 for discharge planning). However, each billed visit must use the modifier "AL" to designate an NP provider. When in doubt about which code to use, check with the person who does the billing or the office manager.

COLLABORATION If your state doesn't have collaboration guidelines for working with a doctor, you must document your scope of practice and indicate what relationships you have in place to deal with patient's needs that fall outside your scope of practice.

Keep in mind that reimbursement for services through Medicare involves sizable deductibles and copayments based on complicated formulas. Also, Medicare reimbursements don't cover the entire cost of services, resulting in large deductibles and coinsurance fees for patients. Because of this, many patients have Medicare supplement plans that provide additional payment. To receive direct reimbursement for these patients, you'll probably have to be listed on the Medicare supplement plan's provider panel.

Finally, when seeking Medicare reimbursement, have patience. HCFA fiscal intermediaries can delay Medicare payments for more than 6 months. Also, third-party reviewers can deny Medicare reimbursement retroactively if they deem the procedure unnecessary.

Managed care and HMOs

To receive direct reimbursement from a managed care organization or health maintenance organization (HMO), you must be listed on that organization's provider panel. Several barriers make this difficult. For instance, doctors sitting on the decision boards of HMO panels may see NPs as competition. In some states, NP groups have successfully fought to be on provider panels. Even so, NPs face drawbacks — for instance, they typically have to agree to provide care and perform procedures at greatly discounted rates or capitation.

ALERT Before signing an agreement to be included on an HMO provider panel and capitation agreement, consult with an experienced health care business attorney; negotiating capitation formulas isn't for novices. Find out exactly what responsibilities and risks you'll face if you're listed on a provider panel.

Medicaid

Many states have direct NP reimbursement programs for several types of services for Medicaid recipients. However, eligibility for patients, preauthorization requirements, NP qualifications, regulations, billing requirements, and reimbursement rates vary from state to state, and welfare reform legislation has resulted in drastic changes in Medicaid. To help you sort out the regulations and requirements, contact your state or regional department of HCFA. You can also log onto *www.hhs.gov/about/regionmap.html* and click on your state or the site closest to you. (See *Regional phone numbers for HCFA.*)

Contracted services and grants

Charitable groups, community organizations, and business-funded grants can reimburse specific NP services, such as physical examinations and services for the underserved. This form of reimbursement typically calls for the submission of a grant proposal in collaboration with another community organization such as a university. Such grant proposals usually require detailed plans for how patients get referred to the practitioner, collaboration relationships with multiple practitioners, and fiscal accountability. The goal is to make sure grant money goes to good use and doesn't serve patients who are already covered.

 COLLABORATION When writing such a grant proposal, consult with an NP group or person who has experience in providing services on a contractual basis or who has received a grant.

Independent practice and private pay

Some states let NPs form their own independent or group practices, and some even allow these practices to incorporate. Such a practice can offer financial and professional rewards, but you'll need business expertise to set up and run the practice. You can set up the practice to accept Medicare or other types of funding but, as mentioned earlier, these forms of reimbursement involve financial risk. Some doctors' practices don't accept Medicare or HMO reimbursement and take only private-pay patients. An NP practice can also be set up to receive private-pay patients, although doing

REGIONAL PHONE NUMBERS FOR HCFA

Office of Health Care Financing Administration (HCFA), by region.

Region 1: 617-565-1188 (Connecticut, Maine, Massachusetts, New Hampshire, Rhode Island, and Vermont)

Region 2: 212-264-4488 (New York, New Jersey, Puerto Rico, and the Virgin Islands)

Region 3: 215-861-4154 (Delaware, Maryland, Pennsylvania, Virginia, and Washington, D.C.)

Region 4: 404-562-7150 (Alabama, Florida, Georgia, Kentucky, Mississippi, North Carolina, South Carolina, and Tennessee)

Region 5: 312-886-6432 (Illinois, Indiana, Ohio, Michigan, Minnesota, and Wisconsin)

Region 6: 214-767-6427 (Arkansas, Louisiana, New Mexico, Oklahoma, and Texas)

Region 7: 816-426-5233 (Missouri, Iowa, Nebraska, and Kansas)

Region 8: 303-844-2111 (Colorado, Montana, North Dakota, South Dakota, Utah, and Wyoming)

Region 9: 415-744-3501 (Arizona, California, Hawaii, Nevada, Guam, Trust Territory of the Pacific Islands, and American Samoa)

Region 10: 206-615-2306 (Alaska, Idaho, Oregon, and Washington)

Additional information at the HCFA Web site: *www.hcfa.gov*

so requires some creative effort. The advantage of such a setup is that it allows NPs to deal with and get paid directly by patients — not third-party payers. To decrease the difficulty of collecting payments, the practice can have a policy that patients must pay at the time of service.

Starting an independent practice involves identifying a specific service

THE LITTLE BLUE BOOK

Listing your name in "The Little Blue Book" is one way to promote your practice and increase the visibility of nurse practitioners (NPs) in the community. This manual contains provider's names (including NPs and physicians' assistants), specialties, contact information, affiliations, and more. It's in many primary care offices and is used by primary care providers and office staff when making referrals. You can submit information on company letterhead by mail and update as needed online at *www.thelittlebluebook.com.* Contact: The Little Blue Book, 302 West Main Street, Suite 206, Avon, CT 06001; phone, 800-345-6865; fax, 860-674-8893

within your scope of practice, setting a price, establishing payment policies, and dealing with other aspects of operating a business. Sometimes, developing a narrow but very needed service can form the basis of an independent practice (for instance, bladder retraining). You also need to develop a referral network.

 COLLABORATION To avoid problems down the road, you may want to consult with experts, such as an attorney and accountant, to help you set up a partnership arrangement and incorporation documents and to help you file documents with state agencies. Topics to discuss include filing papers as a not-for-profit versus a for-profit company, setting up wage-withholding arrangements, dealing with unemployment taxes, and selecting company officers.

When pricing your service, amortize business costs, such as liability insurance, phones, computer equipment, staff wages, office supplies, and reasonable reimbursement for your NP services (including wages, health insurance, retirement, and continuing education). If local zoning ordinances allow it, a home office can help keep overhead costs down. You can find resources for starting your own practice at your local chamber of commerce, Service Corps of Retired Executives, state departments of commerce and business development, and other NPs in private practice. You can also join an Internet discussion group. (See *The Little Blue Book.*) The following Web sites may also help:

• American College of Nurse Practitioners: *www.nurse.org/acnp*
• American Nurses Association: *www.nursingworld.org*
• HCFA: *www.hcfa.gov/medicare.*

ALERT To avoid costly business loans that often overwhelm new businesses, be prepared to pay lower NP salaries for a few years. You can catch up later as your practice gets stronger. Avoid the temptation to go into debt by buying the latest equipment, which the practice really doesn't need.

When you start your practice, have a clear business plan and a vision, but don't let the plan restrict you; a business plan should never be static. Plan how you want to market your independent practice, keeping in mind that word-of-mouth and networking may work better for you than expensive mass advertising that may miss a large part of your potential client base.

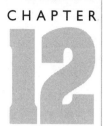

CHAPTER

12

Health promotion
Maintaining health over the lifespan

Current atmosphere

Perfect timing

In recent years, public interest in maintaining a healthy lifestyle has grown dramatically. More and more people are recognizing that their lifestyle directly affects their health. In fact, up to 50% of the deaths from the 10 leading causes of mortality in the United States can be linked to modifiable behaviors such as smoking. As a nurse practitioner, you can help your patients achieve a healthier lifestyle by promoting preventive care.

Guidelines by age

Maternal-neonatal health

Good antepartum care plays a key role in maternal and infant health. It can help decrease the risk of a patient delivering preterm or having a low birth weight baby, two predictors of infant morbidity and mortality. Ideally, a comprehensive prenatal program begins before conception and continues throughout the antepartum period, allowing early detection and treatment of problems. Such a program also gives you the chance to encourage healthy behaviors and prevent disease, teaching mothers about proper nutrition and weight gain; the dangers of smoking, alcohol, caffeine, and illicit drugs; and a host of other factors that might adversely affect the pregnancy.

During the initial prenatal visit, take a complete history and perform a comprehensive physical examination. Also, make sure the patient receives appropriate laboratory and ancillary studies as well as comprehensive risk assessment. Routine prenatal care should focus on the medical, psychosocial, educational, and nutritional needs of the patient and her family. A patient with an uncomplicated pregnancy should generally visit your office every 4 weeks until 28 weeks' gestation, every 2 to 3 weeks until 36 weeks, and weekly thereafter until delivery. However, timing and the specific content of prenatal visits will vary depending on the risk status of the mother and fetus.

History

A complete history includes the patient's current condition as well as her past medical, obstetric, family, and psychosocial history.

History of current condition
The initial history should include:
• date and type (urine or serum) of first positive pregnancy test
• signs and symptoms of pregnancy (amenorrhea, morning nausea and vomiting, breast tenderness)
• date of last normal menstrual period
• contraceptive history
• menstrual history (age at menarche, cycle length, menstrual flow, intermenstrual bleeding).

Previous medical history
This part of the history looks at medical conditions in the parents that may adversely affect the pregnancy outcome, including:
• birth defects
• illnesses (hypertension, diabetes mellitus, thyroid disease, epilepsy, any other major medical illness)
• hospitalizations and surgeries (such as prior abdominal surgery in the mother)
• allergies
• medication use
• immunization status (rubella, varicella)
• recent exposures to infectious disease

• environmental and occupational exposures
• sexual history.

Obstetric history

This part of the history looks at previous pregnancies, including:
• gravidity (total number of pregnancies, including the present one)
• length of labor
• type of anesthesia
• delivery method
• place of delivery
• sex and weight of newborn(s)
• delivery complications
• parity (outcome of each pregnancy)
• full term (births occurring after 37 and before 42 weeks' gestation)
• preterm (births occurring after 20 and before 37 weeks' gestation)
• abortions (elective and spontaneous)
• number of living children
• postterm (births occurring after 42 weeks' gestation).

Family history

Family history should focus on the parents' families and includes:
• physical illnesses (heart disease, congenital anomalies, diabetes, birth defects, any other major family illness)
• psychiatric illnesses
• physical or sexual abuse or domestic violence.

Psychosocial history

This focuses on psychosocial aspects of the family, including:
• nutrition and exercise
• education, occupation, and hobbies
• history of tobacco, alcohol, caffeine, and illicit drug use
• seat belt use
• home environment
• economic situation.

Physical examination

At the first prenatal visit, perform a complete physical examination, especially of the breasts and pelvis. In particular, note the size of the patient's uterus, the contour of her bony pelvis, and her baseline blood pressure and weight. During later routine visits, you only need to check her blood pressure, determine uterine size (by measuring the length of the uterus in centimeters from the pubic symphysis to the top of the fundus), verify fetal cardiac activity, and assess peripheral edema and weight gain.

Testing

The mother and fetus routinely undergo several tests to evaluate their health and detect complications. These include:
• human chorionic gonadotropin levels
• complete blood count
• serum glucose screening
• blood typing and Rh determination
• rubella antibody titer and screening
• hepatitis B and syphilis screening
• urinalysis (microscopic and culture)
• cervical cytology (Papanicolaou test, gonorrhea and chlamydia cultures)
• tuberculosis screening
• toxoplasmosis antibody test (for cat owners)
• maternal serum alpha fetoprotein screening (at 14 to 16 weeks' gestation for women over 35 years and fetuses at risk for neural tube defects)
• chorionic villous sampling (at 10 to 12 weeks' gestation when indicated for congenital anomalies)
• human immunodeficiency virus screening (requires patient consent and counseling)
• genetic screening (if risk factors are present for sickle hemoglobinop-

athies, Tay-Sachs disease, cystic fibrosis, Duchenne muscular dystrophy, fragile X syndrome, α-thalassemia, or β-thalassemia)

• ultrasonography (for dating pregnancy and, at the doctor's discretion, fetal survey; generally for educating parents at 18 to 20 weeks' gestation).

Risk assessment

Risk assessment, another vital part of prenatal care, helps you identify patients at risk for complications. Identifying some patients at risk — such as teenage and single mothers — becomes particularly difficult because they delay prenatal care or don't seek it at all. Although complications can, and do, occur in women without identifiable risk factors, a patient who falls into one of the major risk factor categories — preexisting medical conditions, previous poor pregnancy outcomes, and poor nutrition — is at greater risk. Such a patient stands a much better chance of having a healthy child and remaining healthy herself if she receives appropriate interventions. Risk factors to look for include:

• maternal age under 20 or over 35 years
• single-parent status
• minority status
• low educational level
• low socioeconomic level
• a preexisting medical condition (hypertension; diabetes; renal, cardiac, psychiatric, or pulmonary disease)
• alcohol, drug, or tobacco use
• previous preterm delivery, induced abortion, intrauterine growth restriction (IGR), or fetal death
• risky sexual behavior
• poor nutrition
• cervical or uterine anomalies
• a history of infectious diseases (particularly genitourinary infections).

Nutrition

The pregnant patient needs to understand the crucial role of nutrition in maintaining a healthy pregnancy. Your assessment and counseling can help her deal with such common complaints as nausea and vomiting, pica (a craving for nonfood substances), lactose intolerance, and constipation. You can also help her understand the risks of high caffeine and sodium intake, alcohol and substance abuse, and inappropriate weight gain. Specifically, you can suggest that she:

• eat a well-balanced diet with sufficient protein, carbohydrates, vegetables, fresh fruits (she should wash and dry fruits before eating), and dairy products
• take daily vitamin and mineral supplements (30 mg of ferrous iron and 0.4 mg of folic acid)
• restrict caffeine intake to no more than one cup of coffee, tea, or cola per day
• avoid eating raw or rare meat during pregnancy and practice good hand washing when handling raw meat
• try to maintain an ideal weight gain during pregnancy (which, depending on her body mass index, can vary from 15 to 40 lb); avoid dieting, fasting, and skipping meals; and try not to gain too much weight (which may cause gestational diabetes) or too little weight (which may cause premature labor or IGR)
• avoid excess salt intake, particularly during pregnancy, as it can elevate blood pressure.

Exercise

Although the pregnant patient shouldn't take part in rigorous exercise that causes extreme fatigue, such as prolonged jogging or skiing, she can safely take part in a program geared toward improving muscle strength and flexibility. Such a program may improve muscle tone and posture, which can help reduce some of the discomforts of pregnancy. If she's never exercised, she shouldn't begin a demanding exercise program during pregnancy.

Education and counseling: Alcohol, tobacco, and drug use

One of your most important roles is offering the patient education and counseling about the dangers of alcohol, tobacco, and drugs.

Alcohol

Except for genetic factors, alcohol use during pregnancy ranks as the most common cause of mental retardation. Alcohol acts as a potent central nervous system depressant, and the effects of alcohol on the fetus include prenatal and postnatal growth deficiency, mental retardation, behavioral disturbances, and congenital defects such as craniofacial anomalies (fetal alcohol syndrome). Because it isn't known what level of alcohol can cause fetal malformations, tell the patient—whether pregnant or considering pregnancy—to avoid all alcohol.

Tobacco

Tobacco use in any form during pregnancy—even breathing second-hand smoke—can result in a low birth weight infant. Using tobacco while breast-feeding an infant results in nicotine in breast milk. Suggest that your patient stop using tobacco immediately to avoid its adverse effects, including significant maternal and fetal morbidity.

Drugs

After alcohol and tobacco use, marijuana is the most commonly used recreational drug in pregnancy. The active component, 9-tetrahydro-cannabinol (THC), is a highly active psychotropic compound that is teratogenic in animal models. Although data about the drug's effects on pregnancy outcomes aren't conclusive, some studies suggest it may cause IGR and increased prematurity. Most current data don't suggest an increased risk of major fetal anomalies, but you should still warn your patients against using marijuana during pregnancy.

The two most frequently used addictive drugs during pregnancy are heroin and methadone. These drugs increase the risk of premature labor and delivery, IGR, fetal distress, low birth weight, neonatal infection, and passage of meconium stool. If your patient is taking either drug, refer her to a drug treatment program and an obstetrician experienced in managing pregnancies with addictive disorders.

Infant and child health

Infants and children need a comprehensive primary care program to help them grow into healthy adulthood. Each child in such a program should receive ongoing assessment of his growth and development, preventive care, well-child visits, and scheduled immunizations. (See *Internet resources on immunization*, page 436.) The child's parents also need teaching about nutrition and exercise and guidelines on how to prevent injuries during the accident-prone childhood years.

Growth and development

During infancy and childhood, children grow, develop, and learn new skills, achieving a series of neuro-developmental milestones. The rate at which a child reaches each milestone depends on biological and environmental factors, but every child must follow the same sequence of motor and cognitive development; he must develop basic skills to serve as a foundation for the development of later, more complex skills.

The rate of development is fastest during the first years of life. A newborn starts with the ability to respond to visual, auditory, olfactory, oral, and tactile stimuli. He can signal needs by crying when he's hungry or wet, but he exhibits only disorganized, seemingly purposeless movements when stimulated, which may be primitive reflexes or postural reactions. The primitive reflexes should disappear during the first 6 months of life as normal motor development occurs; persistence of such reflexes may indicate cerebral damage. Postural reactions help the infant maintain orientation of his body in space and serve as building blocks for the development of smoothly integrated motor functions.

Assessing a child's development includes taking a medical and psychosocial history and performing a physical examination. At each well-child visit, you should assess the child's development in each of the five major domains: gross motor, fine motor, language, personal and social, and cognitive. You can use a tool such as the Denver Developmental Screening Test to establish a baseline and assess his progress.

Gross motor skills
Gross motor development starts with head control and progresses in a predictable sequence as the spinal cord matures cephalocaudally. About 90% of healthy children can perform the following tasks at the specified age; inability requires further evaluation. By age 7 months, a child should be able to sit leaning forward on his hands; by 10 months, he should pull himself up to a standing position; and by 12 months he should begin to walk—the primary goal of gross motor development. After developing these fundamental motor skills, he should progress to running, climbing stairs, hopping, and skipping. By age 4, he should be able to pedal a tricycle at least 10′ (3 m) forward.

Fine motor skills
The development of fine motor skills should ultimately lead to the two-finger pincer grasp. However, until about age 3 months, a child's hand only forms a fist. By 6 months, he should be able to transfer objects from one hand to the other. Not until 9 months does the child exhibit the two-finger pincer grasp that allows him to manipulate small objects. Right- or left-handedness may develop at age 3 or as late as ages 4 to 5. By age 5, the child can button clothing; by age 6, he can dress independently.

Language skills

A child normally develops both receptive and expressive language skills. Early receptive milestones include the ability to hear and respond to sound; later milestones include the ability to understand spoken words. Early expressive milestones include basic elements of speech production; later, a child develops the ability to use language to convey his intentions to others.

Specifically, a child should be able to say at least three words (excluding *mama* and *dada*) by age 2 to indicate a specific thing. By age 3, he should be able to name at least one picture when looking at a book; by age 4, he should be able to play games where he takes turns and follows rules. Failure to meet these milestones may indicate developmental delays.

Personal and social skills

The development of personal and social skills allows a child to interact and respond to other people and his environment. Important milestones include the development of the social smile by age 2 months, anticipation of the return of an object when hidden from view by age 1, and the ability to follow rules by about age 4. By age 5, the child shouldn't be too upset when left with a babysitter.

Cognitive skills

Cognitive skills allow children to think, reason, solve problems, and understand their environment. Magical thinking and symbolic play occur from ages 18 months to 5 years. The ability to distinguish fantasy from reality develops later, at about age 5.

Developmental delay

A child who fails to reach a developmental milestone at the expected age is considered developmentally delayed. Such a child may have delays in one or more domains, and the delay may be a fixed or an ongoing process. Because the age at which children reach milestones can vary widely, each child needs ongoing developmental assessment at all well-child visits — using such tools as observation, history taking, physical examination, and screening tests — to assess his overall development over time.

Developmental delay can stem from many causes. Some of the more common include hearing deficits, inadequate environmental stimulation, autism, neuromuscular disease, mental retardation, congenital anomalies, and cerebral palsy.

If you suspect developmental delay, obtain a thorough history of the problem from the child's parents, including age at initial onset, causal factors, and any developmental regression. Also, refer him to the appropriate specialist, agency, or state program for further testing and assessment using standardized, age-appropriate instruments. For example, if the child has gross motor delays, he may need a comprehensive neurologic examination. Language delays merit hearing and speech assessment by an audiologist or speech pathologist, and cognitive delays require formal psychometric assessment.

Nutrition

To develop and grow normally, a child must have proper nutrition. A child grows very rapidly during the first 6 to 12 months and requires high-calorie, high-protein nutrition. Breast milk meets this need the best, but infant formula enriched with vitamins and minerals can also meet the infant's nutritional needs.

Breast-feeding

A healthy, well-nourished mother's breast milk can provide complete nutrition — including vitamins and micronutrients — for her infant during his first 4 to 6 months. For the first 1 to 2 months, the infant usually takes 2 to 3 oz of breast milk every 2 hours (10 to 15 minutes on each breast). After age 3 months, he may take 4 to 5 oz per feeding every 4 to 5 hours. At age 4 to 6 months, the child starts solid foods, but the mother can still breast-feed him. Here are some suggestions you can give new mothers to help them breast-feed successfully.

• Find a comfortable position (sitting or lying down). Hold the baby tummy-to-tummy, with your arm and a pillow supporting his weight. If you've had a Cesarean section, try the football hold so that the baby doesn't come in contact with your stomach.
• Use the baby's rooting reflex to initiate suckling.
• Make sure that the baby's mouth covers the nipple and cups as much of the areola as possible.
• Keep the baby's head higher than his stomach to ensure proper swallowing.
• After the baby finishes, insert one finger into the corner of his mouth between the gums to break the suction. This should help prevent sore nipples.
• Burp the baby before putting him on the other breast to feed. To do this, hold him upright against your shoulder, supporting his head, and gently pat his back.

Formula feeding

If the parents plan to bottle-feed their infant, they can choose from several commercially available infant formulas. Most are made from cow's milk or soy protein. For infants older than 6 months, the parents can choose a weaning formula, but these formulas don't seem to have any advantage over breast-feeding, infant formulas, or iron-fortified solids.

Formulas come in three different preparations. Although less expensive, concentrated and powered formulas require reconstitution. Tell the parents that they must follow the manufacturer's directions when preparing them. The more expensive ready-to-feed formulas come in cans, ready for bottle-feeding. Tell the parents to follow the manufacturer's storage instructions.

Solid foods

Children can begin eating solid foods when they show normal development, usually between ages 4 and 6 months. When the child starts solid foods, suggest to the parents that they limit formula to no more than 32 oz (1 L) per day or slowly decrease the frequency of breast-feeding to supplement solid foods.

Suggest they start the child with one or two feedings a day, beginning with rice and progressing to fruits, vegetables, and meats. They can gradually adjust the schedule so that it eventually matches the family's mealtimes. Tell them to introduce only one new solid food at a time and to wait from 3 to 5 days before adding another food; this allows the parents to note any adverse reactions the child may have. Suggest they offer one-item foods instead of combination foods. Tell them to wait to introduce egg whites, wheat, and fish until the child is much older and to not feed grapes, peanuts, popcorn, hot dogs, raisins, hard candy, and pieces of raw carrots to children under age 4 to avoid choking.

As the child grows, suggest that the parents:
• not insist that the child clean his plate or eat more after he is full (particularly if the child is overweight)

• offer three well-balanced meals a day, being careful not to serve overly large portions
• control portion size rather than denying certain foods
• encourage six to eight glasses of water per day (at least one before each meal if the child is overweight) to flush out waste materials and offer fewer carbonated and high-calorie beverages
• plan meals using the food pyramid
• minimize fried and high-fat foods
• store and eat food only in the kitchen or the dining room
• develop healthy eating habits themselves; this encourages the child to follow his role models.

Exercise

Along with proper nutrition, children need healthy physical activity. Exercise can help children resist temptations, such as eating junk food, taking drugs, and taking part in illegal activities with peers. Suggest to parents that they help their children fill empty time with after-school activities, volunteerism, sports, and spending time with friends and family.

Tell parents not to give a child food as a distraction; they should instead give him something to play with if they can't interact with him. Remind parents that children have more motivation to follow an exercise program or take part in a physical activity if the whole family takes part. Suggest family walks after dinner or games such as tag or basketball; such small changes in regular physical activity burn up calories. As the child gains muscle tone, loses baby fat, and becomes fit, he'll find such exercise less tiring.

Immunization

To decrease the risk of serious illness, children — ideally, all children —

should receive the recommended immunizations. Beyond just protecting individual children from a disease, widespread immunization aims to wipe out the disease itself.

Unfortunately, some groups, such as rural poor and inner-city children, have a relatively low level of immunization coverage. For example, in the United States, 12 cities have immunization rates for 2-year-olds below 75%. What makes such statistics even more distressing is that immunizations save money. Every dollar spent on polio vaccine saves more than $6 in direct medical care costs; every dollar spent on the measles, mumps, rubella (MMR) vaccine saves more than $21; and every dollar spent on the diphtheria and tetanus toxoids and pertussis (DTP) vaccine saves more than $30. The 1989-1991 measles outbreak alone came to an estimated $100 million in direct medical care costs.

Types of immunization

Two types of immunizations exist. In *active immunization,* the patient receives a vaccine that contains all or part of a microorganism or a modified product of that microorganism (toxoid or purified antigen), and has an immunologic response to the vaccine but develops no significant clinical illness. Protection takes a while to develop but lasts lifelong.

In *passive immunization*, the patient receives a vaccine made up of preformed human or animal antibodies. This type of vaccination provides immediate, short-term protection to patients who have been exposed or are at high risk for exposure.

A child can receive a vaccination as soon as his body can mount a protective immunologic response to the vaccine. This varies for each vaccine and for immunocompromised children. The United States currently requires children to receive immunizations from birth until they enter school. For the recommended schedule of immunizations as approved by the American Academy of Pediatrics (AAP), see *Recommended childhood immunization schedule*, pages 442 to 445. These vaccinations include hepatitis B virus (HBV); DTP/DTaP (acellular); inactivated poliovirus vaccine (IPV); *Haemophilus* b conjugate vaccine (Hib); MMR; and varicella-zoster vaccine (VZV). Many of these vaccines come in combination forms, and some require more than one dose.

ALERT Be aware that the rotavirus vaccine was voluntarily withdrawn from the market in October 1999 because of an association with bowel obstruction.

Administering immunizations
In children, you'll usually give subcutaneous and I.M. injections in the anterolateral upper thigh. If a child doesn't have enough muscle mass, use the deltoid area. To avoid sciatic nerve damage, don't inject into the buttocks. Use a 20G or 22G 1¼" needle for I.M. injections in infants and children; use a 25G ¾" needle for subcutaneous injections.

After administering the immunization, tell the parents that common adverse effects include redness, swelling, and tenderness at the injection site and low-grade fever (100.4° F [38° C]), especially following DTaP immunization; rarely, anaphylactic reaction may occur.

Keep in mind that the pertussis vaccination isn't routinely recommended for children age 7 years or older, and the Hib vaccine isn't essential after age 5. Also, an interruption in the immunization schedule doesn't warrant restarting the entire schedule; immunizations may pick up from where they left off. Finally, if a child has an unknown or undocumented immunization status, he should receive all appropriate vaccinations.

Testing

Starting at birth and continuing through childhood, children should undergo various screening tests. Metabolic screening tests in newborns, for example, allow early detection and treatment of more than 50 disorders. However, the specific tests each state requires vary widely, although all states require testing for congenital hypothyroidism and phenylketonuria. To help ensure that each newborn receives the appropriate tests, make sure you obtain a blood sample from full-term newborns just before discharge and a second sample at age 1 to 2 weeks (preterm and sick infants should be screened by 1 week of age).

Of particular concern are hemoglobinopathies, a major cause of illness and death in the United States. It's estimated that sickle cell disease (SS, SC, and SB-thalassemia) affects 1 out of every 400 African-American newborns. Although a National Institutes of Health consensus conference recommended universal newborn screening for hemoglobinopathies, screening guidelines differ from state to state. Heel-stick and cord blood samples examined by electrophoresis allow screening for abnormalities.

Vision and hearing screening
Children should also receive routine age-appropriate vision screening at each well-child visit, starting with the newborn examination. Your assessment should include a gross eye inspection followed by evaluation of the red reflex and fundus, pupillary light reflex, ability to track and follow objects, and position and symmetry of the corneal light reflex. Any abnor-

malities warrant a referral to an ophthalmologist so that early detection and treatment can help ensure normal visual development. When a child reaches age 3, you can use a Snellen alphabet chart, Allen picture cards, or instrumented screening equipment to test his vision. In preschoolers, a visual acuity of 20/40 or worse warrants further evaluation, as does an acuity of 20/30 in a 5- or 6-year-old.

As recommended by the AAP, children should also receive hearing screening starting in infancy. It's hoped that such screening allows detection of abnormalities by 3 months, with intervention starting no later than 6 months. Measuring techniques include brain stem response testing and otoacoustic emissions testing. Risk factors for hearing impairment include a family history of childhood hearing deficits; history of congenital infection or bacterial meningitis; anatomic malformations of the head, neck, or ears; low birth weight; low Apgar scores; and use of ototoxic medications. At-risk children should undergo a regular program of selective screening.

Other screening tests
Starting at age 3, children should undergo routine blood pressure screening at least once a year; children at risk for hypertension may require more extensive monitoring. Normal blood pressure for a child is defined as systolic and diastolic readings that fall below the 90th percentile for age and gender. A child age 2 or older who has a family history of atherosclerotic disease occurring before age 55 should also be screened for lipid abnormalities using a fasting (12-hour) serum lipid profile. If the child's family history isn't known but he has cardiovascular risk factors (obesity, smoking, hypertension, physical inactivity, diabetes), he

may need a nonfasting total serum cholesterol screening; if the screening shows any abnormal values, he'll also need follow-up.

Starting at age 6 months and continuing to 6 years, all children should receive blood lead screening to detect levels of 10 μg/dl or higher. Risk factors include living in a home built before 1960 that is falling apart or being renovated, having physical contact with known lead poisoning articles, having family members in lead-related occupations or hobbies, and living near lead smelters, battery recycling plants, or businesses that emit atmospheric lead.

Children don't need to undergo routine urinalysis unless disease is suspected or a child has an increased risk of renal abnormalities. Also, it's no longer recommended that low-risk, asymptomatic children who live in areas where tuberculosis isn't prevalent receive yearly tuberculin testing. However, if the child has one or more risk factors, he should receive screening based on his degree of risk. If he has no high risk factors and lives in an area where the disease is prevalent, he should be screened periodically from ages 4 to 6 and again from ages 11 to 16.

Education and counseling: Injury prevention

One of the greatest risks children face is the risk of accidental injury or death. The most common cause of accidental death is motor vehicle accidents followed, in order, by drowning, fires, and all burns. Falls, poisoning, aspiration, suffocation, and firearm accidents account for most of the remaining unintentional injuries or deaths in children. Children also

(Text continues on page 444.)

RECOMMENDED CHILDHOOD IMMUNIZATION SCHEDULE

This schedule shows the recommended age for routine administration of currently licensed childhood vaccines. Shaded bars indicate range of acceptable ages for vaccination. Shaded ovals indicate vaccines to be assessed and administered.

Some combination vaccines are available; you can use them whenever administration of all components of the vaccine is indicated. Consult the manufacturers' package inserts for detailed recommendations. For more information about vaccinations, you can also visit *www.aap.org.*

Vaccine	Birth	1 month	2 months	4 months	6 months
Hepatitis B (HBV)[1]		HBV			
			HBV		
Diphtheria, tetanus, pertussis (DTP); diphtheria, tetanus, acellular pertussis (DTaP); or tetanus diphtheria (DT or Td)[2]			DTP/DTaP	DTaP	DTaP
Haemophilus influenzae type b (Hib)[3]			Hib	Hib	Hib
Inactivated poliovirus vaccine (IPV)[4]			IPV	IPV	IPV
Measles, mumps, rubella (MMR)[5]					
Varicella zoster (VZV)[6]					

Range of acceptable ages for vaccination.

Vaccines to be given if previously recommended doses were missed or given earlier than the recommended minimum age.

1. Hepatitis B

Blood should be drawn at the time of delivery to determine the mother's hepatitis B surface antigen (HBsAg) status; if it's positive, the infant should receive hepatitis B immune globulin (HBIG) as soon as possible (no later than 1 week of age). The dosage and timing of subsequent vaccine doses should be based upon the mother's HBsAg status.

Infants born to HBsAg-negative mothers should receive 2.5 μg of Recombivax HB vaccine or 10 μg of Engerix-B vaccine. The second dose should be administered at least 1 month after the first dose. The third dose should be given at least 2 months after the second, but not before age 6 months.

Infants born to HBsAg-positive mothers should receive 0.5 ml of HBIG within 12 hours of birth, and either

Approved by the Advisory Committee on Immunization Practice (ACIP), the American Academy of Pediatrics (AAP), and the American Academy of Family Physicians (AAFP)

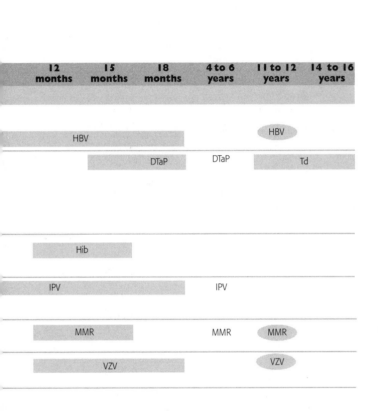

12 months	15 months	18 months	4 to 6 years	11 to 12 years	14 to 16 years
HBV				HBV	
		DTaP	DTaP	Td	
	Hib				
IPV			IPV		
MMR			MMR	MMR	
VZV				VZV	

5 µg of Recombivax HB or 10 µg of Engerix-B at a separate site. The second dose is recommended at 1 to 2 months of age and the third dose at age 6 months.

Infants born to mothers whose HBsAg status is unknown should receive either 5 µg of Recombivax HB or 10 µg of Engerix-B within 12 hours of birth. The second dose of vaccine is recommended at age 1 month and the third dose at age 6 months.

Children and adolescents who haven't been vaccinated against hepatitis B (HBV) in infancy may begin the series during any visit. Those who haven't previously received three doses of HBV vaccine should initiate or complete the series during the 11- to 12-year-old visit, and unvaccinated older adolescents should be vaccinated whenever possible. The second dose should be administered at least 1 month after the first dose, and the third dose should be administered at least 4 months after the first dose and at least 2 months after the second dose. *(continued)*

2. Diphtheria, tetanus, and pertussis

Diphtheria and tetanus toxoids and acellular pertussis vaccine (DTaP) is the preferred vaccine for all doses in the immunization series, including completion of the series in children who have received one or more doses of whole-cell diphtheria-tetanus-pertussis vaccine (DTP) vaccine. Whole-cell DTP is an acceptable alternative to DTaP. The fourth dose (DTP or DTaP) may be administered as early as age 1, provided 6 months have elapsed since the third dose and if the child is unlikely to return at age 15 to 18 months. Tetanus and diphtheria toxoids (Td) vaccine is recommended at ages 11 to 12 if at least 5 years have elapsed since the last dose of DTP, DTaP, or DT. Subsequent routine Td boosters are recommended every 10 years.

3. *H. influenzae* type b

Three *H. influenzae* type b (Hib) conjugate vaccines are licensed for infant use. If PRP-OMP (PedvaxHIB and COMVAX) is administered at ages 2 and 4 months, a dose at age 6 months isn't required. Because clinical studies in infants have demonstrated that using some combination products may induce a lower immune response to the Hib vaccine component, DTaP/Hib combination products shouldn't be used for primary immunization in infants at ages 2, 4, or 6 months, unless Food and Drug Administration-approved for these ages.

4. Poliovirus

IPV is recommended by ACIP, AAP, and AAFP at ages 2 months, 4 months, 6 to 18 months, and 4 to 6 years. Use of inactivated vaccine is particularly important for immunocompromised persons and their household contacts.

---

face the risk of intentional harm. In fact, in 1996, suicide was the fifth leading cause of death in children ages 5 to 14.

In recent years, the emphasis has shifted from changing individual behaviors to changing the surroundings — for instance, requiring the use of seat belts for children — to make children safer. You can teach parents the importance of creating a safe environment for their children. Suggest that parents use the following guidelines from the AAP to help keep their children safe. Where appropriate, teach children how to keep themselves safe and healthy.

For infants and preschoolers
• Use infant and child car seats.
• Use home smoke detectors (change batteries once yearly).
• Keep hot tap water temperatures at a safe level. Set your water heater no higher than 130° F (54° C).
• Install window screens and stairway guards or gates to prevent falls.
• Erect sturdy fences and safety guards around any swimming pools.
• Don't use an infant walker.
• Use a crib with slats 2″ apart, with a firm, snug-fitting mattress; keep the sides of the crib raised.
• Empty water out of all buckets, tubs, and wading pools.
• Keep all drugs (such as ipecac syrup) and household products marked poisonous out of reach of children.
• Keep up-to-date on immunizations.
• Place infants on their side or back to sleep.

According to these panels, OPV is no longer recommended because of the associated risk of paralytic polio in the recipient or someone who has been in contact with the recipient. OPV is acceptable only for special circumstances, including parents who fail to complete the recommended number of injections, late initiation of immunization that would require an unacceptable number of injections, and imminent travel to polio-endemic areas. If someone is inadvertently given OPV, the recipient should avoid close physical contact with immunosuppressed persons for 6 weeks after vaccination.

5. Measles, mumps, rubella

The first dose is recommended at age 12 to 15 months. The second dose of vaccine for measles, mumps, and rubella (MMR) is recommended routinely at ages 4 to 6 years but may be administered during any visit, provided at least 1 month has elapsed since the first dose, and that both doses are administered beginning at or after age 1. Those who haven't previously received the second dose should complete the schedule no later than the 11- to 12-year-old visit.

6. Varicella

Susceptible children may receive varicella-zoster vaccine (VZV) at any visit after the first birthday. Those who lack a reliable history of chickenpox should be immunized during the 11- to 12-year-old visit. Susceptible children ages 13 or older should receive two doses, at least 1 month apart.

• Never leave infants unattended in the care of young siblings.
• Don't drink hot liquids or smoke while holding an infant.
• Feed children age-appropriate foods, and offer age-appropriate toys for play.
• Watch infants at mealtimes and while they're in the bathtub or pool.
• Put sunscreen on children, and don't expose them to too much sun.
• Learn cardiopulmonary resuscitation (CPR).

For school-age children

• Use booster seats or seatbelts, depending on a child's age.
• Make sure children wear bicycle helmets.
• Insist on protective equipment for in-line skating and skateboarding.
• Install home smoke detectors in strategic areas.
• Follow pedestrian safety rules.

• Remove firearms from the home, or unload all guns and keep guns and ammunition locked in separate cabinets.
• Put sunscreen on children, and don't expose them to too much sun.
• Learn CPR.
• Assess the child's readiness for sexual development counseling by keeping lines of communication open.
• Discuss home safety rules about visitors, telephone use, and responses to fires and other emergencies.

Adolescent health

By the time they reach adolescence, many young people already have risk factors for chronic diseases that increase the risk of morbidity and mortality in adults. Obesity, for instance, is at an all-time high in children and adolescents. However, adolescents still have a chance to develop healthy habits that can carry into adulthood. School and after-school activities can still shape habits, and even the adolescent's keen awareness of body image can help. Obsession with body image can cause problems; dysfunctional body image is common by fifth grade, especially in girls. Parents, teachers, and health care providers can also use body image awareness to steer adolescents to healthier lifestyle choices.

Nutrition

Nutrition can pose a particular problem in adolescence, when eating disorders may become a problem. Recognizing and treating such disorders early on can prevent them from becoming critical. Here are some steps you can take.

• Encourage parents to make healthy foods readily available to their teenagers, and discourage foods high in fat, sodium, and added sugars. Suggest the family pick certain days to share in the joint activity of making salads and other healthy meals.

• Discuss healthy eating habits and physical activity with the adolescent. Explain the effects that diet and physical activity have on his current and future health and activities.

• Put up posters that encourage adolescents to make healthy eating and activity choices, and keep a list available of local options for activities, individual and team sports, and volunteering.

• Ask the adolescent to list his own reasons to adopt healthy eating and physical activity habits.

• Teach the adolescent how to identify healthy foods that fit specific needs. For instance, vitamins improve vision; protein builds muscles; meat and dark green, leafy vegetables rich in iron build red blood cells and maintain warmth and energy levels; and calcium builds strong bones. Teach him how to identify foods high and low in fat, saturated fat, cholesterol, sodium, and added sugars. Show him the fat in a potato chip by wrapping it in a paper towel for a few minutes and letting him see the fat that the paper absorbs. Teach him how to read food labels and evaluate diet claims.

• Teach the importance of balancing food intake and physical activity; suggest three meals a day and at least three half-hour exercise periods each week.

• Teach the dangers of unsafe weight-loss methods (weight-cycling, decreased metabolism, electrolyte imbalance, and energy loss) and the benefits of a safe weight-loss program that includes three meals a day, nutritious snacks, and regular exercise.

• Encourage the patient to value his health and take control of his food selection and preparation. Increase his confidence in his ability to eat healthy foods by reinforcing positive behaviors.

• Help the patient examine what motivates good and bad eating habits. If the patient has an eating disorder, suggest keeping a food diary and recording the cues that affect eating behavior (for instance, mood, hunger, stress, or other persons). Refer the patient to counseling to develop alternative coping mechanisms.

ALERT Never remove a patient's coping mechanisms without ensuring that he has effective coping skills. Doing so may lead to further problems. (For instance, don't prescribe appetite suppressants for a patient who may overeat to suppress thoughts of violence that stem from a long history of abuse.)

Exercise

Healthy exercise patterns established in adolescence can carry into adulthood, resulting in a lower risk of such chronic diseases as hypertension and cardiovascular disease and lower mortality rates. Unfortunately, while more physically active than adults, many young people still don't engage in moderate or vigorous physical activity at least 3 days a week, and physical activity tends to decline steadily during adolescence.

You can take several steps to encourage adolescent patients to get the exercise they need. Suggest that they take part in activities with peers and friends. Remind parents that they can act as role models by keeping fit themselves and by arranging family activities that encourage fitness. Also, suggest that they provide appropriate sports equipment, take their children to sports and fitness programs, and make sure children have access to play areas; all of these actions help promote physical activity.

You can also use well-child visits to generate a positive attitude toward healthy behaviors and help adolescents learn how to establish and maintain a physically active lifestyle. Providing the adolescent patient with a list of local options may be all that is needed to foster an interest in a physical activity that will remain a lifelong habit. Try to link teenagers to community physical activity programs that might interest them, and use community resources to support such extracurricular programs. Help your patient see that physical activity is fun and that, whatever his background, he can gain skills and confidence in himself. Promote such skills as self-assessment, self-monitoring, decision making, goal setting, identifying and tackling barriers, reinforcement, and communication to help your patient adopt and maintain a healthy lifestyle that includes regular physical activity.

Immunization

In the United States, disease levels are near record low levels because of the highest immunization coverage levels in history. In 1990, for example, over 27,000 cases of measles occurred at the height of the measles resurgence, whereas only 89 cases of measles were reported in 1998. Yet adolescents continue to suffer from such diseases as varicella, hepatitis B, measles, and rubella, with over 40 million adolescents at risk for vaccine-preventable diseases. The 10 adult and adolescent vaccine-preventable diseases are tetanus, diphtheria, hepatitis A, hepatitis B, influenza, pneumococcal pneumonia, measles, mumps, rubella, and varicella. Because adolescents and adults are less likely to schedule well visits, assess immunization status at each encounter. (See *Adolescent immunization schedule [ages 11 to 18]*, page 448.)

Testing

Like younger children, adolescents should undergo certain screening tests. These include blood pressure measurement and dyslipidemia risk assessment (screening for low-risk patients; lipid panel for those at higher risk). You'll also need to assess the vision of adolescents at risk for vision loss and assess hearing for those at risk for hearing loss. Do a purified protein derivative (PPD) test to screen for tuberculosis. Check lipid levels and hematocrit or hemoglobin levels (in girls) for at-risk patients, including those with heavy menstrual bleeding or poor dietary intake of iron.

ADOLESCENT IMMUNIZATION SCHEDULE (AGES 11 TO 18)

Vaccine	Indications	Timing
Hepatitis B (HBV)	Adolescents not vaccinated previously for hepatitis B	Three doses: second dose 1 to 2 months after first; third dose 4 months after first dose
Measles, mumps, and rubella (MMR)	Adolescents not vaccinated previously with two doses of MMR vaccine at ages 1 or older	One dose*
Tetanus-diphtheria (Td)	Adolescents not vaccinated within previous 5 years	A booster dose and then one every 10 years through age 50, plus p.r.n.
Varicella zoster (VZV)	Adolescents not vaccinated previously and who have no reliable history of chickenpox	Ages 11 to 12 get one dose; ages 13 and older get two doses: second dose 1 month after first dose†
Influenza	Adolescents who are at increased risk for complications caused by influenza or who have contact with persons at increased risk for these complications	Annually (September to December); now available in intranasal form
Pneumococcal	Adolescents who are at increased risk for pneumococcal disease or its complications	One dose (A repeat dose 5 years later may be given to those at highest risk.)
Lyme disease (LYMErix)	Adolescents who are at increased risk for infected tick bite. Consider geographic (Canada, northern and mid-Atlantic U.S.) and behavioral risks.	Ages 15 and older: three doses required; second dose after 1 month; third dose 1 year after first dose. Vaccine administration should be timed so that second dose of the vaccine and third dose are administered several weeks before the beginning of the *Borrelia Burgdorferi* transmission season, usually April.
Hepatitis A (HAV)	Adolescents who are at increased risk for hepatitis A infection or its complications	Two doses, 6 to 18 months apart

* Shouldn't be given to pregnant adolescents or those considering pregnancy within 3 months of vaccination.

† Shouldn't be given to pregnant adolescents or those considering pregnancy within 1 month of vaccination.

Excluding typhoid, never restart a series.

Ensure at least 1 month between doses, excluding typhoid. Early dosing is more significant (if dose is given within 1 month, it may not boost immunity and so may need repeating). Extra doses not contraindicated.

All vaccines can be given simultaneously but not in the same syringe.

If the patient is on pulse steroids, wait 1 month to immunize (inhaled and topical steroids have no impact). For long-term steroid use, consult with a pediatric infectious disease specialist.

DTaP-HIB (TriHIBit) vaccine only used as fourth dose in United States because of possibly lower immunity conferred.

Adapted from recommendations of the Advisory Committee on Immunization Practices, Centers for Disease Control and Prevention.

During the physical examination, determine the patient's body mass index; assess for scoliosis, acne, and Tanner maturation stage; check the teeth; and look for signs of abuse. Teach adolescent girls how to examine their breasts; if they're sexually active, perform an annual pelvic examination. Teach adolescent boys at high risk for testicular cancer or who have a history of undescended testes or a single testicle how to perform a testicular self-examination. Also assess adolescent boys for hernias and gynecomastia. If you detect enlargement and tenderness in one or both breasts, reassure the patient that this occurs transiently in many males between ages14 and 20 and usually resolves within 2 years; however, tell them to watch for signs of testicular cancer or hypothyroidism. Check all sexually active patients for condylomata, and screen them for gonorrhea and chlamydia (from 50% to 75% of patients with infection have no symptoms). Screen high-risk patients for syphilis and human immunodeficiency virus (HIV) infection.

Education and counseling

Adolescents face many challenges and risks, from the risk of violence, to the temptation to smoke or take drugs, to the dangers of high-risk sexual behaviors. They need education and counseling to learn how to deal with these risks. You can start such teaching by offering some basic guidelines that all adolescents can follow.
• Listen to good friends and valued adults, and trust their feelings.
• Seek help if you frequently feel angry, depressed, or hopeless.
• Set reasonable but challenging goals for yourself.
• Learn how to handle peer pressure and how to say no.

• Respect the rights and needs of others, and be sure that yours are also respected.
• Take an active role in identifying and seeking help to meet your goals and plans (such as obtaining financial assistance and college referrals).

Injury and violence prevention
Unintentional and intentional injuries are the leading cause of death for both children and adolescents. Every day, some 60 children die from injuries, and countless others are injured and disabled. Such injuries not only take a huge emotional toll on victims and their families, but they also result in enormous medical expenses and the less obvious costs of the loss of years of potential life and productivity.

Violence, particularly homicide, is the second leading cause of death in 15- to 24-year-olds. For every violence-related death, at least 100 people suffer nonfatal injuries. Young people who experience violence as victims, witnesses, or perpetrators suffer serious short-term and long-term consequences — cognitively, emotionally, and developmentally.

Adolescents also face the risk of suicide — a risk that increases with age. Suicide ranks as the third leading cause of death in 15- to 24-year-olds, up from the fifth leading cause in children ages 5 to 14.

Suggest that adolescents use the following safety guidelines from the American Academy of Pediatrics:
• Use seat belts and follow speed limits.
• Avoid alcohol while driving or participating in water-related sports.
• Wear motorcycle or bicycle helmets; use mouth guards and protective sports gear.
• Use protective equipment for in-line skating and skateboarding.
• Use personal flotation devices when boating.

- Use sunscreen and minimize exposure to the sun; avoid tanning salons.
- Ask your parents to remove firearms from the home, or unload all guns and keep guns and ammunition locked in separate cabinets. This can help decrease the risk of impulsive or unplanned suicide, homicide, and other serious injuries.
- Learn how to protect yourself from abuse, deal with anger, and resolve conflicts. Know where to go for help. Options include peer groups, trusted adults like relatives or teachers, and professional counselors.
- Learn cardiopulmonary resuscitation.
- Seek counseling from parents or other trusted adults for help with puberty issues and sexual development and behavior.
- Discuss home safety rules about visitors, telephone use, and responses to fires and other emergencies.

Smoking and substance use

Tobacco use in adolescents keeps rising, even though it's clear that using tobacco causes harm. Nearly 3,000 children take up smoking each year, and one in three teenagers who do smoke will die prematurely from tobacco use. If an adolescent can resist the temptation to use tobacco, his chances of becoming an adult user drop to 10% — meaning that he probably won't become one of the more than 400,000 Americans who die from tobacco-related illnesses each year. You can help adolescents resist tobacco and drug use, using their interest in body image to help you.

- Remind teenagers that smoking causes yellow teeth, bad breath, a stale smoke smell that clings to clothes and hair, and wrinkles.
- State firmly that smoking, spitting tobacco, and using of alcohol, drugs, diet pills, or steroids will damage their health.
- State that first time use is enough to cause active addiction to drugs or alcohol in some individuals.
- Ask about the patient's long-term goals and relate abstinence or temperance to realize those goals.
- Teach adolescents to avoid situations where drugs or alcohol are present.
- Remind patients to support and spend time with friends who choose not to develop harmful habits.

High-risk sexual behaviors

Adolescents face danger not only from tobacco and substance abuse but also from high-risk sexual behaviors. Consequences include adolescent pregnancy, sexually transmitted disease (STD), and HIV infection. You can help adolescents by counseling them on responsible sexual decision making, beginning with abstinence, which guarantees protection from STDs and pregnancy. Emphasize that the patient doesn't need to have sex if he doesn't want to and that everyone has the right to take the time to think before making a decision. Use a nonjudgmental or neutral manner when issues of homosexuality arise and guide patients to informed resources as indicated, such as the Sexual Minority Youth Assistance League at Web site *smyal.org*.

For sexually active patients, offer confidential contraceptive services and screening for STDs. Explain what safer sex is — limiting the number of sexual partners and using condoms correctly — and emphasize its benefits. If the patient wants further instructions on correct condom use, he can call the Centers for Disease Control and Prevention's (CDC) National Prevention Information Network, 800-342-2437, or the CDC National STD Hotline, 800-227-8922.

Adult health

Even in adulthood, patients need support to maintain health. As adults age, they face chronic diseases that can lead to earlier death, such as stroke and heart disease. They also face changes that decrease quality of life, such as chronic pain or decreased vision and hearing. Even previously life-threatening illness such as heart disease are less likely to kill and more likely instead to affect quality of life. You can help these patients make lifestyle choices to improve their quality of life. Through proper nutrition and exercise, up-to-date immunizations and testing, and education and counseling, adults can continue to maintain a healthy lifestyle.

Nutrition

To maintain proper nutrition, adult patients need to choose healthy foods to fit their needs. The guidelines for adolescent nutrition also work well for most adults (see "Nutrition," page 446). Teach patients how decreasing metabolism, more sedentary lifestyle, and fat redistribution (all common with advancing age) affect the body. Emphasize the importance of nutritious food in proper portions and routine exercise.

Exercise

Proper exercise plays a key role in weight control, muscle tone, physical endurance, glucose metabolism, and energy levels. Suggest to your adult patients that they exercise at least half an hour three or more times a week. If they haven't exercised much before, suggest starting slowly to increase enjoyment and compliance and decrease discomfort. Recommend activities that also offer other rewards, such as biking with a friend, walking the dog, or joining the neighborhood Town Watch; studies show that physical activities that offer secondary rewards are more likely to persist.

Immunizations and testing

Your adult patients need to understand the rationale for immunization and what options they have. For instance, you can explain that although the pneumococcal vaccine isn't effective against all forms of pneumonia, it's effective against some of the most serious types. Emphasize to the patient that if he skips the immunization, he may have serious complications — especially because antibiotic resistance to pneumococcal infections is growing. (See *Adult immunization schedule [over age 18]*, page 452.)

The specific testing your patient may need depends on his history and physical examination as well as problems that affect the particular population or geographical area where he lives. A basic adult health maintenance schedule can guide your care, tailored to the individual needs of each patient. (See *Sample health maintenance schedule for normal adults*, page 453.)

Education and counseling

Like younger patients, adults also need education and counseling. Specific areas include stress reduction, smoking and substance abuse, and sexual practices.

Stress reduction

Stress plays a significant role in many disorders, including hypertension, cardiac disease, GI upset, and constipation. Many adults try to relieve stress with methods that actually cause long-term harm — smoking,

(Text continues on page 454.)

ADULT IMMUNIZATION SCHEDULE (OVER AGE 18)

Vaccine	Timing and considerations
Hepatitis A (HAV) for those at risk	Two doses 6 to 12 months apart to provide long-term protection; first dose 4 weeks before departure to endemic countries
Hepatitis B (HBV) if never had initial series	Three doses: second dose at least 1 month after first; third dose 5 months after first dose
Measles, mumps, and rubella (MMR)	Two doses 1 month apart if born after 1957 and immunity can't be proved*
Tetanus-diphtheria (Td) if never had initial series	Three doses: second dose after 1 month, third dose 6 to 12 months after second; booster for all patients every 10 years
Varicella-zoster (VZV)	Two doses for those who haven't had chickenpox; second dose 1 month after first dose†
Influenza (Flu)	Annually before flu season (U.S.: September-December); now available in intranasal form, especially for ages 65 and older and those with medical problems (heart or lung disease, diabetes, chronic conditions) and those who work or live with high-risk individuals
Pneumococcal	One dose at age 65; also recommended for persons with chronic disease (see indications for influenza) and those with kidney disorders and sickle cell anemia; possibly a repeat dose 5 years later for those at highest risk may be given any time of year
Lyme disease (LYMErix)	For those at high risk because of geography (Canada, northern and mid-Atlantic U.S.) and behavior; ages 15 to 70, three doses: second dose after 1 month, third dose 1 year after first dose; vaccine administration timed so that the first dose and third dose are administered several weeks before the beginning of the *Borrelia burgdorferi* transmission season, usually April

* Shouldn't be given to pregnant patients or those considering pregnancy within 3 months of vaccination.

†Shouldn't be given to pregnant patients or those considering pregnancy within 1 month of vaccination.

Early dosing is more significant (if dose is given within 1 month, it may not boost immunity so may need repeating). Extra doses not contraindicated.

All vaccines can be given simultaneously but not in the same syringe or site.

If the patient is on pulse steroids, wait 1 month to immunize (inhaled and topical steroids have no impact). For long-term steroid use, consult with an infectious disease specialist.

Adapted from recommendations of the Advisory Committee on Immunization Practices, Centers for Disease Control and Prevention.

SAMPLE HEALTH MAINTENANCE SCHEDULE FOR NORMAL ADULTS

Evaluate	Ages 19 to 39	Ages 40 to 49	Over age 50
Diet, physical activity	Each visit	Each visit	Each visit
Substance use or abuse (herbals or supplements)	Annually	Annually	Annually
Sexual behavior risks	Each visit	Each visit	Each visit
Weight, blood pressure, skin	Annually	Annually	Annually
Digital rectal examination		Annually	Annually
Fecal occult blood test			Annually
Sigmoidoscopy			Every 5 years
Breast examination	Annually	Annually	Annually
Papanicolaou test	Annually	Annually	Every 1 to 3 years
Pelvic examination	Annually	Annually	Annually
Mammography	Once after age 35	Every 2 years	Annually
Prostate specific antigen	Annually	Every 1 to 3 years	Annually
Testicular examination	Annually	Every 1 to 3 years	Every 1 to 3 years
Serum cholesterol		Every 5 years	Every 5 years
Thyroid-stimulating hormone			Every 5 years
Hearing and vision		Every 5 years	Annually
Fasting blood glucose to assess risk for type 2 diabetes mellitus	Every 5 years	Every 2 years after age 45	Every 2 years

High-risk populations screened as indicated: sexually transmitted diseases (STDs) annually and p.r.n. (sexually active without condom use); for any STD, discuss human immunodeficiency virus testing; tuberculosis every 2 years and p.r.n. (substance abuse, in prison or residential facility, chronic contact); electrocardiogram every 2 to 5 years if negative (but has a family or personal cardiac history); lipid panel for presence of risk factors for dyslipidemia; fasting blood glucose annually. Major risk factors for type 2 diabetes include (1) family history of diabetes; (2) obesity (more than 20% over recommended desired body weight); (3) African American, Hispanic American, Native American, Asian American, or Pacific Islander descent; (4) age 45 or older; (5) previously identified impaired glucose tolerance (certain prescription drugs, including glucocorticoids, furosemide, thiazides, estrogen-containing products, beta-adrenergic blockers, and nicotinic acid may produce hyperglycemia); (6) hypertension (140/90 or over); (7) high-density lipoprotein-cholesterol level 35 mg/dl (0.90 mmol/l) or less and triglyceride level 250 mg/dl (2.82 mmol/l) or more; (8) physical inactivity; (9) in women, a history of gestational diabetes mellitus or delivery of babies over 9 lb.

alcohol consumption, overeating, taking pills, or taking their aggressions out on someone else. You can help your patient by teaching him how the body and mind work together so that relaxing one helps relax the other.

Talk about the common stress-reducers people use without even thinking about it, including talking about a problem, crying, and exercise. Explain how exercise can help relieve tense muscles and use up some of the adrenaline rush and pent-up energy that results from the fight-or-flight response — a response that is linked to stress. Also teach stress-reduction exercises, including slow deep breathing, progressive muscle relaxation, and imagery. Explain that these options require a quiet, comfortable place where he can be alone for about 20 minutes.

Smoking and substance abuse

If your patient is a smoker or substance abuser, research has demonstrated the significance of a health care provider who keeps telling him the importance of quitting and offers help. Keep reminding him of the consequences of his behavior, including impotence, greater risk of stroke and heart attack, loss of license — or even his life — for drunk driving. In a matter-of-fact way, tell him how the behavior affects his health. For instance, remind him that upper respiratory infections last longer in smokers and that alcohol and smoking elevate blood pressure.

Sexual practices

Adolescents may run the highest risk for contracting sexually transmitted diseases (STDs), but adults are also at risk, particularly older men, many of whom contract an STD from a prostitute. Also, an adult who has gone through a drastic change in a relationship with a primary sexual partner — because of death, discontent, or divorce, for example — is likely to develop different sexual practices that may put him at risk.

Appendix A:
Normal laboratory test values

Hematology

Activated partial thromboplastin time
    25 to 36 seconds

Bleeding time
    Modified template: 2 to 10 minutes
    Template: 2 to 8 minutes
    Ivy: 1 to 7 minutes
    Duke: 1 to 3 minutes

Clot retraction
    50%

Erythrocyte sedimentation rate
    Males: 0 to 10 mm/hour
    Females: 0 to 20 mm/hour

Fibrin split products
    Screening assay: < 10 µg/ml
    Quantitative assay: < 3 µg/ml

Fibrinogen, plasma
    195 to 365 mg/dl

Hematocrit
    Males: 42% to 54%
    Females: 38% to 46%
    Neonates: 55% to 68%

Hemoglobin, total
    Males: 14 to 18 g/dl
    Males after middle age: 12.4 to 14.9 g/dl
    Females: 12 to 16 g/dl
    Females after middle age: 11.7 to 13.8 g/dl

Platelet aggregation
    3 to 5 minutes

Platelet count
    140,000 to 400,000/µl

Platelet survival
    50% tagged platelets disappear within 84 to 116 hours; 100% disappear within 8 to 10 days

Prothrombin consumption time
    20 seconds

Prothrombin time
    10 to 14 seconds; INR for patients on warfarin therapy, 2.0 to 3.0 (those with prosthetic heart valve, 2.5 to 3.5)

Red blood cell count
    Males: 4.5 to 6.2 million/µl venous blood
    Females: 4.2 to 5.4 million/µl venous blood

Red cell indices
    Mean corpuscular volume: 84 to 99 fl
    Mean corpuscular hemoglobin: 26 to 32 fl
    Mean corpuscular hemoglobin concentration: 30 to 36 g/dl

Reticulocyte count
    0.5% to 2% of total red blood cell count

Thrombin time, plasma
    10 to 15 seconds

Blood chemistry

Acid phosphatase, serum
    0.5 to 1.9 U/L

Alanine aminotransferase
    Males: 10 to 35 U/L
    Females: 9 to 24 U/L

Alkaline phosphatase, serum
    Males ≥ 19 years: 98 to 251 U/L
    Females 24 to 65 years: 81 to 282 U/L
    Females ≥ 65 years: 119 to 309 U/L

Amylase, serum
    ≥ 18 years: 35 to 115 U/L

Arterial blood gases
    pH: 7.35 to 7.45
    PaO_2: 75 to 100 mm Hg
    $PaCO_2$: 35 to 45 mm Hg
    O_2CT: 15% to 23%
    SaO_2: 94% to 100%
    HCO_3^-: 22 to 26 mEq/L

Aspartate aminotransferase
    Males: 8 to 20 U/L
    Females: 5 to 40 U/L

Bilirubin, serum
    Adults: direct < 0.5 mg/dl; indirect, ≤ 1.1 mg/dl
    Neonates: total, 1 to 12 mg/dl

Blood urea nitrogen
    8 to 20 mg/dl

Calcium, serum (atomic absorption)
    Males ≥ 22 years: 8.9 to 10.1 mg/dl
    Females ≥ 19 years: 8.9 to 10.1 mg/dl

Carbon dioxide, total, blood
  22 to 34 mEq/L
Cholesterol, total, serum
  0 to 240 mg/dl
C-reactive protein, serum
  Negative
Creatine, serum
  Males: 0.2 to 0.6 mg/dl
  Females: 0.6 to 1 mg/dl
Creatine kinase, isoenzymes
  CK-BB: none
  CK-MB: 0 to 7 U/L
  CK-MM: 5 to 70 U/L
Creatine kinase, total
  Males ≥ 18 years: 52 to 336 U/L
  Females ≥ 18 years: 38 to 176 U/L
Creatinine, serum
  Males: 0.8 to 1.2 mg/dl
  Females: 0.6 to 0.9 mg/dl
Free thyroxine, serum
  0.8 to 3.3 ng/dl
Free triiodothyronine
  0.2 to 0.6 ng/dl
Gamma-glutamyltransferase
  Males: 8 to 37 U/L
  Females <45 years: 5 to 27 U/L
  Females ≥45 years: 6 to 37 U/L
Glucose, plasma, fasting
  70 to 100 mg/dl
Glucose, plasma, oral tolerance
  Peak at 160 to 180 mg/dl, 30 to 60
  minutes after challenge dose
Glucose, plasma, 2-hour postprandial
  <145 mg/dl
Hydroxybutyric dehydrogenase (HBD)
  Serum HBD: 114 to 290 U/ml
  LD/HBD ratio: 1.2 to 1.6:1
Iron, serum
  Males: 70 to 150 µg/dl
  Females: 80 to 150 µg/dl
Lactate dehydrogenase (LD)
  Total: 48 to 115 IU/L
  LD_1: 14% to 26%
  LD_2: 29% to 39%
  LD_3: 20% to 26%
  LD_4: 8% to 16%
  LD_5: 6% to 16%
Lactic acid, blood
  0.93 to 1.65 mEq/L
Lipase
  <300 U/L
Lipoproteins, serum
  HDL cholesterol: 29 to 77 mg/dl
  LDL cholesterol: 62 to 185 mg/dl

Magnesium, serum
  1.5 to 2.5 mEq/L
  Atomic absorption: 1.7 to 2.1 mg/dl
Phosphates, serum
  1.8 to 2.6 mEq/L
  Atomic absorption: 2.5 to 4.5 mg/dl
Potassium, serum
  3.8 to 5.5 mEq/L
Protein, serum
  Total: 6.6 to 7.9 g/dl
  Albumin fraction: 3.3 to 4.5 g/dl
  $Alpha_1$-globulin: 0.1 to 0.4 g/dl
  $Alpha_2$-globulin: 0.5 to 1 g/dl
  Beta globulin: 0.7 to 1.2 g/dl
  Gamma globulin: 0.5 to 1.6 g/dl
Sodium, serum
  135 to 145 mEq/L
Thyroxine, total, serum
  5 to 13.5 µg/dl
Triglycerides, serum
  Males: 40 to 160 mg/dl
  Females: 35 to 135 mg/dl
Uric acid, serum
  Males: 4.3 to 8.0 mg/dl
  Females: 2.3 to 6.0 mg/dl
White blood cell differential, blood
  Neutrophils: 47.6% to 76.8%
  Lymphocytes: 16.2% to 43%
  Monocytes: 0.6% to 9.6%
  Eosinophils: 0.3% to 7.0%
  Basophils: 0.3% to 2.0%

Urine chemistry
Amylase, urine
  10 to 80 amylase U/hour
Bence Jones protein, urine
  Negative
Bilirubin, urine
  Negative
Calcium, urine
  Males: <275 mg/24 hours
  Females: <250 mg/24 hours
Creatinine, urine
  Males: 0 to 40 mg/24 hours
  Females: 0 to 80 mg/24 hours
Creatinine clearance
  Males: 107 to 139 ml/minute
  Females: 87 to 107 ml/minute
Glucose, urine
  Negative
17-Hydroxycorticosteroids, urine
  Males: 4.5 to 12 mg/24 hours
  Females: 2.5 to 10 mg/24 hours

17-Ketogenic steroids, urine
Males: 4 to 14 mg/24 hours
Females: 2 to 12 mg/24 hours
Ketones, urine
Negative
17-Ketosteroids, urine
Males: 6 to 21 mg/24 hours
Females: 4 to 17 mg/24 hours
Protein, urine
≤ 150 mg/24 hours
Red blood cells, urine
0 to 3 per high-power field
Sodium, urine
30 to 280 mEq/24 hours
Sodium chloride, urine
5 to 20 g/24 hours
Urea, urine
Maximal clearance: 64 to
99 ml/minute
Uric acid, urine
250 to 750 mg/24 hours
Urinalysis, routine
Color: straw
Appearance: clear
Specific gravity: 1.005 to 1.035
pH: 4.5 to 8
Epithelial cells: few
Casts: occasional hyaline casts
Crystals: present
Urine osmolality
24-hour urine: 300 to
900 mOsm/kg
Random urine: 50 to
1,400 mOsm/kg

Urobilinogen, urine
Males: 0.3 to 2.1 Ehrlich units
(2-hour collection)
Females: 0.1 to 1.1 Ehrlich units
(2-hour collection)
Vanillylmandelic acid, urine
0.7 to 6.8 mg/24 hours
White blood cell count, urine
0 to 4 per high-power field

Miscellaneous
Cerebrospinal fluid
Pressure: 50 to 180 mm H_2O
Appearance: clear, colorless
Gram stain: no organisms
**Lupus erythematosus cell
preparation**
Negative
Occult blood, fecal
<2.5 ml/24 hours
Rheumatoid factor, serum
Negative
Urobilinogen, fecal
50 to 300 mg/24 hours
**Venereal Disease Research
Laboratory, serum**
Negative

Appendix B:
Crisis values of laboratory tests

Test	Low value	Common causes and effects	High value	Common causes and effects
Calcium, serum	< 7 mg/dl	Vitamin D or parathyroid hormone deficiency: tetany, seizures	> 12 mg/dl	Hyperparathyroidism: coma
Carbon dioxide/bicarbonate, blood	< 10 mEq/L	Complex pattern of metabolic and respiratory factors	> 40 mEq/L	Complex pattern of metabolic and respiratory factors
Creatinine, serum			> 4 mg/dl	Renal failure: coma
Glucose, blood	< 40 mg/dl	Excess insulin administration: brain damage	> 300 mg/dl (with ketonemia and electrolyte imbalance)	Diabetes: diabetic coma
Hemoglobin	< 8 g/dl	Hemorrhage, vitamin B_{12} or iron deficiency: heart failure	> 18 g/dl	Chronic obstructive pulmonary disease: thrombosis, polycythemia vera
Partial thromboplastin time			> 40 sec > 70 sec (for patient on heparin)	Anticoagulation factor deficiency: hemorrhage
Pco_2, arterial	< 20 mm Hg	Complex pattern of metabolic and respiratory factors	> 70 mm Hg	Complex pattern of metabolic and respiratory factors
pH, blood	< 7.2	Complex pattern of metabolic and respiratory factors	> 7.6	Complex patterns of metabolic and respiratory factors
Platelet count	< 50,000/µl	Bone marrow suppression: hemorrhage	> 500,000/µl	Leukemia, reaction to acute bleeding: hemorrhage
Po_2, blood	< 50 mm Hg	Complex pattern of metabolic and respiratory factors		

Test	Low value	Common causes and effects	High value	Common causes and effects
Potassium, serum	< 3 mEq/L	Vomiting and diarrhea, diuretic therapy: cardiotoxicity, arrhythmia, cardiac arrest	> 6 mEq/L	Renal disease diuretic therapy: cardiotoxicity, arrhythmia
Prothrombin time			> 14 sec > 20 sec (for patient on warfarin)	Anticoagulant therapy, anticoagulation factor deficiency: hemorrhage
Sodium, serum	< 120 mEq/L	Diuretic therapy: profuse sweating, GI suctioning, diarrhea, vomiting, burns	> 160 mEq/L	Dehydration: vascular collapse
White blood cell count	< 2,000/µl	Bone marrow suppression: infection	> 20,000/µl	Leukemia: infection
White blood cell count, CSF			> 10/µl	Meningitis, encephalitis: infection

Appendix C: Simplified charting

One format you can use for focused visit charting involves using standard abbreviations for listing findings, some general negatives for all systems, plus significant negatives for systems related to the chief complaint. Organizing your data in this shorthand fashion helps you avoid omitting key data points for a complete patient record.

Charting model for focused visit history

C/O: (what × how long)
HPI: (age, sex, PMH)
Per pt: (list of all complaints plus any elicited abnormalities)
Pt. denied: trauma, incontinence, blurry vision, H/A, neck/back pain, sore throat, chest pain, SOB, abd. pain, N/V/D, change in voiding or BM, no bloody stools/urine, no numbness/tingling in Ext. ROS otherwise unremarkable.
Allergies: Meds: (prescription, OTC, personal [caffeine, nicotine, alcohol, others])
SH:
Fhx:
Labs:

Charting model for systems that are nonaffected, noncontributory to chief complaint

PE: WD, WN
HEENT: NCAT
Neck: full ROM
Lungs: CTA
Cor: S1/S2 (−) M/G/A
Abd: soft, NT, no organomegaly, (−) CVA tenderness
Ext: (−) C/C/E
Neuro: strength +4/4, even gait

Charting model for systems related to chief complaint

Document all abnormal findings (one to two negatives per system if no abnormal findings).

PE: AA&O × 3, WD, WN
Color: pink conjunctiva
Skin: warm/dry, rapid/mobile
Neck: supple, full ROM, (−) JVD, trachea midline and mobile, (−) thyromegaly
Vertebra: NT, full ROM, (−) contusions
H: NCAT
E: all landmarks V
E: pupils ____mm, OU, EOMI, fundoscopic, no hyphema/field cuts/papilledema
N: patent
T: clear. Oropharynx: (−) exudate/ulcerations/broken teeth/erythema/cobblestoning/edema/tonsils; post. pharynx not injected
Chest: symmetrical, no accessory muscle usage
Lungs: CTA&P
Cor: S1/S2 (−) M/G/A
Abd: soft, NT, (+) BS, (−) Murphy's/Psoas/Kern's/Balance, (−) rebound/CVA tenderness/fluid wave/striae
Ext: (−) C/C/E. Full ROM at hip/knee/ankle. (−) straight leg raises, (−) Patrick's, Anterior/Posterior Drawer, Ballotment, Bulge Valgus, Adduction Stress, Abduction Stress, and Lachman's. Pulses: _____
Adnexae: (−) masses/tenderness
Pelvic: ext. genitalia without lesions. Vagina: (−) lesions/discharge. Cervix: (−) CMT, pink, firm, dilated ____mm. Uterus A/V (or R/V), smooth, size
Rectovag: neg.
Rectal: (−) ext. hemorrhoids/mass/prostate/hemoccult

KEY:
AA&O: awake, alert, and oriented
all landmarks V: all landmarks visualized
BM: bowel movement
BS: bowel sounds
C/C/E: cyanosis, clubbing, or edema
C/O: complained of
CMT: cervical motion tenderness
Cor: coronary
CTA&P: clear to auscultation and percussion
CTA: clear to auscultation
CVA: costovertebral angle
EOMI: extraocular movements intact
Ext: extremities
Fhx: family history
H/A: headache
HEENT: head, eyes, ears, nose, and throat

HPI: history of present illness
JVD: jugular vein distention
M/G/A: murmur, gallop, or arrhythmia
N/V/D: nausea, vomiting, and diarrhea
NCAT: normocephalic atraumatic
NT: nontender
OTC: over-the-counter
OU: bilateral eyes
PE: physical examination
PMH: past medical history
Pt: patient
ROM: range of motion
ROS: range of symptoms
SH: social history
SOB: shortness of breath
Uterus A/V or R/V: uterus anteverted or retroverted
WD, WN: well developed, well nourished

Selected references

American Academy of Pediatrics and The American College of Obstetricians and Gynecologists. *Guidelines for Perinatal Care,* 4th ed. Elk Grove Village, Ill.: American Academy of Pediatrics, 1997.

Barker, L.R., et al. *Principles of Ambulatory Medicine,* 5th ed. Philadelphia: Lippincott Williams & Wilkins, 1999.

Behrman, R.E., et al. *Nelson Textbook of Pediatrics,* 16th ed. Philadelphia: W.B. Saunders Co., 2000.

Behrman, R.E., and Kliegman, R.M. *Nelson Essentials of Pediatrics,* 3rd ed. Philadelphia: W.B. Saunders Co., 1998.

Colyar, M.R. *Ambulatory Care Procedures for the Nurse Practitioner.* Philadelphia: F.A. Davis Co., 1999.

Dambro, M.R. *Griffith's 5 Minute Clinical Consult,* 7th ed. Philadelphia: Lippincott Williams & Wilkins, 1999.

Ezell, S.L., Kobernick, et al. "Arthrocentesis," in *Clinical Procedures in Emergency Medicine.* Edited by Hedges, R., et al. Philadelphia: W.B. Saunders Co., 1997.

Fauci, A.S. *Harrison's Principles of Internal Medicine,* 14th ed. New York: McGraw-Hill Book Co., 1998.

Fenstermacher, K., and Hudson, B.T. *Practice Guidelines for Family Nurse Practitioners.* Philadelphia: W.B. Saunders Co., 1997.

Fitzpatrick, T.B., et al. *Color Atlas and Synopsis of Clinical Dermatology,* 3rd ed. New York: McGraw-Hill Book Co., 1997.

Gamponia, M.J., and Herting, R.L. "Office and Hospital Procedures: Arthrocentesis," in *University of Iowa Family Practice Handbook,* 3rd ed. Philadelphia: Mosby—Year Book, Inc., 1997.

Hacker, N.F., and Moore, J.G. *Essentials of Obstetrics and Gynecology,* 3rd ed. Philadelphia: W.B. Saunders Co., 1998.

Hay Jr., W.W., et al. *Current Pediatric Diagnosis and Treatment.* Stamford, Conn: Appleton & Lange, 1997.

Hector Dunphy, L.M. *Management Guidelines for Adult Nurse Practitioners.* Philadelphia: F.A. Davis Co., 1999.

Hedges, J.R., et al. *Clinical Procedures in Emergency Medicine,* 3rd ed. Philadelphia: W.B. Saunders Co., 1998.

Larrabee, R.J. *The Annual Family Practice Review, Workshop #78, Basic Principles of Suturing.* Philadelphia: Temple University School of Medicine, 1997.

Otten, E.J. *Clinical Procedures in Emergency Medicine.* Philadelphia: W.B. Saunders Co., 1997.

Richards, C. "Ankle, soft-tissue injuries," in *EMedicine: Emergency Medicine (online medical reference).* Boston: Boston Medical Publishing Corp., 1999. http://www.emedicine.com.

Robinson, D.L., and McKenzie, C. *Procedures for Primary Care Providers.* Philadelphia: Lippincott Williams & Wilkins, 1999.

Rudolph, A.M., and Kamei, R.K. *Rudolph's Fundamentals of Pediatrics,* 2nd ed. Stamford, Conn.: Appleton & Lange, 1998.

Schumacher, H.R. "Arthrocentesis of the Knee," *Hospital Medicine* 33(7):60-64, July 1997.

Schumacher, H.R. "Arthrocentesis of the Shoulder," *Hospital Medicine* 33(8):57-60, August 1997.

Tierney, L.M., et al. *Current Medical Diagnosis & Treatment 1999,* 38th ed. Stamford, Conn.: Appleton & Lange, 1999.

Wu, K. *Techniques in Surgical Casting and Splinting.* Philadelphia: Lea & Febiger, 1987.

Index

i refers to an illustration; t refers to a table.

463

i refers to an illustration; t refers to a table.

i refers to an illustration; t refers to a table.

i refers to an illustration; t refers to a table.